To
Jennifer Nicole Guggenheim
Hannah Carol Guggenheim
Jeanette Weiner

Manual of Psychiatric Consultation and Emergency Care

Edited by
Frederick G. Guggenheim, M.D., and
Myron F. Weiner, M.D.

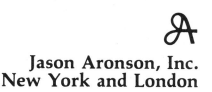

Jason Aronson, Inc.
New York and London

Library of Congress Cataloging in Publication Data
Main entry under title:

Manual of psychiatric consultation and emergency care.

Includes index.
1. Psychiatric emergencies.   2. Hospital patients—
Mental health.   3. Social psychiatry.   I. Guggenheim,
Frederick G.   II. Weiner, Myron F. [DNLM: 1. Crisis
intervention.   2. Mental health services.   3. Referral
and consultation. WM 401 M294]
RC480.6.M35   1984   616.89′025   84-477
ISBN 0-87668-666-8

Manufactured in the United States of America.

MANUAL OF PSYCHIATRIC CONSULTATION AND EMERGENCY CARE

Contents

PART II. MEDICAL/SURGICAL WARDS

Preface

The training of staff to handle consultation and psychiatric treatment of the more severely emotionally disturbed patient has changed significantly in the past two decades. Modern psychiatric trainees are taught a flexible approach to many clinical problems in a broad range of settings, including the general hospital.

The roles played by psychiatric personnel in the general hospital have increased in number and significance, and they continue to amplify. Psychiatrists, psychologists, social workers, and other mental health professionals participate in direct patient care and in creating a therapeutic environment throughout the hospital. Demands for rapid psychiatric assessment and patient care have risen with the growth in psychiatric sophistication of other physicians. Where once mental health professionals were called on to evaluate only the severely psychotic or the suicidal patient, they are now also called upon to help medical patients deal with the psychosocial consequences of illness and to determine the role of emotional factors in patients' medical problems. In addition, the psychiatric staff is now frequently consulted before patients exhibit disturbed behavior, to facilitate the patients, cooperation with complex and often frightening medical procedures.

Advances in modern technology have certainly affected the scope of psychiatric interventions in the general hospital. With techniques for prolonging the lives of the chronically ill, psychiatric consultation is being sought to help in both selecting and managing patients who require complex treatment and support systems. In addition, the policy of deinstitutionalization has placed a greater burden on hospital emergency facilities, where the chronic psychiatric patients are brought when they become unable to cope at home or in their community.

This book is intended as a guide for psychiatrists, psychologists, social workers, and all those who must deal with the wide range of psychiatric problems in the hospital and clinic settings. It should also be useful to the increasing number of medical students whose primary psychiatric clerkship assignment is on a consultation/liaison service. The situations that present most frequently are covered here with an emphasis on practical management. Our aim is to provide an easy reference for staff and trainees under pressure and to facilitate quick action on behalf of patients in situations that are highly stressful and often dangerous.

Contributors

PAUL S. APPELBAUM, M.D.
Assistant Professor of Psychiatry and Law, Western Psychiatric Clinic,
University of Pittsburgh School of Medicine and Law, Pittsburgh, PA

WALTER F. BAILE, M.D.
Assistant Professor of Psychiatry and Medicine,
The Johns Hopkins Medical Institution;
Staff Physician, Baltimore City Hospital, Baltimore, MD

THOMAS P. BERESFORD, M.D.
Chief, Psychiatric Service, V.A. Hospital Medical Center;
Associate Professor of Psychiatry,
University of Tennessee College of Health Sciences, Memphis, TN

NORMAN R. BERNSTEIN, M.D.
Professor of Psychiatry,
University of Illinois College of Medicine, Chicago, IL

STEPHANIE CAVANAUGH, M.D.
Associate Professor of Psychiatry, Rush Medical College;
Director of Consultation/Liaison Service, Department of Psychiatry,
Rush-Presbyterian-St. Luke's Medical Center, Chicago, IL

HAROLD B. CRASILNECK, Ph.D.
Clinical Professor of Psychiatry and Anesthesiology,
The University of Texas Health Science Center at Dallas, TX

JAYE CROWDER, M.D.
Resident in Training in Psychiatry,
The University of Texas Health Science Center at Dallas, TX

REV. ROBERT L. DAVIS
Director of Pastoral Care,
Riverside Methodist Hospital, Columbus, OH

DOUGLAS A. DROSSMAN, M.D.
Assistant Professor of Medicine and Psychiatry,
University of North Carolina School of Medicine, Chapel Hill, NC

MILTON K. ERMAN, M.D.
Assistant Professor of Psychiatry,
The University of Texas Health Science Center at Dallas, TX

BARRY J. FENTON, M.D.
Assistant Professor of Psychiatry,
The University of Texas Health Science Center at Dallas, TX

MICHAEL C. FITZPATRICK, M.D.
Assistant Professor of Psychiatry,
The University of Texas Health Science Center at Dallas, TX

CARL FULTON, M.D.
Assistant Professor of Clinical Psychiatry,
The University of Texas Health Science Center at Dallas, TX

CHARLES M. GAITZ, M.D.
Clinical Professor of Psychiatry,
The University of Texas Health Science Center at Houston;
Head, Gerontology Center, Texas Research Institute of Mental Sciences,
Houston, TX

ROLLIN M. GALLAGHER, III, M.D.
Associate Professor of Psychiatry,
Director of Residency Training, Director of Behavioral Medicine Service,
University of Vermont College of Medicine, Burlington, VT

ROBERT J. GATCHEL, Ph.D.
Associate Professor of Psychiatry,
The University of Texas Health Science Center at Dallas, TX

FREDERICK G. GUGGENHEIM, M.D.
Associate Professor of Psychiatry and Chief, Consultation/Liaison Division,
The University of Texas Health Science Center at Dallas, TX

RICHARD C.W. HALL, M.D.
Chief of Staff, V.A. Hospital Medical Center;
Professor of Psychiatry and Internal Medicine,
University of Tennessee College of Health Sciences, Memphis, TN

NELSON HENDLER, M.D.
Assistant Professor of Psychiatry and Neurology, Johns Hopkins University;
Clinical Director of the Mensana Clinic, Baltimore, MD

THOMAS M. JOHNSON, Ph.D.
Assistant Professor of Anthropology, Southern Methodist University, Dallas;
Adjunct Clinical Assistant Professor of Psychiatry,
The University of Texas Health Science Center at Dallas, TX

ARTHUR KLEINMAN, M.D., M.A.
Professor, Departments of Social Medicine and Anthropology,
Faculty of Arts and Sciences, Harvard Medical School, Cambridge, MA

JOSEPH A. KWENTUS, M.D.
Assistant Professor of Psychiatry,
Uniformed University for Health Sciences, Washington, DC

DON R. LIPSITT, M.D.
Associate Professor of Psychiatry, Harvard Medical School;
Chief of Psychiatry, Mount Auburn Hospital, Cambridge, MA

MERNA P. LIPSITT, M.S.W.
Clinical Instructor, Simmons College of Social Work, Boston;
Clinical Social Work Supervisor, Faulkner Hospital, Boston, MA

ROBERT LOVITT, Ph.D.
Associate Professor of Psychiatry,
The University of Texas Health Science Center at Dallas, TX

DENNIS LOW, M.D.
Clinical Instructor of Medicine,
Stanford University School of Medicine, Palo Alto, CA;
Associate Director, Primary Care Division, Department of Medicine,
Santa Clara Valley Medical Center, San Jose, CA

THOMAS B. MACKENZIE, M.D.
Co-Director of Consultation/Liaison Service, Department of Psychiatry,
The University of Minnesota Medical School, Minneapolis, MN

PAUL C. MOHL, M.D.
Assistant Professor of Psychiatry,
The University of Texas Health Science Center at San Antonio, TX

CAROL C. NADELSON, M.D.
Professor and Vice Chairman, Department of Psychiatry,
Tufts University School of Medicine, Boston, MA

MALKAH T. NOTMAN, M.D.
Clinical Professor of Psychiatry,
Tufts University School of Medicine, Boston, MA

LINDA GAY PETERSON, M.D.
Assistant Professor of Psychiatry,
Director of Consultation/Liaison Service,
The University of Texas Medical Branch at Galveston, TX

MICHAEL K. POPKIN, M.D.
Associate Professor of Psychiatry and Medicine,
Director of Consultation/Liaison Service,
The University of Minnesota Medical School, Minneapolis, MN

DOUGLAS A. PURYEAR, M.D.
Associate Professor of Clinical Psychiatry
The University of Texas Health Science Center at Dallas;
Director of Psychiatric Emergency Services,
Parkland Memorial Hospital, Dallas, TX

A. JOHN RUSH, M.D.
Betty Jo Hay Professor of Psychiatry,
The University of Texas Health Science Center at Dallas, TX

EDMUND C. SETTLE, Jr., M.D.
Clinical Assistant Professor of Psychiatry,
West Virginia University, Charleston, WV

REGE S. STEWART, M.D.
Associate Professor of Clinical Psychiatry,
The University of Texas Health Science Center at Dallas, TX

JOHN A. TALBOTT, M.D.
Professor of Psychiatry, Cornell University, New York, NY

KENNETH TARDIFF, M.D., M.P.H.
Associate Dean and Associate Professor of Clinical Psychiatry,
Assistant Professor of Public Health, Cornell University, New York, NY

DAVID A. WALLER, M.D.
Associate Professor of Clinical Psychiatry,
The University of Texas Health Science Center at Dallas, TX

MYRON F. WEINER, M.D.
Professor and Vice Chairman, Department of Psychiatry,
The University of Texas Health Science Center at Dallas, TX

AVERY D. WEISMAN, M.D.
Senior Professor of Psychiatry, Harvard Medical School, Cambridge, MA

CHARLES A. WELCH, M.D.
Instructor in Psychiatry, Harvard Medical School;
Director of Somatic Therapies Consultation Service,
Massachusetts General Hospital, Boston, MA

THOMAS N. WISE, M.D.
Professor of Psychiatry, Georgetown University Medical School;
Chairman of Department of Psychiatry, Fairfax Hospital, Fairfax, VA

PART I

IN THE EMERGENCY ROOM

The First Five Minutes: Likelihood of Mayhem or Elopement

The emergency room is the most stressful treatment environment encountered by psychiatrists. But such a setting also provides an abundance of learning experiences and a chance to limit the morbidity and mortality associated with acute psychiatric disorders. Clinical effectiveness in the emergency room is limited by the lack of a set of procedural guidelines and a frame of reference for immediate action. Dealing with severely disturbed patients or with patients in need of rapid disposition requires more than empathic reflection and verbal limit setting. Psychodynamically trained psychiatrists tend to flounder in an emergency room situation if they fail to recognize that a dynamic approach can have great benefit on a one-time basis. Moreover, a dynamic approach can be readily combined with various environmental and pharmacological measures to produce a rapid amelioration of patients' symptoms.

From the very outset of work in the emergency room, psychiatrists must be in command of information about several critical topics—taking time out to consult with a supervisor may waste precious moments and precipitate an untoward result. These critical topics are rapid differential diagnosis, recognition and management of violence and suicide risk, crisis-oriented treatment, and rapid neuroleptization. Chapter 1, on differential diagnosis, provides clues to differentiating functional from organic disorders. The next two chapters, on violence to others and suicide risk, point out ways in which clinicians can immediately reduce the danger to patients and hospital staff. Chapter 4, on crisis-oriented treatment, suggests psychological means by which changes can be made in patients' home environments that may increase stability and avoid hospitalization. And the last chapter in this part, on rapid neuroleptization, a recent development in psychopharmacology, details criteria for sedation and management of acutely psychotic patients, with the goal of handling the episode without psychiatric hospitalization.

On the medical/surgical side of the emergency room, the first emphasis is on maintaining an airway, stemming hemorrhage, and monitoring vital signs. On the psychiatric side of the emergency room, the first order of the day is making certain that patients do not elope, inflict injury, or otherwise grossly lose control. With a firm grounding in the topics covered in this section, psychiatrists in the emergency room will be able to respond rapidly. Mastery of these topics benefits not only the psychiatrists and the disturbed patients but also other staff and patients in the emergency room, for all occupants are often overwhelmed by the assaultive, suicidal, or perplexing people who present at a psychiatric emergency service.

F.G.

CHAPTER 1

Rapid Differential Diagnosis

THOMAS N. WISE, M.D.

Psychiatrists seeing emergency room patients for the first time operate very differently from psychiatrists seeing outpatients for the first time. In the emergency room, the psychiatrist begins, not with an open mind, but with suspecting the worst: organic brain disorder, functional psychosis, or danger to self or others. In addition, the primary source of information is often not the patient's accounts of difficulties. Instead, much information is obtained from friends, relatives, peace officers, laboratory studies, and the formal mental status examination. Finally, the psychiatrist in the emergency room may need to perform a physical or neurological examination when a medical consultant is not readily available.

Organic Brain Disorders

Psychiatrists must first rule out an organic mental disorder. They begin their examination by noting vital signs. Fever, abnormality of heart rate or rhythm, and abnormality of blood pressure or respiratory rate all point to physical causes of mental disorder. Even when vital signs are normal, the rule of thumb is to suspect an organic disorder in patients over 50 years of age with no previous psychiatric history. Patients particularly likely to have a toxic organic disorder are adolescents using recreational drugs and older people with no history of psychiatric disorder who have recently started on or changed medication, as illustrated in the following vignette.

Mr. A., a 57-year-old married salesman with a history of heart disease, presented to an emergency room appearing agitated and confused. He stared anxiously about the examining room. According to his wife, his sensorium had been clear and his functioning reasonable until two days before. At that time the patient had been directed to increase his cardiac glycoside. Over the next 24 hours, he became confused and began to complain of men running around his living room. He was brought to the emergency room, agitated and fearful. Physical examination revealed no evidence of cardiac failure or hypoxia. The psychiatric consultant suspected a delirium because the patient had an impaired sensorium and was experiencing visual hallucinations. After admission to the medical service, the patient's delirium was found to have been precipitated by his cardiac glycoside.

Acute organic mental disorders are characterized by disorientation, fluctuating level of consciousness, poor attention span, and impaired recent memory and judgment. The patient who develops an acute organic brain syndrome in response to a trivial insult such as a mild viral pneumonia or a single dose of a sedative hypnotic is likely to have an underlying chronic brain disorder.

The sensorial aspect of the formal mental status examination is helpful in distinguishing an organic disorder from a psychogenic disorder. Brief screening instruments such as the Mini-Mental State Examination allow a rapid, reliable quantitative measure of cognitive impairment. If the patient's lucidity is impaired, friends and family members are good sources of information about fluctuating states of consciousness and impaired memory and judgment.

Anxiety itself can diminish concentration and thereby modify the sensorial examination. Indeed, it can unmask and temporarily exacerbate a mild to moderate dementia. For example, elderly people admitted to the hospital for diagnostic procedures can become confused even before they receive any potentially delirogenic medications, such as anxiolytic, narcotic, and strongly anticholinergic medications.

The emergency room evaluation can serve primarily as a triage process to admit patients for more comprehensive hospital evaluation when the etiology of the underlying organic disorder is unclear.

Functional Psychoses

After ruling out an organic disorder by thorough history taking, mental status examination, physical evaluation, and pertinent laboratory studies, psychiatrists proceed to evaluate for functional psychosis.

The major functional psychotic disorders to be ruled out are schizophrenia and schizophreniform disorders, and the affective disorders. Agitation, mood-incongruent delusions, ideas of reference, and notions of thought broadcasting or thought intrusion point to a major thought disorder. Information from outside informants about a prior psychiatric history and the duration of the present illness is important. Generally, greater disorganization and agitation are associated with acute illness, such as a brief reactive psychosis or a schizophreniform psychosis. People with chronic mental illness are often more alienated from and more alienating to the examiner than are those suffering a first psychotic break.

Profoundly depressed patients may appear organically impaired on mental status examination because of psychomotor retardation, paucity of thought content, and difficulty in making the effort required to cooperate with the examiner. Although suicidal ideation, self-recrimination, and low self-esteem all point to an affective disorder, it is important to remember that a depressive syndrome can be precipitated or aggravated by the cognitive impairment caused by an underlying organic brain disorder. Patients' low self-esteem may be due in part to their real inability to maintain their former level of intellectual functioning.

An irritable, excited manic patient may be indistinguishable in the emergency room from an agitated, paranoid schizophrenic patient. A past history of affective disorder and mood-congruent delusions is helpful in making the diagnosis of mania. The following case illustrates a functional psychosis.

> Mr. B., a 31-year-old single librarian, was brought to the emergency room by police after he was found walking down a crowded street, not wearing any clothes. The patient stated that "the Emperor had new clothes." This statement was followed by his explanation that he was a brilliant inventor who was soon to be crowned Emperor of the World. His mood was euphoric. Past history obtained from a roommate revealed that the patient had cyclical episodes of depression and euphoria accompanied by grandiose thoughts, with previous good response to lithium carbonate.

In this case, the presence of a mood disorder with mood-congruent delusions, a past history of mood disorder, and an absence of a clouded sensorium pointed to a bipolar affective disorder (manic-depressive disorder).

Danger to Self or Others

Psychiatrists next consider the issue of danger to self or others. Evaluation of potential violence to self or others requires direct questioning in a compassionate and sympathetic manner. Questions such as, "Have things ever gotten so difficult that you have considered ending it all?" may elicit more data than directly asking the patient, "Are you going to kill yourself?"

If the first approach yields a positive answer, further questions must delineate the probability of the patient's actually carrying out the behavior.

The rule of thumb in evaluating suicidal patients is *when in doubt, hospitalize*. There are two basic exceptions to this rule. People who are awaiting trial or who have been convicted of a crime are often brought to the emergency room because of a suicide attempt or threats of suicide. They usually claim that if they are kept in jail, they will suicide. This behavior often represents a coercive threat to avoid continued incarceration. An ordinary mental status examination will establish the presence or absence of severe depression or other mental illness.

The other exception is people with borderline personality disorders who have made multiple suicide attempts in order to manipulate others. Some of these people actually do suicide, but it is usually not because they wish to kill themselves but because they have miscalculated the response of a potential rescuer. Here again, the examiner needs to see whether the patient has a complicating psychiatric illness. If the patient meets criteria for a major affective depressive disorder, hospitalization is appropriate. (The issues of violence to self and violence to others are examined more thoroughly in Chapters 2 and 3).

In the following case, a psychiatrist faced with a woman who was threatening self-harm decided against hospitalization because of his concern that a dramatic response to her behavior would reinforce and encourage it.

> Ms. C., a 32-year-old divorced waitress, was seen in a psychiatric waiting room. She had made superficial abrasions on her wrists with a razor blade in a calm, deliberate fashion in the presence of the examining physician and other patients. When interviewed by a psychiatrist, the patient stated that such behavior made her feel more alive. She also admitted to wishing to indicate boldly her displeasure with her own psychotherapist.
>
> The patient had been previously diagnosed as having a borderline personality disorder and had been hospitalized many times. Although it is true that her present lethality was not great, her long-term risk of serious self-harm was considerable. The emergency room psychiatrist felt that her life was not in immediate danger and that her core problem would not be resolved by hospitalization at that time. As a protection for himself, he adequately documented his reasons for discharge on the hospital chart. (For a discussion of legal liabilities in the emergency room, see Chapter 11.)

The potential for harm to others is a constant source of concern in the emergency room. A past history of violent behavior is a useful—in fact, the most useful—historical element in such assessment, but even with this information, psychiatrists' ability to predict future violence is poor. Nevertheless, when confronted with a stridently speaking, posturing individual who is sitting tensely in a chair and gripping the armrest tightly or a person who paces during an interview, psychiatrists should be alerted to the potential for violence in the near future. Individuals suffering from toxic drug or alcohol withdrawal syndromes can also become violent.

Acutely manic patients, hyperactive and delusional, may become violent, particularly if they are restrained. Paranoid individuals can be dangerous when frightened by attempted treatment interventions such as injections. In a setting of potential violence, psychiatrists must always elicit support from emergency room personnel, family members, and guards. Often, it is better to evaluate potentially violent patients in an open area instead of a small, isolated interviewing room.

The Mute, Unresponsive Patient

Mute, unresponsive patients are particularly challenging to psychiatrists in the emergency room. The differential diagnoses of such patients include organic mental disorders (especially those caused by endogenous or exogenous toxins), catatonic schizophrenia, dissociative states, malingering, and elective mutism. The basic rule is to never make a primary diagnosis of a functional psychiatric disorder in the face of abnormal vital signs or lab values.

If an adequate physical examination has not been previously done, the psychiatrist performs or calls for one. Vital signs must be determined to be certain that the patient's life is not in danger because of septic shock, diabetic acidosis, or an intracranial lesion. After the general physical examination is carried out, microscopic hematological examination, blood chemistries, and screening blood tests for exogenous toxins are performed and potential informants are contacted to obtain a history.

Patients' level of consciousness should be determined next. This includes noting the presence or absence of decerebrate or decorticate rigidity, and pathological reflexes, such as Babinski, snout, and suck reflexes. Spontaneous eye movement, pupillary reactions, and response to painful stimuli are noted. Of particular importance in differentiating functional from organic states is voluntary muscle resistance, such as resisting opening of the eyelids or mouth. Such resistance usually points to a functional disorder in the absence of spasticity or overall hypertonus of the voluntary musculature as occurs in tetanus or the neuroleptic malignant syndrome.

Catatonic schizophrenics are usually obviously awake. Their eyes follow objects. They sit or stand mute and unresponsive, and often they will not move their limbs, even when they are placed in awkward positions. Catatonics frequently appear frightened and have dilated pupils and a rapid heartbeat. Their resistance to moving or being moved is also usually quite obvious. Psychiatrists' communicating their awareness that the patients are in distress will often stimulate enough response to permit a tentative diagnosis. An intramuscular injection of haloperidol, 5 mg (given after explaining to the patient that it is a calming medicine), will often relax patients sufficiently to enable them to talk.

Psychiatrists must not assume that an apparent catatonic state or paranoid ideation is a sign of functional disorder. Either one or both often accompany organic brain disorders.

Patients in dissociative states show no physical abnormality and, like malingerers, have obvious secondary gain from their symptoms. Both malingerers and individuals having dissociative episodes tend to recover spontaneously if left essentially alone (with periodic checks of vital signs) for several hours. An Amytal interview (see Chapter 33) is useful for uncovering a dissociative state or elective mutism, but it may not arouse the malingerer who is feigning unconsciousness. Although it may be tempting to inflict pain on obvious malingerers as a means of rousing them from their state, it is best to inform them matter-of-factly that they are being returned to the situation (frequently jail) that they are trying to evade. As they are being helped to walk from the emergency room, they usually recover dramatically.

Reasons for Requesting a Consultation

Because of their exclusively medical focus, primary emergency room physicians frequently fail to recognize the nonmedical problem that brings an ill patient to the emergency room, as seen in this example.

A psychiatric consultant was asked to help manage Mrs. D., an 84-year-old widowed nursing home resident brought in by ambulance. The patient had a long-standing dementia and was not in acute distress. The emergency room intern did not know why she had been brought to the hospital. The psychiatrist talked to her nursing home caretakers and a family member. She learned that Mrs. D. could no longer afford the nursing home. An ambulance had been called by the facility on the pretext that she had become unmanageable. The psychiatrist confirmed the diagnosis of dementia and then worked with the Social Service Department to find an appropriate placement.

The emergency room intern did not understand that the problem was financial and social, not medical. The psychiatrist detected the financial problem and helped initiate steps toward an appropriate disposition.

Patients' and Physicians' Reactions
to the Emergency Room

The diagnostic process is often complicated by patients' and psychiatrists' reactions to the circumstances and the place in which they meet.

Patients who are brought unwillingly to an emergency room are often resentful and angry. To them, the emergency room physicians or psychiatrists are judges or potential jailers. Such feelings can evoke angry, uncooperative attitudes and behavior, which complicate the diagnostic process. By encouraging patients to discuss their feelings about being held and examined against their will, psychiatrists can establish enough rapport to permit an adequate examination and to avoid physical violence.

Psychiatrists' attitudes and reactions can also distort the appraisal of a patient. In a busy and crowded emergency room, physicians and other staff may not agree that the putative complaint that brought the patient to an acute emergency setting warranted such a visit. Psychiatrists' anger at patients or physicians who request a consultation in such situations may be displaced onto emergency room interns or patients. Such feelings clearly bias either diagnostic perception or, as this case history indicates, treatment decisions.

> The emergency room physician requested that a psychiatric consultant evaluate Mrs. E., a 35-year-old housewife recently discharged from the hospital's psychiatric unit. The psychiatrist angrily berated the emergency room physician, stating that since this patient had not followed advice while hospitalized, it was unlikely that she would follow advice now. The emergency room physician listened patiently but became angry and confronted the psychiatrist, stating that it was not his fault that the patient hadn't cooperated and that now he wanted some help in managing her.

The psychiatrist had felt angry and defeated by this patient's prior behavior and displaced some of those feelings onto the emergency room physician. Unfortunately, the psychiatrist's anger exacerbated an already difficult situation and clouded his clinical judgment.

Patients' social class, ethnic background, and disease may also bias the judgment of clinicians. In the next case, the primary care physician reacted to the patient's illness, alcoholism.

> An emergency psychiatric consultation was requested for Mr. F., a 38-year-old married executive who was brought in by his wife for excessive drinking. The emergency room physician called the psychiatrist to evaluate "a loud, crazy drunk." The psychiatrist found the patient to have a bipolar affective disorder that he was medicating with alcohol. The

patient was hospitalized, successfully treated with lithium carbonate and referred to Alcoholics Anonymous, and eventually returned to work for his corporation.

A physician's negative attitude toward alcoholism can prevent proper diagnosis and treatment of individuals who present with high blood levels of alcohol.

In addition to covert phenomena that may bias physicians, there may be overt difficulties in such settings that complement unconscious phenomena. Fear of violent patients, the need to quickly assess suicide potential, the need to make involuntary commitments, difficult dispositions, overwork, constant uncertainty, and the need to make numerous rapid decisions all create tension. Because emergency services rarely have full-time psychiatrists, psychiatric consultants are usually engaged in another task when called into the emergency room, which also increases their sense of being overwhelmed and inconvenienced.

A Final Word

Psychiatrists in the emergency room must remember that the context in which patients are seen is one of urgency. They must therefore begin by assessing rapidly the possibility that there is a problem whose treatment is truly urgent: an acute organic brain disorder, a functional psychosis, or imminent physical danger to self or others. Once these truly urgent possibilities have been ruled out, psychiatrists use their knowledge of psychosocial and intrapsychic issues to deal with other questions, such as the reason an emergency consultation is sought by patient, family, or emergency room physician. Difficulties in rapid differential diagnosis in an emergency room setting are often attributable more to patients' and psychiatrists' emotional reactions to the setting than to the actual task itself.

Suggested Readings

American Psychiatric Association. (1980). *Diagnostic and Statistical Manual of Mental Disorders*, 3rd ed. Washington, D.C.: American Psychiatric Association.

Dubin, W.R., and Stollberg, R. (1981). *Emergency Psychiatry for the House Officer*. New York: Spectrum.

Eisenberg, J.M. (1979). Sociologic influences on decision-making by clinicians. *Annals of Internal Medicine* 90:957–964.

Folstein, M.F., Folstein, S.E., and McHugh, P.R. (1975). "Mini-mental state": a practical method for grading the cognitive state of patients. *Journal of Psychiatry and Research* 12:189–198.

Gerson, S., and Bassuk, E. (1980). Psychiatric emergencies: an overview. *American Journal of Psychiatry* 137:1–11.

Kendell, R.E. (1973). Psychiatric diagnoses: a study of how they are made. *British Journal of Psychiatry* 122:437–445.

McHugh, P.R., and Slavney, P.R. (1982). Methods of reasoning in psychopathology. *Comprehensive Psychiatry* 23:197–215.

Perry, J.C., and Jacobs, D. (1982). Overview: clinical applications of the Amytal interview in psychiatric emergency settings. *American Journal of Psychiatry* 139:552–559.

Sandifer, M.G., Hardern, A., and Green, L. (1970). The psychiatric interview: the impact of the first three minutes. *American Journal of Psychiatry* 126:92–97.

Wise, T.N. (1979). Assessing emotional problems in medical practice. *Primary Care* 6:233–244.

CHAPTER 2

The Violent Patient

KENNETH TARDIFF, M.D., M.P.H.

Approximately 17 percent of patients presenting to an emergency room and 13 percent of patients presenting for admission to psychiatric hospitals are violent. Studies show that among chronic mental patients residing in hospitals, 7 percent physically assault another individual at least once in three months. Furthermore, violence by mental patients can be life-threatening to psychiatrists who treat them. In fact, 40 percent of psychiatrists have reported being assaulted at least once in their careers, and 40 percent of psychiatric residents in one program reported being assaulted at least once during their training.

This chapter considers physical aggression or serious threat of physical aggression toward people or objects, and focuses on evaluating and managing the violent patient in the emergency room, on the wards, and in the outpatient setting. Evaluating and managing the patient after the clinician controls the initial episode are also discussed.

The Biopsychosocial Approach

In determining the etiology and management of violent behavior, psychiatrists must always consider factors or treatments in the biological, psychological, and social spheres. Each violent person has a biological substrate for violence, whether it is the basic biological mechanism located in the limbic system or more unique influences such as genetic inheritance, low intelligence, hormonal influences, gross organic brain lesions, or a major psychiatric disorder. This biological substrate is tempered by learning, modeling, and the influences of family, peers, and society. A violent episode is triggered by various elements, such as stress, frustration, one's financial situation, the physical environment (including heat, crowding, and noise), alcohol or drugs, and conflict with others, whether family members, friends, or treatment personnel. These factors converge in a unique way for each person and lead to the explosion psychiatrists are called on to manage in the clinical setting.

The Setting

When a screaming, violent patient is surrounded by staff, family, other patients, and perhaps police, there is often a vicious cycle of the crowd's struggle with the patient increasing the patient's resistance and violence. The ideal way to interrupt this cycle is for the psychiatrist to deal with the patient alone. But before undertaking a one-to-one encounter, the psychiatrist must make certain decisions.

Will the patient respond with self-control to verbal interaction? Patients least likely to respond to verbal interventions are manics, schizophrenics, and those with organic mental disorders. Patients with personality disorders or other nonpsychotic disorders who are not drug- or alcohol-intoxicated are more likely to respond to a verbal interchange with the clinician.

In these circumstances, clinicians must exercise caution, avoid bravado, and use their intuition. If the clinician feels more comfortable with potential assistance in the same room, he or she should not see the patient alone. It is important for clinicians to be comfortable with violent patients so that they can convey a sense of security and calm competence.

The settings in which a psychiatrist sees patients will vary in their degree of restrictiveness from interviewing the patient in a room alone with the door open or closed, to interviewing the patient in a room with attendants present, to conducting the interview with the patient in restraints.

Patients Who Must Be Restrained

Patients who are not amenable to verbal intervention must often be physically restrained. Action must be rapid, without hesitation, and without further attempts at verbal communication. Implementing restraints places the staff and the patient at risk of injury, and thus it is necessary that facilities have written guidelines for these procedures and that they be rehearsed, observed, and critiqued. The staff should avoid humiliating the patient and should preserve routine and order throughout the procedure.

Adequate staff must be available—at least one person for each limb and one person to lead or coordinate the restraint procedure. Staff members should remove potentially dangerous items from themselves, such as jewelry or glasses, before beginning the procedure. At a predetermined signal from the restraint leader, each staff member seizes and controls the movement of one extremity. The patient is brought to the floor with a backward movement and each limb is restrained, immobilized, across elbow and knee joints. The restraint leader controls the patient's head to prevent biting.

Note that certain techniques are not permissible. A joint should not be bent beyond its normal range of motion, nor should pressure be applied opposite the normal motion of a joint, such as hyperextending the elbow. Undue pressure should not be applied to any part of a patient's body; for example, sitting on the patient. Pulling a patient's hair or choking, hitting, or pinching a patient is also prohibited, as are words, acts, or gestures showing disrespect or lack of concern. The psychiatrist should not be physically involved in applying restraint, because such action may preclude future successful verbal intervention with the patient. After the patient has been restrained, involved staff should meet, evaluate the procedure, and deal with their own emotional reactions.

During the time patients are restrained, they should be observed every 15 minutes by members of the nursing staff. In addition, appropriate vital signs should be determined, and freedom of circulation and respiration should be ensured. At proper intervals, fluids and meals should be given and toileting attended to.

The following case illustrates the use of restraints with a young man suffering from intoxication with an unknown drug.

> Mr. G., a 17-year-old white male, was brought to the emergency room by police. He was very agitated and screamed and struck out wildly at people around him. He was unresponsive to questioning. Three friends who accompanied him said that this was very unusual behavior for him. They had been wandering around the entertainment part of the inner city when they were approached by a person offering to sell them "uppers." The patient had accepted his friends' dare to swallow two of the pills they had purchased. After they had walked around some more and had consumed several beers, the patient had become agitated and belligerent. He was taken into custody by a policeman and was taken directly to the emergency room.
>
> A psychiatrist saw him within minutes of his arrival and immediately instituted four-point restraints. He decided not to use medication, since he could not determine the nature of the drugs ingested. Instead, he stayed with the patient for an hour and assured him that the effects of the drugs would pass. A friend remained with the patient for continued reassurance. When the psychiatrist visited four hours later, the patient was still anxious, but he was able to speak coherently. In the presence of four

attendants, the psychiatrist removed the restraints. The patient remained in the emergency room until the next morning and was then discharged to his parents.

Organic Mental Disorders

Once patients are in restraints or in control of themselves, clinicians must determine whether there is an organic mental disorder and, if so, treat that disorder. Toxic reactions to illicit drugs are a common cause of violence in the emergency room. Violent behavior accompanies the abuse of many drugs, including phencyclidine, LSD, barbiturates, amphetamines, and cocaine. Such patients are often brought to the emergency room by friends, who can give important information about what drug or drugs were consumed and whether they gave medications, such as phenothiazines, to relieve the problem. In toxic drug reactions, supportive verbal therapy is the treatment of choice; tranquilizers should be used with caution. If they are used, oral diazepam should be considered first because the margin between effective sedation and cardiovascular depression may be small with phenothiazines.

Violence can also be associated with alcohol intoxication or alcohol withdrawal. In pathological intoxication, men usually erupt after one or two drinks and attack other men who stare at them or make fun of them in bars. Because alcohol can trigger an epileptic focus, a thorough neurological evaluation of the patient is warranted. In addition, many patients engage in unprovoked assaultive behavior accompanied by amnesia, dizziness, or headache. Temporal lobe epilepsy, an infrequent cause of violence, can be accompanied by depersonalization and dreamlike lapses with nondirected rage. Other organic causes of violent behavior include brain trauma, infection, tumors, and metabolic disorders that result in delirium.

This case illustrates the evaluation and handling of alcohol-associated violence.

Mr. H., a 25-year-old construction worker, arrived in the emergency room accompanied by his wife, who had a swollen, contused area around her right eye. He asked to see a psychiatrist because he was concerned that he was "going crazy." When the psychiatrist arrived, the patient was sitting with his wife in the waiting room. The psychiatrist had been informed of the physical violence between the two. He approached the patient and asked him to follow him into an interview room. The patient's wife was asked to wait.

The interview with the patient revealed a history of alcohol abuse, absenteeism, and frequent automobile accidents. Often, when he returned from drinking, his wife confronted him and argued with him about his drinking. He had struck her more than once. Afterward, she usually left and stayed with neighbors. The next day he ordinarily expressed extreme remorse. He was now concerned because this was the first time she had suffered obvious physical injury. There were no weapons at home.

The psychiatrist asked the wife to join them, and she verified her husband's story. After speaking with the patient and his wife, the psychiatrist decided that both were well motivated for psychotherapy and that the likelihood of a recurrence of violence that day was slight. He arranged an appointment for them in the outpatient clinic for the following day. The patient and his wife were seen in couples therapy, and he was placed on disulfiram to help control his drinking.

The Use of Medication in the Emergency Situation

Neuroleptic medication is usually indicated if an organic brain syndrome has been ruled out and the violent patient appears to be schizophrenic or manic. Intramuscular medication is usually necessary unless the patient has regained control and will voluntarily take oral medication. Rapid neuroleptization may be employed. In this procedure, a drug such as haloperidol is given intramuscularly in a dose of 2.5 to 10 mg every 30 minutes until the violent behavior is controlled. Administration of up to 100 mg in 24 hours has been safe and effective. (For further discussion, see Chapter 5.) As with a patient in restraints, blood pressure, pulse, cardiac rhythm, respiration, and level of consciousness must be carefully monitored, and the psychiatrist must be equipped to manage any drug-related problems as they develop.

If the patient is not psychotic but is actively violent, barbiturates or diazepam should be considered. Slow intravenous administration of either type of drug is indicated. A 10 percent solution of sodium amobarbital in a dose of 200 to 500 mg may be administered [at a rate of 0.5 to 1.0 ml per minute,] or 5 to 10 mg of diluted diazepam may be given slowly intravenously. The total dose used is determined by the patient's reaction. With either medication, one should observe for side effects, such as depressed respiration, laryngospasm, and hypotension, and be prepared to resuscitate the patient.

Speaking with a Patient Who Is in Control

Patients who are in control of themselves can be interviewed alone. An interview room should have easy exit and should not contain objects that could be used as weapons, such as letter openers, bookends, or paperweights.

If there is a desk, it should widely separate the patient and the physician. Decorative cushions in a room can double as protective devices. Ideally, there should be a buzzer or some other device to signal impending danger to people outside the room. Security personnel, nurses, or family members can be asked to wait nearby. This spares the physician great embarrassment and danger should his or her omnipotent fantasy of single-handedly containing the patient not be fulfilled.

When alone with the patient, the psychiatrist sits down and asks the patient to do the same. The patient's anger and hostility are acknowledged in a simple, calm, gentle, and down-to-earth fashion. The patient should be encouraged to express verbally his or her anger. The psychiatrist should ask whether the patient wishes to take oral medication if it is indicated. Derogatory, judgmental, or other questions that attack the patient's self-esteem should be avoided.

The Question of Hospitalization

In evaluating violent patients, psychiatrists must make a decision about hospitalization. This process is analogous to evaluating suicide potential, and takes into account the seriousness of the actual violent episode. Threats of violence must be considered in terms of their planning. For example, a man who has well-formulated plans to kill his employer should be taken very seriously, while someone who makes vague threats about getting even or striking out at others may be taken somewhat less seriously. As with evaluation of suicide potential, the availability of a weapon should be considered. The role of the intended victim and his or her behavior in provoking violence should be considered if the patient is to be returned home.

The use of alcohol or drugs increases the likelihood of impulsive, serious violent behavior. Certain demographic characteristics must be considered. Young patients are more likely to be violent than older patients, and men are more likely to be violent than women. A history of previous violence may be an indicator of future violence, as may a history of being an abused child. Delusional, psychotic individuals must be hospitalized. In addition to considering a patient's potential for violence toward others, a psychiatrist must consider the patient's potential for suicide, which is often associated with other forms of violence.

Hospitalization was deemed necessary in the following case, in which the patient was mentally ill and had purchased a weapon.

Ms. I., a 32-year-old unmarried legal secretary living with her parents, was brought to the walk-in psychiatric clinic by her father, who was concerned because she had recently purchased a gun. Her father described her as a bright woman with few friends and no history of violent behavior. He said she had begun working for a large company immediately after graduation from college.

A psychiatrist interviewed the patient alone in her office. The patient initially stated that she had no problems and had purchased the gun for her own protection. As the interview progressed, she admitted dissatisfaction with her job. Over the previous year or two, she had felt increasingly alienated from her co-workers and believed a number of them talked about her. Recently, she had been denied a promotion, and she blamed the denial on a senior partner. Further questioning revealed that her thoughts were delusional and that she had probably purchased the gun to retaliate against the senior partner and others in the office.

The psychiatrist excused herself, telling the patient that she wanted the father to join them. While outside the office, she alerted the inpatient unit and requested that four male attendants be available in the walk-in clinic. She reentered the office with the patient's father and firmly but compassionately told the patient that she was arranging for hospitalization. The patient at first threatened legal action but finally acquiesced to hospitalization.

The Hospitalized Patient

A number of factors must be considered in managing hospitalized patients. Patients' violence on general hospital wards or psychiatric wards is commonly an expression of their anger toward staff, family, themselves, or their illness. Violence may result from lack of trust resulting from miscommunication between physicians and patients. Instead of striking out at physicians, patients may threaten or strike out against nurses, aides, or family members. By reestablishing lines of communication between patients and their treating physicians, psychiatric consultants can often bring immediate relief to both patients and staff.

Countertransference problems of physicians and other treatment personnel may compound problems of violence. Staff members may be irrationally afraid of a patient because of their own past experiences with violence, or physicians may be inappropriately angry with patients because of their past experiences with violent patients or with aggression by significant people in their lives.

Violent patients may also evoke a positive countertransference reaction, which also interferes with treatment. Physicians with personal conflicts regarding aggression may overidentify with violent patients. Physicians should not act out their own hostilities through patients, and may become aware of such tendencies while exaggerating patients' dangerousness to colleagues. Clinicians' use of denial to handle their conflicts about violence is very dangerous because this may prevent them from taking proper precautions for their own and others' safety.

Countertransference reactions of staff produce a number of counterproductive patterns on inpatient units. In staff conferences, the staff's views of violent patients' dangerousness may polarize meetings and produce conflict on the inpatient unit. As in the rest of psychiatric practice, having emotional reactions to violent patients is not poor practice, but not understanding them and not acting objectively is.

In sum, not all violent behavior is preventable, but there are indicators of potential violence and specialized techniques for dealing with patients who are violent or who are threatening violence. Astute clinicians, by maintaining vigilance and by taking prompt action, can often prevent patients' violent feelings from becoming violent behavior.

Suggested Readings

Donlon, P.T., Hopkin, J., and Tupin, J.P. (1979). Overview: efficacy and safety of the rapid neuroleptization method with injectable haloperidol. *American Journal of Psychiatry* 136:273–278.

Edelman, S.E. (1978). Managing the violent patient in a community mental health center. *Hospital and Community Psychiatry* 29:460–462.

Lion, J.R. (1972). *Evaluation and Management of the Violent Patient*. Springfield, Ill.: Charles C Thomas.

Madden, D.J., Lion, J.R., and Penna, M.W. (1976). Assault on psychiatrists by patients. *American Journal of Psychiatry* 133:422–425.

Rada, R.T. (1981). The violent patient: rapid assessment and management. *Psychosomatics* 22:101–109.

Ruben, I., Wolkon, G., and Yamamoto, J. (1980). Physical attacks on psychiatric residents by patients. *Journal of Nervous and Mental Disease* 168:243–245.

Skodol, A., and Karasu, T. (1978). Emergency psychiatry and the assaultive patient. *American Journal of Psychiatry* 135:202–204.

Tardiff, K., and Maurice, W. (1977). The care of violent patients by psychiatrists: a tale of two cities. *Canadian Psychiatric Association Journal* 22:83–86.

Tardiff, K., and Sweillam, A. (1980). Assault, suicide, and mental illness. *Archives of General Psychiatry* 37:164–169.

Tardiff, K., and Sweillam, A. (1982). The occurrence of assaultive behavior among chronic psychiatric inpatients. *American Journal of Psychiatry* 139:212–215.

CHAPTER 3

Management of Suicide Risk in the Psychiatric Emergency Room

FREDERICK G. GUGGENHEIM, M.D.

Assessing suicide risk is a challenging task. It demands an accurate forecast of dangerousness to self; and predictions of dangerousness are notoriously difficult to make. Determining whether and when a suicide will occur is problematic because there are so many variables involved. However, knowledge of psychodiagnostic and sociodemographic factors does enhance clinical judgments about suicidal patients.

General Considerations

Making a psychiatric diagnosis, evaluating psychosocial support systems, and assessing psychodynamic issues are important aspects of the evaluation of suicide risk.

Psychiatric Diagnosis

Of foremost importance in assessing suicide risk is determining the presence of a psychiatric disorder. Some disorders are associated with a high suicide rate. One in six people with recurrent affective disorders die of suicide, and a similar proportion of those with alcoholism also die from an active attempt at suicide. Among depressives, those with a bipolar disorder are much more self-lethal than are those with a unipolar disorder. One in ten schizophrenics perishes of suicide. One of every twenty individuals with a personality disorder dies of suicide. Death from suicide is rare for individuals suffering anxiety disorders or somatoform disorders. Among those few patients with borderline personality disorders who commit suicide, some do so by miscalculation; the remainder probably have a complicating affective disorder. Death by suicide is extremely rare in the absence of a psychiatric disorder. Knowledge of the type of psychiatric disorder and its appropriate treatment is therefore essential. Perhaps *nonmedical* psychotherapists' initial problem in assessing and managing severely suicidal people is that their clinical training is not focused on recognizing specific psychiatric disorders.

Psychosocial Support Systems

Weighing the noxious psychosocial forces against the supportive forces is often crucial in determining suicide risk for an individual who is struggling with the decision to live or to die. Families can support, but if chronically overwhelmed, they can also scapegoat and exclude. The reality of this external milieu, complementing the patient's own internal milieu, is of fundamental importance when the clinician is considering discharging an individual with a potential for suicide back into the community.

Psychodynamic Issues

A third essential element in assessing suicide risk is evaluating meanings, associations, and feelings linked with relevant biological events, interpersonal relationships, and intrapersonal configurations. A person usually becomes suicidal in a setting of hopelessness associated with some real or imaginary loss. That loss can be biological, interpersonal, or symbolic. When losses are both intrapersonal and interpersonal, the patient may feel like giving up and feel that he or she has been given up on. This is a potentially lethal set of circumstances.

Life events have a unique meaning for each person. Some people are impelled toward suicide after financial loss. Others manage such circumstances with equanimity but are drawn to suicide after the loss of a love object or after experiencing public humiliation. Familial disruptions are important prelethal events for children and teenagers as are loss of love objects for teenagers and for those in their twenties, economic setback for those in their thirties, forties, and fifties; and failing health in later life. Nevertheless, these statistical relationships may have little specific value when assessing the suicide potential of a particular individual.

Evaluating the Patient

Neophyte clinicians fear that asking depressed patients if they are thinking of killing themselves may alienate the patients, or even implant the idea and drive them toward suicide. The considerable experience of the Los

Angeles Suicide Prevention Center is that no patients have been harmed by being tactfully asked that important question. However, patients and emergency room psychiatrists can be harmed if that question is *not* asked. Physicians who fail to ask patients about suicide, and/or who do not document patients' responses in the chart, may be held liable for negligence if a patient commits suicide shortly after the interview.

Mental Status Examination

A focused mental status examination is crucial to the evaluation of suicidal patients. It is important to determine rapidly whether the patient is psychotic. In psychotic patients, suicidal ideation, or even a trivial gesture, needs to be managed differently from suicidal ideas in, say, borderline patients. Psychotic patients with suicidal ideation are at great risk, especially if command hallucinations are of recent onset. Suicidal ideation in patients with organic brain disease also represents a high risk, as the ego strength necessary to deal with such intrusive thoughts (whether they be ego-alien or ego-syntonic) is considerably decreased.

The phase of the specific disorder is also important. For example, severely depressed individuals may be at less risk for suicide as they become more depressed and develop psychomotor retardation. Conversely, the risk of suicide may increase as the depression begins to recede, leaving patients dysphoric and still perceiving their situation as hopeless but with an abundant store of energy to develop and implement a suicide plan. Similarly, the severity of the disorder may be relevant to predicting suicide. For example, individuals may have recurrent unipolar depressive episodes but be suicidal only during the most profound of these episodes.

The emotional tenor of suicidal individuals is another important factor to assess. Some suicide-prone people are looking for release and relief. Others are looking for revenge. The emotions most often associated with actual suicide are hopelessness, helplessness, exhaustion, and feelings of failure. The expression "I just want out" has a particularly ominous ring, as does conveying a sense of inner emptiness. The danger of immediate or subsequent lethal behavior is generally less when the predominant affect is anger, rage, or frustration. The venting of feelings during the psychiatric emergency room evaluation often decreases the suicidal inclination seen with acute anger. But since the affect of acute depression in suicidal patients often lasts longer and is less readily discharged in a benign manner, there is greater potential for it to be lethal. Similarly, if patients being evaluated have already made a premeditated (rather than an impulsive) suicide attempt, the risk of a subsequent suicide attempt is increased.

The final component of the mental status evaluation to be considered is the presence or absence of the presuicidal syndrome. In this highly lethal condition, patients feel constricted. Life has them boxed into a no-win situation, values seem useless, human relationships empty. Patients' behavior begins to manifest a fixed patterning; free associations are monotonous. The depressed mood "hangs on," heavily. Time stands still. Decisions are seen as either black or white. Patients feel restless, although outwardly they may appear calm.

Suicide Plans

Clinicians need to ask patients about future plans for life, and for death. The suicide plan, implemented or not, is one element in the assessment of risk. Certain patients will admit to a vague plan that on further assessment turns out to be only mildly lethal. But with patients who have meticulously detailed plans, further assessment usually determines that they are at high risk. When suicidal patients focus more on the impact of a potential suicide on others than on its actual implementation, the risk of subsequent lethality is somewhat diminished, especially if nonlethal methods are being considered.

The Help Repudiator

The patients who are the most suicide-prone are often the least cooperative in delineating the extent of their own lethality. When people have actually decided to end their lives, help repudiation often becomes an important implementing tactic. Thus, suicidal individuals may lie on direct questioning about the extent of their lethality, the nature of their suicide plans, and other details that might frustrate a lethal outcome. In such circumstances, an indirect approach may generate meaningful information. For example, in assessing individuals who have made a near-lethal suicide attempt, the best question to ask is: "Are you surprised that you survived?" The individuals are likely to respond honestly to this question because they do not view surprise as being related to the intent and seriousness of lethality, whereas such questions as "Did you plan to die during the attempt?" and "Do you plan to try to take your life in the near future?" may be dealt with less honestly.

Occasionally, individuals with lethal intent may make a moderately risky preliminary suicide attempt concealing from all the true extent of their imminent lethality. Then, having worked out the tactics, they execute the plan successfully.

Fortunately, most people who come or are brought to a psychiatric emergency room for evaluation do not grossly distort the extent of their lethal intent. Indeed, a clear majority of suicide attempters seen in the emergency room make their attempt as a desperate cry for help. Statistics show that if clinicians were to discharge without follow-up all patients brought to the psychiatric emergency room for therapeutic assessment of suicide potential, 95 percent would probably survive the year. High-risk patients have a mortality rate of about 5 percent per year, and low-risk patients have a mortality rate of about 1 percent per year.

Claims, Suspicions, Acts

Clinicians assessing suicide risk in the psychiatric emergency room must evaluate three different clinical situations: (1) patients who claim to be suicidal, whether or not they have made any suicide attempt, (2) patients who, on the basis of statements or actions, are suspected by family members or health care providers of having strong suicide potential, and (3) patients who have just attempted suicide. When these three clinical situations occur simultaneously, the initial assessment of the patient is simple. The relevant parties concur that the individual is at risk, the extent of the risk can be determined (high or low), and the clinical care (as an inpatient or an outpatient) can be planned accordingly. When only one or two of these conditions are present, the evaluation of the patient and the formulation of a care plan will involve at least some conjecture. The care plan for the suicidal patient also assumes that the psychopathological and sociodemographic risk factors will remain stable or improve with clinical intervention.

Risk and Rescue Factors

After concluding that a patient is suicidal, the next issue is the determination of the extent of the suicide risk. High risk suggests a serious suicide attempt or dying of suicide in the future. The suicide attempts of high-risk individuals actually put their lives in jeopardy. In the case of wrist-slashing, there are multiple deep cuts, with severing of arteries and tendons. If carbon monoxide is used, the level is greater than 30 mg percent. If a drug has been ingested, there is loss of consciousness. If a gun is used, the bullet actually enters the cranial, abdominal, or thoracic cavity. If a single-car accident, there are no brake marks before impact. Such pieces of evidence all indicate high risk, and this information is almost always on the admission medical chart.

Just as important in calculating lethality are the rescue factors involved in a suicide attempt. By contrast, these are rarely spelled out on the admission medical chart. High-risk cases usually make efforts to avoid rescue. For example, a patient might go to a motel under an assumed name and ingest medication, drive to a deserted place and do violence to himself or herself, or lie to family about going somewhere with friends and then sneak off to make the attempt. A highly lethal method coupled with planning of low rescuability clearly indicates high risk. Typically, four times more low-risk than high-risk patients are seen in a psychiatric emergency room. Still, clinicians should remember that the likelihood of suicide in a low-risk patient is 1,000 times greater than it is in the general population.

Managing the Crisis

After a patient in the emergency room is identified as a potential suicide risk, the clinician's first task is to ensure the patient's physical safety. Individuals who have recently attempted suicide will not usually try to take their lives in the emergency room or even in the intensive care unit after awakening from a coma. Occasionally, however, such behavior does occur. Those with agitated melancholia or with the command hallucinations of schizophrenia are especially at risk, even in a hospital environment. It is always possible to smash an intravenous bottle and inflict lacerations; a needle can be swallowed; surgical knives and other surgical instruments can be used to produce penetrating wounds. Also, unattended patients may use a concealed weapon or poison.

The best precaution against suicide is the constant vigil of an appropriate caregiver. Strict suicide precautions, that is, one-to-one precautions, can be lifesaving. At times when the medical staff cannot be utilized, clinicians may have to rely on the help of hospital security forces or family members. But in all instances, backup staff must be close at hand. The consultants themselves may need to stay with patients until physical, chemical, or interpersonal restraints have secured patients' safety.

Strict suicide precautions need not always be instituted following an attempt or a threat. For example, following a suicide gesture with high manipulative intent (low risk, high rescuability), patients may have gained considerably because grievances have been effectively communicated and there are prospects of some gratifying shift in family dynamics. After matters have stabilized, even basic suicide precautions—observing the patient every 15 minutes and making certain that no potentially lethal objects are present —may not be necessary. After patients' safety has been assured, clinicians begin or continue the information-gathering process.

Management of Perturbation

The development of a therapeutic alliance will at times be thwarted if the patient experiences a high degree of perturbation. Psychomotor agitation, intense dysphoria, and the inability to concentrate may all be alleviated by the steadying interest and concern of the clinician. Psychoactive medications will rarely be required during the interview. When agitation is truly life threatening, 5 to 20 mg of diazepam may be given slowly intravenously. If a suicidal patient is extremely agitated and psychotic, a neuroleptic such as haloperidol may be given orally or parenterally. Patients who have recently self-overdosed usually need no additional medication until the delirium and lethargy have cleared. Occasionally, when patients have ingested a tricyclic antidepressant, they may develop an anticholinergic psychosis. In such circumstances, intravenous physostigmine, 1 to 2 mg, may reverse the agitation and delirium for up to four hours.

Criteria for Hospitalization

Despite the psychiatrist's best efforts at learning all relevant facts, the time pressures of a busy psychiatric emergency room and the long-standing feelings and private agendas of the familial participants sometimes make adequate assessment nearly impossible. Nonetheless, clinicians need to decide whether to hospitalize or to discharge patients.

If discharged, will the patient's social network taunt and molest him or her? Or will it be warm, supportive, understanding, and ever-present? Unfortunately for the clinician, there are no simple means to assess the adequacy of psychosocial supports. But if a patient has made a recent near-lethal suicide attempt that has not accomplished its goal—for example, reunion with a loved one, revenge on a significant key person, or escape from despair—the available community outpatient support system may not suffice. In general, high-risk cases are hospitalized voluntarily or involuntarily, and low-risk cases are discharged to appropriate outpatient care.

There are absolute and relative indicators for hospitalization. Absolute indicators are any of the following: (1) psychosis (even if the suicide attempt was trivial or the suicidal ideation is at a low level), (2) patient age 40 or older (unless there is a long history of manipulative suicide gestures without any increase in the degree of risk taken or attempts to avoid rescue), and (3) a premeditated near-lethal attempt. Because of medical complications of a near-lethal attempt, such survivors are often hospitalized for several days or weeks on a medical/surgical service, thus allowing for unhurried evaluation and initiation of appropriate treatment. When this occurs, transfer to a psychiatric service is often not necessary.

Relative indicators for hospitalization are (1) the presence of a major untreated or undertreated suicide-prone psychiatric disorder, (2) precautions taken to avoid being rescued alive, (3) regret of survival and/or demonstration of a rising level of perturbation in the hospital, (4) refusal of help, (5) signs and symptoms of the presuicidal syndrome, and (6) living alone, unemployed and without a social support system.

Implementing the Disposition

The decision to send a suicidal patient to a psychiatric unit is always a difficult one to make. The psychiatrist wants neither to facilitate a suicide nor to subject a person in a brief, self-limited crisis to a stigmatizing unneeded psychiatric hospitalization. Moreover, the psychiatrist wants to avoid rewarding crisis-seeking, histrionic behavior by authenticating the patient's sick role and providing the wished-for secondary gain.

When clinicians do decide to psychiatrically hospitalize the patient, they must be prepared to help patients accept that judgment. Acceptance of hospitalization is often gradual. Clinicians whose patients are most apt to accept hospitalization mention hospitalization early in their evaluation and work on the issue during the entire interview of patients and their families.

Outcomes

Most suicidal patients who arrive at the psychiatric emergency room go home the same day. One study of 100 patients who were alive when brought to a hospital emergency room revealed that 67 percent went home the same day, 11 percent signed out against medical advice or eloped, 5 percent later died in the hospital of medical/surgical complications of their attempt, and 17 percent were sent to a psychiatric unit. Using a standardized risk/rescue ratio, lethality was judged to be high for 8 percent, moderate for 45 percent, and low for 47 percent.

At times, suicide attempts are not perceived as such by the medical/surgical house staff. Physicians' chart notes sometimes include such euphemisms as "drug ingestion," "drug intoxication," or "toxic metabolic coma" when the issue is self-induced poisoning. Self-laceration is sometimes considered accidental; jumping under a subway train has been described on the chart as merely "crush amputation, left leg"; carbon monoxide poisoning may be signed out as "cerebral anoxia secondary to carbon monoxide"; and gunshot wounds witnessed by others as self-inflicted and intentional may be signed out as "G.S.W., left chest, accidental." The wish not to see behavior as deliberately self-inflicted is strong both in medical and nonmedical personnel. The number of these psychiatrically nonreferred patients with medically serious suicide attempts that are later referred for psychiatric evaluation varies from institution to institution. Subsequent psychiatric consultations on the wards, changes in psychosocial circumstances, the passage of time, and a renewal of hope all tend to lessen the suicidal behavior in these patients, and suicide attempts in the hospital itself for these attempters are rare.

Mr. J., a 54-year-old airline pilot, abruptly unemployed three months earlier when his company went bankrupt, was rushed to the emergency room, accompanied by his wife and his mother. They had discovered him retching profusely in the bathroom, having apparently ingested a bottle of 25 prescribed sleeping tablets and consumed a pint of vodka. The family gave no history of prior mental illness or alcoholism until his layoff, but they had noted he had become increasingly despondent since that time and had said that he was unemployable and that his continued existence would be a burden to the family. During the preceding sleepless week, he had begun avoiding friends, and had become increasingly anorectic, irritable, and agitated, especially after his wife began working at a downtown bakery. On the day of the attempt, he had told family members he was going to a suburban employment agency, but instead returned home, parked his car on a nearby street, entered the home by a side door, and made his suicide attempt. His wife, who had forgotten her lunch, had returned home for it and heard him retching.

On examination in the emergency room, the patient was severely depressed and showed little spontaneity. He adamantly denied that he was still suicidal, saying, "I learned my lesson." He did, however, admit to surprise at surviving, the alcohol apparently having induced an acute gastritis.

Further questioning by the psychiatrist revealed that the patient did indeed have the manifestations of a severe depression, and the family was helped to understand this. With support, they were able to fill out forms for a mental illness warrant to permit involuntary hospitalization, in spite of the patient's wrenching pleas that such a hospitalization would "ruin any further chances for gainful employment."

He was hospitalized in a psychiatric unit. Imipramine helped induce a complete remission of symptoms within four weeks. He admitted that if he had been discharged that first day to the custody of his wife and his mother, he would have used the gun in the bedside nightstand to terminate his painful existence as soon as his wife had fallen asleep that night.

Suggested Readings

Berman, A.L., and Cohen-Sandler, R. (1982). Suicide and the standard of care: optimal versus acceptable. *Suicide and Life-Threatening Behavior* 12:114–122.

Farberow, N.L., and Schneidman, E.S. (eds.) (1965). *The Cry for Help*. New York: McGraw-Hill.

Guggenheim, F. G., and Weisman, A. D. (1974). Suicide in the subway: psychodynamic aspects. *Suicide and Life-Threatening Behavior* 4:43–53.

Guggenheim, F. G. (1978). Suicide. In *Massachusetts General Hospital Handbook of Consultation-Liaison Psychiatry*, ed. T.P. Hackett and N.H. Cassem, pp. 250–263. St. Louis, Mo.: C.V. Mosby.

Kuesper, D.J. (1982). A study of referral failures for potentially suicidal patients: a method of medical care evaluation. *Journal of Hospital and Community Psychiatry* 33:49–52.

Miles, C.P. (1977). Conditions predisposing to suicide: a review. *Journal of Nervous and Mental Disease* 164:231–246.

Ringel, E. (1976). The presuicidal syndrome. *Suicide and Life-Threatening Behavior* 6:131–149.

Weisman, A.D., and Worden, J.W. (1972) Risk-rescue rating in suicide assessment. *Archives of General Psychiatry* 26:553–560.

CHAPTER 4

Crisis Intervention

DOUGLAS A. PURYEAR, M.D.

Crisis intervention is a technique by which individuals or families in crisis are assisted efficiently in using their own resources to reestablish their previous psychological equilibrium.

Principles, Steps, and Techniques

The five main principles of emergency room crisis intervention are: setting limited goals, employing focused problem solving, expecting the individuals or family to take some action on their own behalf, providing support for that action, and building self-reliance and self-esteem.

These principles are employed in six basic steps: establishing rapport, taking charge, assessing the patient or family's problems and assets, closing, and follow-up. In the examples that follow, specific techniques, such as assigning tasks, active listening, positive reinforcement, reversing, and reframing, are employed to help mobilize people in crisis.

As part of establishing rapport, the psychiatrist quickly takes charge of the interview, meets everyone in the family, organizes the beginning of the interview, and starts by getting to know each person. Through controlling the process, the psychiatrist makes sure that everyone is heard, that no one is attacked, and that feelings are ventilated in a controlled and productive fashion. The psychiatrist becomes established as a resource to assist the family's work in solving their problems, but does not take direct responsibility for the family or for solving their problems.

Assessing the problem involves looking for a critical sequence of events that led up to the crisis state and focusing on specific facts and behaviors instead of accepting generalizations, accusations, or feelings. The psychiatrist helps the family to focus on a manageable piece of the problem and does not allow the interview to become diffuse. Issues that must be evaluated are sequentially addressed (for example, assessing the presence of suicidal intent, psychosis, or organic mental disorder) while the psychiatrist continues the intervention along the track of the problem-solving process. Assets and resources are evaluated early in the interview. The psychiatrist inquires about other family members in the community, church membership, and other helping professionals who may be involved. The family's own resources are used as plans are developed. As issues are resolved, and the situation and the specific problems to be worked on are established, the family members are helped to plan for dealing with them. The psychiatrist asks about different options that may have been considered. The technique of reversing (telling the family to do the opposite of what they might expect) may be used; the psychiatrist may ask the family not to try to do too much at once, may mention what other people have found helpful, or may simply leave the room and by letting some time elapse, may begin to mobilize the family. In these ways, responsibility is left with the family, and they are expected to deal with the problem. The mobilization is enhanced by the psychiatrist's support, which may include giving family members written tasks and making clear the intention to follow up and find out how they were performed.

By focusing on a limited problem, discussing possibilities for the future, and having expectations of the family, the psychiatrist makes it clear from the beginning that this is a time-limited interaction, and thus begins to close. If a referral is set up, a phone call is made after the time of the appointment, to see how it went. Usually the psychiatrist makes at least one follow-up telephone call.

Active listening involves more than receptiveness. An active listener reflects the patient's statements in ways that vigorously convey understanding and nonjudgmental acceptance. In reframing, a situation is cast in a way that gives it an entirely different meaning. For example, a mother's overcriticism of her child is reframed as an indication of her caring.

The principles, steps and techniques of crisis intervention are illustrated in the two vignettes that follow. Each is taken from situations that might otherwise have culminated in hospitalization.

Mrs. J., a 47-year-old housewife and grandmother, was brought to the emergency room by her husband and a good friend. She was agitated at first. She stuttered when she tried to speak, and looked about wild-eyed.

The psychiatrist began taking charge by inviting the trio into the interview room and asking them to sit down. He controlled the interview while meeting each person, learning their identities, occupations, and roles. Only after taking charge and establishing rapport did the psychiatrist ask the patient what had been happening. The entire interview was structured to keep all three people involved, emphasizing each one's perceptions and avoiding centering on the patient. Although the patient was agitated, stuttered, and sometimes spoke disjointedly, her communications were relevant. Active listening in the interview gave her the opportunity to ventilate in a controlled fashion, and her feelings and perceptions were clarified. As a result, she became calmer and more articulate.

The patient had worked hard most of her life. Fifteen years earlier she had had a similar episode from which she recovered without treatment. Two months earlier she had suffered a back injury, which kept her out of work, and afterward developed insomnia and irritability. Three days before coming to the emergency room, she and her husband had had a serious argument about disciplining their 13-year-old granddaughter, who lived with them. The patient's symptoms of agitation, stuttering, and disorganization began after that argument.

The patient complained that her husband had never taken responsibility for the children, was quite indulgent, and would never say no. If she said no to them, they went to him and received a yes. Three days before, her granddaughter had stayed away from the house for 12 hours. The patient did not know where the granddaughter had gone or with whom. While relating this, the patient became angry and more agitated. The psychiatrist intervened, focused on facts, and questioned the patient and the friend about the argument. The patient calmed down, and the psychiatrist then reframed the argument by asking, "Was it a good argument?" He wondered aloud if the argument had clarified or resolved some issues, or had merely stirred up anger and ended with nothing being worked out. The patient and her husband felt the argument had not been very productive but had clarified certain issues.

The psychiatrist then positively reinforced their strength and their basic good will. He emphasized the strain the couple had been under. He suggested that the wife had been worrying about her husband's carrying the load alone while she was unable to work and that the husband had been worrying about his wife's back injury and her recent upset. They also were raising a young granddaughter and struggling financially. The psychiatrist emphasized the value of the good friend who was able to provide support for the patient without taking sides.

At that point, the psychiatrist asked to see the patient alone. Her comments suggested that she felt unimportant and that her husband and granddaughter were colluding to act against her wishes. She wanted her husband to start saying no, but she had been unable to ask him directly to do this.

The psychiatrist evolved a plan and presented it to the husband, the wife, and the friend. He emphasized that the patient, a very hard worker, was understandably having difficulty being out of work and having time on her hands. He encouraged her to become more active in her church and in her granddaughter's PTA. Since the psychiatrist thought it was unlikely that the husband would change and begin to say no to his granddaughter, he took an indirect approach with him. The psychiatrist referred to the granddaughter as a vulnerable adolescent and expressed his concern that she might not be receiving all the female guidance she needed. He suggested that when the husband gave the granddaughter permission to go out or was going to take her out himself, he tell her to consult with her grandmother about her clothing, to see if she was dressed appropriately. The psychiatrist emphasized that dress was important and that a young woman needed much guidance about proper attire. The friend agreed to stay with the patient for the next few days. A follow-up emergency room visit and telephone contact were arranged for further support.

The foregoing crisis intervention used a family/network approach. It focused on the patient's feeling unimportant and on her husband's indulgent attitude toward the granddaughter. To maintain rapport and to increase the chance of success, an indirect approach was used with both. Limited goals were set, and there was no direct involvement with other issues, such as sexuality or the patient's long-smoldering resentment or other marital problems. The review of systems and mental status examination did not suggest medical or organic mental problems, and the diagnostic questions of psychosis and/or agitated depression remained unanswered. The patient improved and was referred for follow-up treatment. Her needs for a sense of value and for power were partially deflected from her husband and granddaughter to her church and PTA, where they could be partially satisfied. Her self-esteem was supported by the psychiatrist's focusing on the whole family, minimizing her status as "the patient" and emphasizing understandable life problems and reliance on the family's resources to deal with them. The working hypothesis was that the patient was a strong woman who denied dependency needs, needed to feel important and in control, and was temporarily derailed by her back injury. Aside from chronic marital problems, she generally functioned without overt symptoms until meeting those needs was threatened.

In dealing with a crisis, the psychiatrist attempts to focus on one component of the situation as the problem to be solved. Resolving that problem will relieve some of the tension in the family and enable them to get back to dealing with their own problems. Moreover, beginning to work on a problem helps them to get organized, to begin moving, and to develop a sense of hope, and thus restores their feelings of potency. It is therefore critical to select a problem that can be resolved, or to break a large problem into small manageable ones. The psychiatrist rejected the patient's definition of the problem as "my husband won't say no," because it was doubtful that this problem could be resolved. Instead, the problem was reframed as, "Your granddaughter needs more guidance and direction from her grandmother." Something could be done about this, and it would meet some of the patient's needs without provoking her husband. By taking small steps and making small changes in direction, the chances of success are greater than if large steps or larger changes are attempted.

The members of a family in crisis are demoralized. They are uplifted by the psychiatrist's working with them in a way that shows that they are expected to participate, to come up with useful information and ideas, and to carry out tasks. Beginning work on a problem conveys the notion that the problem is solvable and that the crisis can be resolved.

Action is important in crisis intervention. The family members are actively employed in planning what action is needed and in selecting tasks to be performed. The family's energy has been depleted and the members depend on expert support to get them started. That support is offered by problem solving with them and by showing empathy and respect. It is continued with follow-up visits and phone calls. For example, if the psychiatrist sets up a clinic appointment for the family, he or she makes a phone call after the appointment time, to be sure that everything went as planned. At the same time, the psychiatrist draws other supports in from the family's own network and from the community.

It is most important for the psychiatrist to maintain the family's self-reliance and self-esteem by having them do what they can for themselves, beginning with small tasks. They are treated as capable of functioning adequately and with the expectation that they will do so. The family's ideas are utilized, choices are offered, and options are explored; giving directives or advice is avoided.

The following is an example of a crisis intervention with a potentially suicidal person.

Mr. K., a 43-year-old single unemployed executive, came to the emergency room alone, stating that he feared he might kill himself. He said he had left a good position in Massachusetts because of family problems and had come to Dallas seven months before. He had been unable to find the type of work he wanted and had lost a lesser job two months earlier. Since then, he had failed to find employment. He was living with a man he had met in Dallas. He had kept the apartment clean and had cooked. Cleanliness and neatness were very important to him. Because they were unable to pay their rent, he and his friend had moved to what he described as a shack. He reported increasing depression and had given up trying to keep house because there were too many roaches and living conditions were so terrible. Being out of money, he could no longer keep his clothes clean and had also given up looking for work.

The patient's attitude was sullenly passive, as though saying, "There's nothing I can do; it's up to you." Otherwise his mental status examination and a review of systems were unremarkable. He appeared more frustrated than depressed and did not meet DSM-III criteria for a major depressive disorder. A formal assessment of suicide risk was postponed until later in the interview because the psychiatrist sensed that the patient might be promoting hospitalization as a means to escape his situation.

In crisis intervention, it is often better not to deal with the patient's initial request or assess suicide risk early in the interview. During the interview, it may be possible to mobilize the patient, instill some hope, and make it clear to the patient that he or she will not go away empty-handed. This may change the entire clinical picture. In addition, the patient may then be more responsive, even if the initial request is not granted.

Active listening (and responding) to Mr. K. went along the following lines.

"You're really feeling terrible."

"This is extremely frustrating for you."

"You have always been a hard-working man with high standards."

"Cleanliness and neatness are very important to you; when your house isn't clean, you feel even worse."

No suggestions were made during this phase. The patient became more responsive and revealed more information. His visit appeared to have been precipitated by his roommate's developing a friendship with a Mexican-American man who lived nearby. Each evening they conversed in Spanish and excluded the patient. He felt hurt and rejected.

The psychiatrist used reversal, stating, "You probably wouldn't feel like doing anything right now, even if I made some suggestions." He then began to explore possibilities with the patient and focused on the patient's feeling very depressed at the condition of the house. The patient indicated that cleaning it was hopeless and he had given up. The psychiatrist agreed that it probably was hopeless but stated that the lack of effort was probably making the patient more depressed. He asked the patient which was the dirtiest and which the most important room in the house, and the patient indicated the kitchen on both counts. The psychiatrist suggested that even though it was impossible, it would be worthwhile for the patient to clean the kitchen as well as possible, recognizing that it wouldn't ever look good or meet his standards. He then suggested that the task might be too hard right then and that the patient might instead focus his attention on either the stove or the refrigerator to see how clean he could get it. Mr. K. replied that the task was not too hard and that he could try to clean the whole kitchen. The psychiatrist then suggested that the patient not try to do that all at once but that he break it into separate tasks and try to do one of them each day. The patient thought he could do the whole kitchen but said that plan might be reasonable. They agreed that the following day, the patient would clean the refrigerator and then decide if he wanted to do more.

The psychiatrist then asked if the patient felt he could benefit from some support or someone to talk to, as he was estranged from his family. They agreed that the Suicide Prevention Center's hot line might be useful, and the psychiatrist gave the patient that phone number, explaining its 24-hour availability and the nature of the service. He asked the patient if he would be able to call. The patient thought so. The psychiatrist then handed him the phone, saying, "Here, I'll dial for you." While dialing, the psychiatrist suggested that the patient explain the situation to the suicide prevention worker, and ask if he could call once a day for the next four days to report how he was doing. The patient was startled, but accepted the assignment. He began talking to the volunteer who answered the telephone. The psychiatrist said that he had to leave the room for a time, but would be back shortly.

In helping people to undertake tasks, it is important to make the tasks specific and immediate. People will agree to perform assigned tasks but may not follow through. After maneuvering patients into agreeing to call for a clinic appointment or to call the Suicide Prevention Center, it is often useful to push them into doing it on the spot instead of leaving it as a vague possibility. Thus patients are already taking some action in their own behalf.

Sometimes it is useful to leave patients alone to think about what has been said, to mull over various possibilities, or merely to stew for a time if they have not made any positive movement during an interview. Such a break also gives the psychiatrist time to think over the situation, a chance to consult with a colleague, or time to see another patient if the work load is great.

When the psychiatrist returned, Mr. K. was talking to the Suicide Prevention Center volunteer and the conversation seemed to be going well. After hanging up, he appeared to be in a much better mood. The psychiatrist, again using reversal, said, "I've been thinking about your job situation. It sounds pretty bad. It's going to be hard for you to look for a job without money for clean clothes." The patient agreed. The doctor said, "You might pick up a few dollars at a labor pool or some kind of menial job—just to get enough to get your clothes clean for job hunting—but I think you probably really don't feel up to that at this point." The patient thoughtfully said that it might be worth a try but remained noncommital. The psychiatrist then said, "You've got this other problem with your friend and the guy across the way. What if you just went to him on your own and asked him to give you Spanish lessons." The patient looked dubious but said, "It might be worth a try."

The psychiatrist shifted gears and proceeded to assess suicide risk, mentioning in passing (using reversal again), "We don't like to have to put people into mental wards, even when it is for their own protection." Assessment suggested that there was some suicide risk but that it was relatively low. The patient appeared to feel better and said he felt better.

The psychiatrist repeated what they had decided on, obtained agreement, and then wrote on a card:

1. Keep the kitchen as clean as possible.
2. Call the Suicide Prevention Center once daily for four days.
3. Consider labor pool.

He then asked what the patient had thought about asking for Spanish lessons, and the patient agreed to try it. The psychiatrist then asked if the patient wanted to ask about lessons that day or the day after. Mr. K. settled on the day after. That was added to the card along with a final instruction to return to the emergency room or to call the psychiatrist if needed. A follow-up call was not arranged because the patient had a firm contact with the Suicide Prevention Center.

Uses, Limitations, and Requirements

The crisis intervention approach cannot be used in every crisis situation in the emergency room. Sometimes psychiatrists do not have time, and sometimes cases are not suitable. However, the principles, steps, and techniques can be usefully applied in almost every case. For example, they can be used to engage the family and assist the members in dealing with a psychotic person for whom the primary treatment is rapid neuroleptization.

In order to practice crisis intervention in an emergency room, certain resources are necessary. The psychiatrist must have sufficient time. An average initial crisis intervention interview takes about an hour. The psychiatrist can handle most aspects of the case alone; this entails the patient and the family's initial visit, one or two brief follow-up visits to the emergency room, and several phone calls. The first interview may result in immediate referral, in which case the psychiatrist may need only to make one or two follow-up phone calls. The demand on the physician's time may be as much as eight hours spread over several weeks, but most cases are handled in much less time.

Other resources necessary for crisis intervention include a telephone, the psychiatrist's periodic availability over several weeks, and a relatively quiet, private place in which a family can be interviewed. It is also helpful if the facility's other personnel and administration are aware of the approach and agree with it.

Some patients of families become engaged in ongoing therapy as a positive outcome of their crisis. However, most people in crisis who present at the emergency room are not interested in therapy and wish only a quick resolution of their pain. Attempting to push or coerce them into therapy frequently backfires, building up even more resistance to therapy and damaging the rapport necessary for the crisis intervention. Instead of regarding patients or their families as ill, the psychiatrist regards them as temporarily overwhelmed by problems and in need of help to resolve them.

Crisis intervention offers treatment instead of triage. It helps families restabilize with minimum disruption, often averts hospitalization, and thereby protects the patient's sense of competence. Its effectiveness justifies the extra expenditure of time and effort.

Suggested Readings

Caplan, G. (1981). Mastery of stress: psychosocial aspects. *American Journal of Psychiatry* 138:413–420.

Haley, J. (1976). *Problem Solving Therapy.* San Francisco: Jossey-Bass.

Langley, D.G., and Kaplan, D.M. (1968). *The Treatment of Families in Crisis.* New York: Grune & Stratton.

Puryear, D.A. (1979). *Helping People in Crisis: A Practical Family-Oriented Approach to Effective Crisis Intervention.* San Francisco: Jossey-Bass.

CHAPTER 5

Rapid Neuroleptization

EDMUND C. SETTLE, JR., M.D.

Rapid neuroleptization refers to the frequent intramuscular administration of high-potency neuroleptic medications to quell acute psychotic symptomatology. Rapid neuroleptization is important because psychotic patients are unpredictable; they can be assaultive or belligerent, and they may suddenly lose control of their behavior. Therefore, acute treatment can be lifesaving.

Basic Principles and Pharmacokinetics

High-potency, low-dose neuroleptic agents are usually the drugs of choice for rapid neuroleptization. They cause less sedation, less alpha-adrenergic and cholinergic blockade, and fewer cardiovascular side effects than lower-potency compounds. Haloperidol, thiothixene, fluphenazine, and loxapine are particularly good agents for rapid neuroleptization.

Orally administered neuroleptics take about 1½ hours to appear in the serum; peak levels are obtained in 4 to 6 hours. In contrast, intramuscularly administered neuroleptics are rapidly absorbed, with peak blood levels occurring in about 30 minutes.

Due to incomplete absorption and the "first-pass effect," representing initial deactivation by the liver, only about 60 percent of an oral dose of a neuroleptic reaches the systemic circulation. Because bioavailability differs significantly among subjects, initial oral dosage is also relatively imprecise.

Intramuscular administration achieves much higher blood levels than oral administration during the initial dosing sequence. Multiple sequential oral doses are necessary before adequate blood levels are reached, but with intramuscular administration, adequate blood levels are reached almost immediately. After approximately 24 hours, plasma levels of drugs administered either orally or parenterally become more equal. Oral neuroleptization is therefore not the method of choice for acute situations.

Phases of Rapid Neuroleptization

A major difficulty with rapid neuroleptization is the use of inflexible regimens. Unfortunately, rapid neuroleptization is sometimes viewed as a standardized method of treatment rather than as a precise, symptom-specific adjunct to initiating neuroleptic agents. Due to the pharmacokinetic properties of neuroleptic agents and to the typical progression of symptom resolution in psychotic patients, rapid neuroleptization can be divided into two treatment phases. The division between phase I and phase II is at about 24 hours of treatment. Patient assessment and optimal medication usage differ significantly between these two treatment phases.

During the initial 24 hours, intramuscularly administered neuroleptics are needed for acute, rapidly effective drug action. During this initial phase, target symptoms include acute agitation, hostility, overactivity, and other objective behavioral manifestations. During phase II, oral medication is effective for most patients. Typical target symptoms during phase II are thought disorganization and lower-grade psychotic activity.

Phase I

As stated, intramuscular neuroleptics are used in phase I of neuroleptization. Parenteral administration of low-potency agents should generally be avoided because of their side effects, including local irritation, orthostatic hypotension, and oversedation. Low-potency agents should not be totally excluded, however, as will be discussed later.

Haloperidol or thiothixene, 2 to 5 mg, fluphenazine, 5 mg, or loxapine, 25 mg, when administered every 30 to 60 minutes, give good results. Higher doses cause extrapyramidal symptoms, occasional slight hypotension, and some sedation. There is no clear correlation between dose size and frequency and the amount of extrapyramidal side effects. Also noteworthy is the extremely wide variation in individual dosage requirements.

Phase I Problems

EXCESSIVELY HIGH DOSAGES.   Large doses every ½ to 4 hours are usually not necessary for adequate symptom control. Some doses reasonable for physically healthy patients are:

		CHLORPROMAZINE EQUIVALENCE
Haloperidol	2–10 mg	100–500 mg
Thiothixene	2–10 mg	100–500 mg
Fluphenazine	2–10 mg	100–500 mg
Loxapine	25 mg	100 mg

When possible, the smaller doses should be utilized. Wide individual variation is seen. Rigid protocols such as "haloperidol, 10 mg every 30 minutes until calm" should be avoided.

OVERLY AGGRESSIVE DOSE ESCALATION.   Patients who respond poorly to a neuroleptic regimen may be treated by rapidly increasing the dose. Not all patients respond to every neuroleptic. In some cases, it may be wise to change the neuroleptic agent instead of increasing the dosage.

Many clinicians find that a subgroup of highly agitated and aggressive young healthy manics respond poorly to all high-potency neuroleptics but do well on lower-potency compounds. Loxapine, a moderate-potency compound with greater sedative properties, may be useful in these patients. In some cases, intramuscular chlorpromazine (25 to 50 mg) can be of marked benefit.

SIDE EFFECTS.   Many neuroleptic-induced side effects can occur during intramuscular usage. Akathisia may be misinterpreted as worsening agitation. A potentially lethal side effect is laryngeal dystonia. An order for a parenteral anticholinergic agent as needed should be written and patients closely observed by a well-trained nursing staff. The use of parenteral neuroleptics calls for the highest degree of cooperation between physicians and nursing staff. Specific education and close observation are essential if potentially dangerous side effects are to be avoided.

MEDICATIONS GIVEN WITHOUT IDENTIFYING SPECIFIC TARGET SYMPTOMS.   Ordering intramuscularly administered neuroleptics for patients "until calm" or "until agitation subsides" invites disaster. Specific target symptoms must be identified and closely monitored. Phase I target symptoms include agitated sleeplessness, belligerence, and psychotically driven motor behavior. Resolution of all signs of psychosis is not the goal of intramuscular administration of neuroleptics.

INTRAMUSCULAR ADMINISTRATION CONTINUED WHEN ORAL ADMINISTRATION HAS BECOME APPROPRIATE.   As soon as patients can reasonably cooperate with oral administration, routine intramuscular use should be stopped. Usually this occurs after 24 hours. During the first few days of phase II oral treatment, additional infrequent, smaller doses of intramuscular medication may be necessary for optimal symptom control.

Phase II

Oral neuroleptics are used in phase II of neuroleptization. Phase II continues in the acute phase until patients are well stabilized on an oral regimen, typically requiring several days up to several weeks. It is important to achieve rapid stabilization since some psychotic symptoms will persist following initial intramuscular treatment. For most patients, large oral doses have no great advantage over moderate doses. Likewise high intramuscular loading doses provide no advantage during phase II.

A dosage equivalence of at least 300 mg per day of chlorpromazine is necessary for acute treatment response; a dosage equivalence range of 300 to 600 mg per day of chlorpromazine is adequate for most patients. Little is gained by increasing daily dosage beyond 1,000 mg of chlorpromazine equivalence.

It is advisable to use the same neuroleptic when converting from successful phase I parenteral treatment to phase II oral treatment. Requirements vary, but a rough rule is to use a total daily oral dose of double the parenteral dose given over the preceding 24-hour period. Initially oral medication should be given three or four times a day, gradually decreasing the total dose, and eventually giving it twice a day or once daily at bedtime.

Phase II Problems

INTRAMUSCULAR ADMINISTRATION CONTINUED OVER MANY DAYS.   Parenteral administration is a prelude to oral use; it does not replace it. Patients should be started on oral medicine as soon as they can cooperate, although occasional use of intramuscular doses may be necessary early in oral treatment.

EXCESSIVE INITIAL ORAL DOSES.   Large oral doses are of no advantage in most patients. Neuroleptics have long half-lives and accumulation of repeated high doses can produce problems of extended duration.

OVERLY AGGRESSIVE TREATMENT.   Time is our ally during phase II treatment since there is much less potential for loss of behavioral control. A structured and supportive inpatient milieu can be of great benefit and can lessen medication requirements if the medication is first given time to take effect. Total symptom resolution in the first few days is not to be expected or attempted by pushing medication dosages.

PATIENTS DISCHARGED PREMATURELY.   Early in phase II treatment, obvious psychotic symptoms disappear. Psychotic thinking may then be disavowed but is not likely to have been eliminated. Premature discharge can result in a rapid return of these symptoms. Early discharge is advisable only for compliant patients with very supportive and cooperative families.

The following case illustrates the positive effects of rapid neuroleptization.

Mr. L., a 51-year-old single white unemployed man, presented to the emergency room with complaints typical for angina. He was sweating profusely and appeared to be in some distress. Vital signs were within normal limits except for a pulse rate of 90 with frequent premature ventricular contractions. It was immediately noted that the patient was probably psychotic. His thoughts were very disorganized and he was unable to give a coherent history because of his idiosyncratic and discursive speech. He was fearful, had frankly paranoid delusions, and was mistrustful of emergency room staff. His fear increased with his delusional misperceptions of the medical care necessary. He declined to cooperate with either blood drawing or EKG. He believed the emergency room personnel were trying to harm him, and he became restless and agitated. At that point, an emergency psychiatric consultation was obtained.

Initially, little history could be obtained from the patient except that he had been hospitalized several times in the past for "nerves." He had been prescribed a "nerve medicine" as an outpatient but had not taken it for some time. Although very disorganized, the patient showed no symptoms of a delirium, and his sensorium was intact as far as could be tested.

Haloperidol, 5 mg IM, was given immediately. One nursing staff member was assigned to the patient to reduce the stimulation of contact with multiple persons in the emergency room. Within 30 minutes, the patient's agitation and paranoid thinking diminished to the point that he allowed medical testing. The EKG revealed frequent premature ventricular contractions and evidence of ischemia. Soon after these tests were performed—about an hour after the initial injection of medication—the patient's paranoid thinking and agitation slowly began to return. At that point, a second 5-mg injection of haloperidol was given.

Improvement again took place rapidly. More history and the phone number of a close relative were obtained from the patient, who was now much more cooperative. The patient's past psychiatric history and treatment were very compatible with a diagnosis of schizophrenia. The patient was then admitted, without objection, to the coronary care unit. About six hours later, his agitation and fear again increased, and he became preoccupied with the monitors at his bedside. A third 5-mg injection of haloperidol was given, again with good results. The patient fell into a light sleep for the next several hours.

Repeat EKG and cardiac enzymes showed no evidence of an actual infarction, and the patient's pain lessened dramatically. His PVCs were also much reduced, and his vital signs remained stable.

The next morning, about 24 hours after initial presentation, the patient was in good behavioral control, without agitation. He remained somewhat suspicious and guarded, however, and, in a more thorough interview, delusional ideation was still noted. The patient was begun on haloperidol, 5 mg PO q.i.d. He did well with this medication, and no further injections were necessary. He later tolerated transfer to a medical unit and further cardiac testing without incident.

Although it was not practical to admit the patient to a psychiatric unit, he was closely followed by the consultation service. Discussions were held with the CCU nursing staff regarding possible difficulties and symptoms. Later transfer to the psychiatric inpatient unit was not necessary because of the marked improvement in the patient and supervision by the consulting psychiatrists.

Rapid neuroleptization has been a major advance in the treatment of acute, severe psychosis. It should be used flexibly, with adequate regard to the basic underlying treatment principles. Clinicians should familiarize themselves with neuroleptic pharmacokinetics, the typical progression of psychotic symptom resolution, and specific dosage regimens. Finally, psychiatrists must not view this very effective treatment as a replacement for treatment staff or adequate inpatient treatment facilities and procedures.

Suggested Readings

Anderson, W.H., Kuehnle, J.C., and Catanzano, D.M. (1976). Rapid treatment of acute psychosis. *American Journal of Psychiatry* 133:1076–1078.

Dean, G.A., and Gallant, D.M. (1979). Intramuscular loxapine: rapid tranquilization of acutely disturbed schizophrenic patients. *Current Therapeutic Research* 25:721–725.

Donlon, P.T., Hopkin, J., and Tupin, J.P. (1979). Overview: efficacy and safety of the rapid neuroleptization method with injectable haloperidol. *American Journal of Psychiatry* 136:273–278.

Donlon, P.T., Meadow, A., Tupin, J.P., and Wahba, M. (1978). High vs. standard dosage fluphenazine HC1 in acute schizophrenia. *Journal of Clinical Psychiatry* 39:800–804.

Ericksen, S.E., Hurt, M.A., and Chang, S. (1978). Haloperidol dose, plasma levels, and clinical response: a double-blind study. *Psychopharmacology Bulletin* 14:15–16.

Forsman, A.O., and Ohman, R. (1977). Applied pharmacokinetics of haloperidol in man. *Current Therapeutic Research* 21:396–411.

Linden, R., Davis J.M., and Rubinstein, J. (1982). High vs. low dose treatment with antipsychotic agents. *Psychiatric Annals* 12:769–781.

Neborsky, R., Janowsky, D., Munson, E., and Depry, D. (1981). Rapid treatment of acute psychotic symptoms with high- and low-dose haloperidol. *Archives of General Psychiatry* 38:195–199.

Reschke, R.W. (1974). Parenteral haloperidol for rapid control of severe, disruptive symptoms of acute schizophrenia. *Diseases of the Nervous System* 35:112–115.

Settle, E.C. (1982). Rapid neuroleptization in a rural setting. *Psychiatric Annals* 12:788–795.

Other Crises
in the Emergency Room

After the truly urgent issues have been dealt with, less urgent ones can be tended to. As important as rapidly assessing patients for violence or suicidal behavior are ruling out or treating physical illness, establishing the exact type of depressive syndrome in the depressed patient, giving adequate support to the rape victim, investigating the psychological circumstances of the geriatric patient, looking beyond the diagnosis of the chronic mentally ill person, and being aware of the legal issues for patients presenting voluntarily or involuntarily for emergency psychiatric care.

Detecting medical illness requires that psychiatrists retain their medical skills and have a high index of suspicion for possible medical disorders, especially when patients are confused, agitated, or depressed. Making a diagnosis of depression is insufficient; clinicians must assess need for hospitalization and determine the type of treatment indicated. This calls for an up-to-date awareness of the depressive syndromes and their diagnosis and treatment.

Highly vulnerable patients, whose conditions give rise to a variety of charged feelings, need especially prompt and skilled interventions. Rape victims, elderly patients, and the chronic mentally ill often arouse stereotyped reactions in regular staff and consultants. Rape victims elicit the need to protect and blame and may become further traumatized if psychiatrists do either one to excess. Elderly people are often seen as ill merely because of their age, and insufficient attention is paid to reversible medical and psychiatric disorders. The chronic mentally ill are often written off by those who view them only in terms of their need for hospitalization or medication and give insufficient attention to remediable environmental or interpersonal factors. Adequately paying such attention may obviate the need for rehospitalization or for altering previously prescribed medication. Finally, psychiatrists in the emergency room must realize that they function as an interface between the medical and the legal systems, and that the best medical care can be given only if psychiatrists know how to operate medically within the context of each community's laws.

M.W.

CHAPTER 6

Diagnosis and Treatment of the Depressed Patient

A. JOHN RUSH, M.D.
CARL FULTON, M.D.
JAYE CROWDER, M.D.

Depression is a common disorder for which emergency psychiatric care is sought. Prompt, effective treatment requires an adequate differential diagnosis, an estimate of the severity of illness, knowledge of practical treatment measures, and means to evaluate the results of the treatment.

Diagnosis of Depression

A major depressive disorder consists of persistent, intense dysphoria nearly every day for at least two weeks. The dysphoria, usually expressed as sadness, may also be expressed as irritability, anxiety, loss of interest or pleasure, indifference, or general feelings of being upset. In addition, a descriptive diagnosis of depression requires four or more of these eight symptoms: poor appetite or significant weight loss, or increased appetite or significant weight gain, insomnia or hypersomnia; psychomotor agitation or retardation; loss of interest or pleasure in usual activities or decrease in sexual drive; loss of energy or easy fatigability; feelings of worthlessness, self-reproach, or excessive or inappropriate guilt; difficulty concentrating, slowed thinking, or indecisiveness; and recurrent thoughts of death, suicide, or suicidal action.

A major depressive syndrome may also be associated with depressed appearance, tearfulness, feelings of anxiety, fear, or brooding, excessive concern with physical health, panic attacks, and phobias. In prepubertal children, separation anxiety may develop; children may cling, refuse to go to school, or fear that they or their parents will die. In adolescence, negativistic or antisocial behavior may appear. Aggression, sulkiness, withdrawal, and school difficulties are likely. Substance abuse may develop. In the elderly, symptoms suggesting dementia, such as slowed thinking, memory loss, distractibility, apathy, and inattentiveness may occur.

Depressions may or may not arise in response to clear environmental precipitants. Mood-congruent psychotic features may be present, including delusions or hallucinations whose content involves themes of personal guilt, sin, poverty, nihilism, inadequacy, or depreciation.

Types of Depression

Depressive disorders may be bipolar or unipolar and may appear as a single episode or be recurrent. Bipolar depressions have an earlier age of onset, a higher frequency of affective illness in extended families, and higher family suicide rates.

Unipolar depression can occur at any age. Predisposing factors include chronic physical illness, alcohol dependence, and cyclothymic and dysthymic disorders. Frequently, the depression follows a psychosocial stressor. The course of illness is variable, but functioning usually returns to premorbid levels between episodes. However, in 20 to 35 percent of the cases there is a chronic course, with mild to severe symptomatic and social impairment. In some cases, suicide results.

Major depression with melancholia is characterized by a full depressive syndrome plus loss of pleasure in all or almost all activities, as well as lack of reactivity to usually pleasurable stimuli and at least three of the following: distinct quality of depressed mood (different from feelings of grief or mourning), depressed mood that is worse in the morning, early morning awakening (at least two hours before usual awakening time), marked psycho-motor retardation or agitation, significant anorexia or weight loss, and excessive or inappropriate guilt. These depressions usually require biological treatment.

A minor depressive episode (dysthymia) is expressed as a disorder of at least two years' duration (one year for children and adolescents), with either a sustained or an intermittent mood of depression or a loss of interest or pleasure in almost all usual activities and pastimes. Dysthymia may be relatively persistent, or it may be separated by periods of normal mood lasting from a few days to a few weeks, but no more than a few months at a time.

The bipolar counterpart of dysthymia is cyclothymic disorder, an illness of at least two years' duration involving numerous periods of mild depression and mild hypomania. During the symptomatic periods there are signs of depression and hypomania.

In an atypical affective disorder, depression is accompanied by hypersomnolence instead of insomnia, and by overeating instead of anorexia. Mood is not constant and can lift in response to some events; diurnal variation is usually not experienced.

Rating the Severity of Depression

Descriptive diagnoses are based both on patients' immediate observable and reportable signs and symptoms and on their past histories. From the point of presentation to the emergency room, psychiatrists work backward in time to determine when the current signs and symptoms began. A lifeline methodology is used, and various episodes of depression and other symptomatology are sought by careful questioning on a year-by-year basis. Thus the number and length of episodes, and the symptomatology and severity of each episode, lead to a descriptive diagnosis.

Psychiatrists can also employ rating scales to measure current symptom severity, confirm clinical impressions, and objectify distress to help them in decision making.

The most widely used rating scale for depression is the Hamilton Rating Scale for Depression (HRS-D), consisting of 17, 21, and 24 items, depending on the format. Each item is rated on a 3- or 4-point scale. The sum of the items indicates the severity of the depression. The scale allows differentiation of clinically depressed from clinically nondepressed patients. Moreover, it is clinically sensitive to changing levels of affect in the same patient. The 17-item version elicits primarily neurovegetative signs and symptoms.

Another widely used and clinically helpful rating scale is the Beck Depression Inventory (BDI), an easy and quickly administered self-report measure. It consists of 21 items (range of scores: 0 to 63) with 4 possible alternatives for each item group. Patients select one statement under each item group that best describes them for a selected time interval (usually the preceding 7 days). The BDI contains a greater number of "cognitive" items and fewer "vegetative" symptom items compared to the HRS-D. The BDI correlates significantly with the HRS-D and is a sensitive measure of changes in symptoms. Patients with HRS-D scores of 20 or higher, or BDI scores of 26 or higher, are usually severely depressed and may require hospitalization.

Biological Tests for Depression and Mania

The psychiatrist in an emergency room setting needs to make a careful general medical assessment of patients with depressive symptomatology, because many medical disorders can imitate psychiatric disorders (see Chapter 10, "Commonly Missed Medical Diagnoses"). From 10 to 20 percent of all depressed patients have a medical disorder that causes or maintains their emotional symptomatology. In addition, physical illness is a common cause of severe depression (see Chapter 22). In such cases, treatment of the physical illness relieves the depression.

A careful medical history, physical examination, and selected laboratory tests help to exclude medical disorders such as thyroid, adrenal, and parathyroid dysfunctions, pernicious anemia, viral infections, cancer, epilepsy, vitamin deficiency, autoimmune diseases, rheumatoid arthritis, Parkinson's disease, Huntington's disease, and others. Finally, a number of medications are known to cause depression; among these are reserpine, alpha-methyldopa, propranolol, birth control pills, and steroids.

The subtyping of depressive disorders has been advanced by the development of biological measures, including the dexamethasone suppression test (DST), sleep EEG, and the thyrotropin-releasing hormone stimulation test (TRH-ST). Of these, the DST is the most simple and useful. When used in an emergency room follow-up or outpatient setting, these procedures do provide some clarification of clinical issues, but currently their use is more for research purposes than for clinical clarification.

DST nonsuppression occurs in 30 to 40 percent of outpatients and in 50 to 75 percent of inpatients with the melancholic subtype of major depression. However, a normal DST result does not rule out major depression or melancholia. DST nonsuppression is not found in schizophrenia. Thus the DST can help differentiate schizophrenia from psychotic depression. Effective treatment normalizes the DST. Failure of DST normalization suggests an incomplete resolution of underlying pathophysiological processes; these patients are at risk for early relapse or suicide. A number of medical conditions and medications, however, produce false positives, so DST results must still be interpreted cautiously.

Treating Depression

Most treatments for depression require one to two weeks before substantial symptom relief begins. Because patients' cooperation with the treatment plan is needed, therapists' initial approach is very important.

The first question to be answered concerns treatment locale. Inpatient treatment is indicated for patients at high risk for suicide (see Chapter 18), who have medical illnesses complicating treatment of their depression (see Chapter 22), who require rapid or sophisticated psychiatric/medical workup, or whose depressive symptoms such as weight loss or psychosis require close attention. Strong social or family support can sometimes decide the issue in favor of outpatient care. Such caregivers must fully understand their roles and should be assigned specific tasks, such as monitoring sleep or medication. In addition, they must be emotionally supported for their efforts.

As in all therapeutic relationships, acceptance, empathy, and understanding help establish rapport. Acceptance is particularly important because depressives often feel unacceptable and undeserving of help. Acceptance is the first of a series of interventions designed to instill a measure of hope and thereby to engage patients in treatment, increase compliance, and help ward off suicide. In addition to their accepting demeanor, therapists' availability in person and by telephone is important. Depressive symptoms appear infinitely pervasive and uncontrollable to patients. Explaining to patients that their mood is part of a treatable disorder helps to confine their anxiety. When giving this rationale, special care must be taken not to exacerbate the pathological guilt and anxiety of severely depressed persons. Specific reassurance is justified in light of the large number of highly efficacious interventions for depression. General reassurances such as, "I'm sure you'll do better," are to be avoided in favor of more specific ones such as, "Studies show that 90 percent of depressed people improve with treatment." Finally, providing the concrete details of the treatment program and where and when the treatment will be provided will affirm patients' relationship to a source of help and will reemphasize that relief is in sight.

Medication

Many depressive disorders respond to medication. The disorders that respond best are accompanied by terminal insomnia, anorexia, and anhedonia. The two main classes of established drugs, tricyclic antidepressants (TCAs) and monoamine oxidase inhibitors (MAOIs), are compared in Table 1.

Initially, antidepressants should be prescribed in small amounts to reduce the danger of overdosing and to ensure patients' return for monitoring of symptoms and dosage and for supportive psychotherapy. Guilt-ridden, depressed patients often have difficulty returning for treatment because they feel that they are unworthy or that they might prevent a truly deserving person from receiving treatment.

TRICYCLIC ANTIDEPRESSANTS. Tricyclic antidepressants affect primarily the central catecholamine (norepinephrine and dopamine) and indoleamine (serotonin, 5HT) neurotransmitter systems. Melancholic and nonmelancholic depressions respond to TCAs. The most common side effects of TCAs are sedation and dry mouth. Other side effects include constipation, blurred vision, orthostatic hypotension, palpitations, urinary retention, and weight gain, all probably related to the drugs' anticholinergic properties. TCAs are contraindicated during the acute recovery period following a myocardial infarction. Other patients at risk from TCAs are the elderly, in whom orthostatic hypotension, lower-extremity tremors, and proneness to confusion are more likely and more dangerous, and those with underlying

TABLE 1.

Established Antidepressants

DRUG	ANTICHOLINERGIC SIDE EFFECTS	SEDATION	THERAPEUTIC ADULT DAILY DOSAGE RANGE: ACUTE	THERAPEUTIC ELDERLY DAILY DOSAGE RANGE
Amitriptyline	+3	+3	150–300 mg	20–100 mg
Doxepin	+3	+3	200–400 mg	30–200 mg
Imipramine	+2	+2	100–300 mg	20–100 mg
Nortriptyline	+2	+2	75–150 mg	10–75 mg
Desipramine	+1	+1	100–300 mg	20–100 mg
Protriptyline	+2	0	30–60 mg	10–30 mg
Phenelzine	+1	0	60–90 mg	30–60 mg
Tranylcypromine	+1	0	40–60 mg	20–30 mg

0 = least potent.
+4 = most potent.

cardiovascular disease, cardiac conduction defects, and congestive heart failure.

Generally, TCAs are begun at low doses (50 to 75 mg/day). The dose is increased gradually (by 25 to 50 mg every 2 or 3 days) until a dose in the therapeutic range is reached, usually by the end of the first week. Then, on the basis of clinical effect, the dose is increased to the maximum indicated for each drug. Young patients (under 16 years of age) and elderly patients generally require about half the ordinary adult dosage. Patients must remain on therapeutic doses for three to four weeks for a full therapeutic trial. Clinicians need to be particularly alert to the issue of suicide around the tenth day of treatment with TCAs. By this time, the patient's energy level will have increased, and patient and family expectations will also be augmented, but the dysphoria may not yet have been eliminated. As a precaution against patients' taking a lethal overdose of antidepressants, no more than two weeks' supply of the TCAs or the MAOIs should be given. If there is no improvement, another TCA may be tried.

Once patients have responded, they should be continued at the therapeutic dosage for 6 to 12 additional months to prevent relapse. Relapse is common with depressive disorders. Approximately 18 to 40 percent of patients relapse within two years of recovery unless they are maintained on antidepressants.

MONOAMINE OXIDASE INHIBITORS.   Monoamine oxidase inhibitors increase the availability of catecholamine and indoleamine neurotransmitters by inhibiting their metabolic enzymes. The two most commonly used MAOIs are phenelzine (Nardil) and tranylcypromine (Parnate). MAOIs are more stimulating and less sedating than TCAs, and they have fewer anticholinergic side effects than TCAs. Their most common side effects are hypotension, loss of appetite, and insomnia.

The most important adverse effect of MAOIs is a hypertensive crisis caused by an interaction with tyramine and other amines found in fermented foods and beverages and in certain drugs. Patients taking MAOIs should avoid all sympathomimetic amines (dopamine, amphetamine, methylphenidate), as well as many over-the-counter cough, cold, and "sinus" remedies and nasal decongestants. In addition, they should avoid meperidine and TCAs. Patients should avoid beer, liquors, red wine, aged cheese, fermented foods and excessive chocolate. Phentolamine (Regitine), an alpha-adrenergic blocker, is given intravenously or orally (25 to 50 mg) to treat severe hypertensive reactions. If phentolamine is not available, chlorpromazine (Thorazine), which also has some alpha-adrenergic blocking activity, can be given intramuscularly (25 mg) or orally (25 to 50 mg).

Markedly anxious, fearful, panicky, phobic, or nervous depressed patients often respond well to MAOIs. Other patients who respond well to MAOIs have atypical features such as reversed diurnal mood variation (mood worse in the evening), hypersomnolence or initial insomnia, hyperphagia with weight gain, extreme sensitivity to perceived rejection, and hyperreactivity of mood (increased irritability and emotionality). The MAOIs require two to six weeks at therapeutic doses to produce a full therapeutic effect. Once this acute response is obtained, MAOIs also prevent relapses if continued on a regular basis.

NEW ANTIDEPRESSANTS. The information in Table 2 compares four new antidepressants. Maprotiline (Ludiomil) is a tetracyclic noradrenergic with moderately low cardiovascular and anticholinergic side effects. Seizures may occur, however, with therapeutic doses above the recommended level or with a previous history of loss of consciousness.

Amoxapine (Asendin), a tricyclic compound, is the demethylated metabolite of the neuroleptic loxapine. It has noradrenergic effects similar to imipramine, but its serotonergic effects are only a tenth as potent. A metabolite of amoxapine also has dopamine-receptor blocking and neuroleptic properties. Its therapeutic effect may have a more rapid onset (4 to 7 days) than the older TCAs, and it has fewer anticholinergic effects.

Trazodone (Desyrel) blocks serotonergic re-uptake. It has few anticholinergic properties and low cardiotoxicity. In addition, it may have definite antianxiety effects equal or superior to chlordiazepoxide without significant tachyphylaxis.

Alprazolam (Xanax), a triazolobenzodiazepine, is an anxiolytic with some antidepressant activity at higher doses. It does not have anticholinergic or cardiotoxic side effects. Its only important side effect is drowsiness or

TABLE 2.
New Antidepressants

DRUG	ANTICHOLINERGIC SIDE EFFECTS	SEDATION	THERAPEUTIC ADULT DAILY DOSAGE RANGE: ACUTE	THERAPEUTIC ELDERLY DAILY DOSAGE RANGE
Maprotiline	+1	+2	150–300 mg	50–100 mg
Amoxapine	+1	+2	200–400 mg	50–150 mg
Trazodone	0	+3	100–600 mg	50–200 mg
Alprazolam	0	+4	4–12 mg	2–6 mg

0 = least potent.
+4 = most potent.

sedation. Although not yet approved by the FDA as an antidepressant, it may be helpful in nonmelancholic or anxious depressions. Because of its rapid onset of action (one week) and its mild side effects, alprazolam may prove useful in treating geriatric depressions. The question of long-term dependence and tolerance has yet to be clarified.

The most common causes of medication failure are incorrect diagnosis and failure to titrate the dose to obtain maximal clinical response. This latter difficulty can be reduced by employing a clinician-completed or self-report scale, such as the HRS-D or BDI described earlier, to rate symptom severity. If complete symptom remission is not obtained, the diagnosis may be incorrect, the patient may be in need of alternative medication, or medication should be supplemented by additional or different psychotherapeutic interactions.

It is important to emphasize that drug treatment must be balanced by attention to patients' psychological makeup, as the following case illustrates.

Mrs. M., a 31-year-old married dental hygienist and office practice manager with a prior episode of suicidal depression and brief hospitalization, was brought to the emergency room for treatment after four months of depressed mood, self-castigation, suicidal ideation, decreased sexual interest, and decreased interest in work and family. She had also experienced a slight weight gain and had a tendency to oversleep. An internist had begun treating her with no substantial help with doxepin, 50 mg a day, at the time she sought psychiatric help. The psychiatrist suggested she increase the doxepin to 150 mg and take it at bedtime. The psychiatrist explored the patient's expectations of herself and found her to be exceedingly self-critical. She demanded of herself a rigorous schedule, similar to that of a colleague who comfortably saw many more patients a day, even though the patient was uncomfortable doing the brief examinations required by such a volume of patients.

The daily dose of doxepin was rapidly pushed to 250 mg, but four weeks after treatment had begun, a breakthrough of depressive symptoms occurred and the patient again became suicidal. As an alternative to hospitalization, her medication was changed from doxepin to phenelzine, which was quickly increased within a week to 60 mg per day. By then, the patient was more comfortable, but two weeks later a breakthrough of depressed symptoms occurred, and she was again suicidal. At this point, finding that the patient was again attempting to meet her unrealistic work expectations, the psychiatrist advised her firmly to slow down. The patient, who was desperate, took the advice, slowed down, calmed down, and continued to do well on a dose of medication that was reduced when she began modifying her pattern of activities to better meet the needs of her personality style instead of her overly strict conscience.

Electroconvulsive Therapy

Electroconvulsive therapy is the treatment of choice for patients with melancholic, psychotic, or treatment-resistant depression. ECT is safer and more effective than antidepressants, especially for pregnant women, the elderly, and patients with heart disease or other significant medical illnesses. ECT is also effective in cases of mania. Present-day methods of administration are safe and, as indicated in Chapter 23, have few side effects.

Psychotherapy

The management of major depression almost always involves supportive psychotherapy in addition to medication. Examination of motives and deep feelings is unwise initially because it may increase the patient's feelings of anxiety, guilt, and desperation. In treating depression, therapists actively focus on specific goals and explain to patients that they are ill. Care is taken to form a collaborative, supportive alliance. The therapist-patient relationship then serves as a model for problem solving and ultimately for more productive relationships.

Physicians should provide general information and support to their patients undergoing antidepressant therapy to ensure compliance with treatment, to help modify the consequences of the depression, and to help reduce countertherapeutic attitudes among family members.

Psychotherapy should be considered as a primary treatment when there is a chronic course, when the patient has a nonmelancholic symptom picture, when interepisode recovery is only modest, when personality difficulties are present, when the patient is demoralized, discouraged, or despairing because of a long or chronic illness, or when there is a clear-cut psychological pattern to environmental events associated with the onset of each depressive episode.

A reeducative psychotherapy, such as cognitive therapy, may help in mild to moderate depressions, may improve the quality of remissions, and may even protect against future relapses.

Predictors of clinical response

Melancholic features predict positive response to somatic therapy. ECT is the treatment of choice for melancholic patients. Less severe melancholic features often predict a positive response to TCAs. Nonmelancholic patients who meet the criteria for major depression may respond to antidepressant medication, to psychotherapy, or to combined treatment. A family history of major depression in first-degree relatives may also predict a positive response to somatic therapy.

It is not known whether current descriptive diagnostic syndromes predict the type or efficacy of a specific form of psychotherapy. Psychotherapy alone should not be used with hallucinating or delusional patients. However, psychotherapeutic methods to improve reality testing and foster a positive doctor-patient relationship will help in obtaining compliance with treatment.

Suggested Readings

American Psychiatric Association. (1980). *Diagnostic and Statistical Manual of Mental Disorders*, 3rd ed. Washington, D.C.: American Psychiatric Association.

Greist, J.H., Jefferson, J.W., and Spitzer, R.L. (1982). *Treatment of Mental Disorders*. New York: Oxford Press.

Kalinowsky, L.B., Hippius, H., and Klein, H.E. (1982). *Biological Treatments in Psychiatry*. New York: Grune & Stratton.

Klein, D.F., Gittelman, R., Quitkin, F., and Rifkin, A. (eds.) (1980). *Diagnosis and Drug Treatment of Psychiatric Disorders: Adults and Children*, 2nd ed. Baltimore: Williams & Wilkins.

Paykel, E.S. (ed.) (1982). *Handbook of Affective Disorders*. New York: Guilford Press.

Rush, A.J. (ed.) (1982). *Short-Term Psychotherapies for Depression*. New York: Guilford Press.

Rush, A.J., and Beck, A.T. (1978). Adults with affective disorders. In *Behavior Therapy in the Psychiatric Setting*, ed. M. Hersen and A. Bellack, pp. 286–330. Baltimore: Williams & Wilkins.

Rush, A.J., and Fulton, C.L. (1982). Affective disorders. In *Handbook of Medical Psychology*, ed. R.J. Gatchel, A. Baum, and J.E. Singer, pp. 431–463. New York: Springer.

Rush, A.J., Schlesser, M.A., Fulton, C.L., and Allen, M.A. (1983). Biologic basis of psychiatric disorders. In *Clinical Neurosciences*, ed. R. Rosenberg. London: Churchill-Livingston.

CHAPTER 7

Urgent Psychiatric Problems of Elderly Patients

CHARLES M. GAITZ, M.D.

Because of their physical and emotional fragility, elderly people's psychiatric problems usually require immediate attention. The possibility of rapid decompensation adds a sense of urgency to these situations, and prompt intervention may avert serious consequences. Elderly patients who present with seeming psychiatric problems often have a combination of other medical and social problems. Planning for treatment, therefore, must be based on an exploration of the potentially remediable factors, as illustrated here.

Mrs. N., an 80-year-old widowed apartment manager who lived alone, was brought into the psychiatric emergency room one evening by her family. Two weeks previously her internist had found no significant physical disorder on extensive workup for the patient's failing health. Referral to the emergency room had been precipitated by her daughter, when she learned that the patient was seeing visions of her long-deceased mother and a small child. The patient had been preparing food for these imaginary people and communicated with them by means of facial expressions. She talked freely about her hallucinatory experiences. Although she admitted that the two visitors were not real, she persisted in preparing food for them.

In the psychiatric emergency room, the psychiatrist found the patient to be a gracious, well-groomed, and frail but healthy-looking woman. She was oriented to place and date, but made several incorrect guesses about the year. She admitted to having great recent difficulty keeping up with her tenants, supervising personnel, and balancing her checkbook, which she had previously kept meticulously. Her work had become more stressful, but she had not asked for help. She denied fears or feelings of harrassment. She had decided to tell her daughter about her visions as she approached her eightieth birthday, when she also began to realize she was "showing her age." She was not depressed and still had work and hobbies to keep her occupied. Her sleep pattern had not changed over the previous three years. She was not agitated. She felt that the haloperidol, 1 mg b.i.d., given her several days earlier by her internist had decreased slightly the vividness of her visions as well as her level of tension. The examining psychiatrist made the diagnosis of a mild to moderate organic brain syndrome, explained the nature of the problem to the family, and informed them of the potential benefits of the medication in this case.

Two subsequent interviews revealed that the patient had had a close relationship with her own mother. Her associations to her hallucinations suggested two possible derivations. She had sought support from her mother at times of crisis. She had also become concerned about her own death and afterlife. She was well aware that dead people do not need food, but that did not stop her from preparing food for her visitors. Seeing only portions of her mother's and the child's bodies, she was fascinated by such questions as: Does mother eat? Does she sleep? Does she wash? Does she change clothes?

The psychiatrist continued the patient on small doses of haloperidol. The patient began to accept help from her daughter and other family members, who took over management of the apartments. Within three weeks, her visions stopped and she enjoyed having real visitors and turning her attention away from herself. She had no symptoms of depression, but her need for help in managing day-to-day affairs was evident.

In this case, active intervention clarified stresses that could be relieved and brought a favorable response with little investment of the psychiatrist's time and energy. Together, the patient and her family agreed on ways to alleviate pressure and provide support for the patient, at the same time allowing her to maintain as much independence as was compatible with her abilities.

The principle that psychiatric disorders have multiple etiological factors is especially helpful in understanding elderly people's psychopathology and in planning for their treatment. Biological and social factors should be considered with patients of all ages, but elderly patients who present psychiatric problems require a special evaluation that considers many factors as potentially significant.

Psychiatric disorders in the elderly may not pose serious problems unless the patients' behavior interferes considerably with ongoing social systems. For example, negativism and combative, aggressive behavior certainly can be disruptive. Many elderly patients manifest passivity, dependency, and withdrawal symptoms that do not hinder others but that detract from their own quality of life—resulting in either poor self-care or a poor patient-caregiver relationship. One also should remember that both the so-called health providers and the recipients of care may behave in ways that are not helpful as the delicate balance of family dynamics disintegrates.

Critics of hospital care often describe staff members' poor, inadequate, or stereotyped reactions to patients' needs. For example, autocratic and irritable behavior by staff members antagonizes patients who want to participate in making decisions that affect them. Similar situations are seen in patients' interactions with family members or friends. Elderly people living alone may develop disturbing behavior toward their neighbors. Such behavior can be a plea for help, a reaction to what is or is not being done, or a response to a developing organic brain syndrome. Extremes of either passive or aggressive behavior may signal urgent psychiatric problems.

Some Relevant Characteristics of Aging

Aging and being old affect adjustment, behavior, and treatment. The elderly have learned to cope with stress, but the cumulative effects of their life stresses may have finally taken their toll. Furthermore, some stresses are unique to the late stages of life, when individuals' coping strengths may have diminished.

As people age, they experience numerous losses as significant individuals die or become less able to help. The death of a spouse may precipitate a major crisis. Changes in social roles affect social relationships. Retirement from work produces psychological changes as well as a new financial status. Retirees are likely to spend more time with their spouses, a change in life style that may cause tension.

Aging also produces important changes in one's sense of self. Older people normally experience some sensory deficits and loss of motor ability. Hearing and visual impairments and slowed locomotion may restrict some sources of satisfaction, though many elderly people find pleasure and contentment by substituting one type of activity for another. The elderly also respond to social stereotypes. Our society has fixed expectations and ideas about people of various ages. If the elderly accept these concepts, they may find themselves struggling needlessly with negative self-images, feelings of inadequacy, low self-esteem, and other feelings that lead to depression and social withdrawal. Correction of sensory impairments may lead to more socialization and interaction. On the other hand, a person's acceptance of some degree of impairment may lead to a more reasonable life style and may reduce accidents.

Health problems also increase with age. A psychiatrist's failure to recognize this point can lead to misdiagnosis, with an overemphasis on social factors and psychological conflicts. Physical illness often affects the mental status of elderly people. They may maintain a reasonable level of functioning under ordinary conditions but become quite upset when they must adapt to moving or to different living conditions. Those whose adjustment is fragile may decompensate when their external situation becomes more demanding. A minimally demented person may, for example, become quite disoriented, have hallucinations, and become paranoid when hospitalized for cataract surgery, prostatectomy, or a myocardial infarction. Such a patient requires careful, patient, concrete explanations of the therapeutic efforts being made. Physicians who understand the fragile adjustment of elderly people will make certain that both patients and family are informed about what is being done and that their cooperation is enlisted.

Noncompliance with treatment, whether active or passive, may be psychologically determined. But in the elderly it more likely results from a combination of biomedical, social, economic, and psychological factors. A patient with a mood disturbance may not take an antidepressant that has been prescribed because of the mood itself, because of impaired locomotion, or because of a shortage of funds.

Family relationships are important. Relatives with unresolved antipathies may be unwilling to share their resources with elderly patients who need help. Social isolation grows out of a host of socioenvironmental factors, such as lack of transportation or fear of being assaulted and robbed, or out of physical impairments that limit activity. Isolation may also be symptomatic of a mood disturbance. A treatment plan for an elderly patient with an emotional disturbance, then, should take into account the probability that the patient also has social and physical health problems.

Elderly people often do not know what services are available, and they will obtain a service only if given exact direction. Moreover, a person's connection to social support systems can be disrupted when the caregivers involved develop their own medical or social problems. The daughter of an elderly person, for example, may become ill or lose access to a car, thus producing a barrier to care for the elderly person. Caregiving changes may bring about disruptive behavior or noncompliance in elderly people, and may prompt their being brought in for medical attention.

Mental Disorders in Old Age

Mental disorders in old age fall into two broad categories, those with onset in the young adult or mid-life years and those with late-life onset. Elderly patients often continue to manifest mental illnesses that developed decades earlier. But we also recognize that the social, neurological, and other medical changes of old age may contribute to the onset of mental disorders.

Every elderly person manifesting untoward behavior or cognitive changes must be suspected of having an organic brain syndrome.

Organic brain disorders in the elderly are usually slow-developing, irreversible dementias. Most demented patients have Alzheimer's disease. The second and much less frequent cause of dementia is multi-infarct dementia, which usually results from small cerebrovascular accidents associated with generalized arteriosclerosis. Not infrequently, however, elderly patients present with the acute onset of confusion, and workup reveals a reversible etiology related to medications, systemic disorders, or substance abuse. Other causes may also be implicated; quite frequently these problems have multiple origins.

Dementia is a frequently encountered impairment of elderly people. Its manifestations and severity vary. Elderly people may show very little evidence of dementia in a protected environment, where needs are met and demands are few. The same people, if expected to take on more responsibility because of changes in their life situations, may be unable to do so.

Demented people require more time and explanation to ensure their comprehension of and cooperation with instructions. How demented patients respond to simple or complex interventions depends on the level of understanding they can attain. Dependency on others increases when intellectual capability declines. When the relationship between demented people and their caregivers is trusting and confident, stress can remain low and fewer problems will arise.

Brief Dementia Workup

An exhaustive routine diagnostic evaluation is not cost-effective, and it often alienates elderly people with dementia. A careful history, physical examination, and appraisal of mental status are essential. Collateral information from caregivers and additional medical and social history are often helpful. Psychiatrists, consulted before or after a medical evaluation, are uniquely qualified to determine whether a patient's abnormal behavior is related to a physical disorder.

It is all but impossible to specify absolute essentials of a diagnostic appraisal. The art and skill of individual physicians determine what information is needed. The objective of a diagnostic evaluation is to discover intra- and extra-cranial conditions that contribute to the disordered mental state, and to uncover abnormal conditions that can be reversed with appropriate treatment.

Having an adequate history and the results of a physical examination, physicians must then consider diagnostic possibilities to be confirmed with testing. Priority must be given to lifesaving measures. (A patient who is unable to swallow can wait to have psychological tests!) Routine medical evaluations for such patients often include a complete blood count, urinalysis, electrocardiogram, electroencephalogram, and tests of electrolyte levels, blood urea nitrogen, fasting blood sugar, thyroid and liver function, and vitamin B_{12} and folate levels. Physicians should use clinical judgment in evaluating the risks to the patient of an invasive technique such as cerebral arteriography. Less dangerous procedures such as computerized tomography often may be used first. Sophisticated, expensive studies may or may not be necessary once the history and physical findings are reviewed.

It is impossible to establish a minimum, standard diagnostic approach; physicians must weigh the possibilities and probabilities in each individual case. Optimistic therapists who recognize the potential of rehabilitating elderly patients will ultimately strike a happy balance. Conscientious practitioners will prefer doing extra examinations to uncover a remediable condition rather than fail in providing their patients the best possible care, but they must also reckon with cost factors. Ultimately, clinicians must decide which evaluations are essential to define remediable conditions and to gain information for accurate treatment and prognostic judgments.

Mental disorders with prominent affective and paranoid symptoms are common. These syndromes may be related to organic brain syndromes or to functional disorders. Somatoform disorders, including hypochondriasis, and atypical somatoform disorders are also seen in elderly people, and may be caused by a flare-up of social stress. Posttraumatic stress disorders may occur after burglaries and robberies.

In sum, when patients are elderly, differential diagnosis can be complicated because of overlapping mental illness, normal aging, and the psychiatric manifestations of neurological or other physical disorders. Consequently, patients with urgent problems and considerable distress may or may not have a primary psychiatric illness.

Evaluation and Treatment Issues

Elderly people are likely to have a combination of problems that interact in a number of ways. A diagnostic evaluation should aim to uncover remediable conditions. Treatment for congestive heart failure, for example, may resolve symptoms of apathy and withdrawal. A delirious patient with uremia and hyponatremia will improve mentally when these abnormalities are identified and treated. A frail, anxious person may respond better after moving to an emotionally supportive and physically secure environment.

Because so many factors affect the mental status of elderly people, they benefit from a team approach. Even when teamwork is not possible, psychiatrists must pay attention to interacting factors. Expecting a patient to comply with a treatment plan requires evaluation of the patient's cognitive and affective state and consideration of the available caregiving from family members, friends, and community agencies.

The timing of intervention also deserves some attention. In certain situations, the psychiatrist may activate a protective service approach. An elderly person's judgment may become so impaired that there is no alternative. Compliance, however, is more likely when a patient has been included in planning and has a sense of participating in and controlling what is being done to and for him or her. Similarly, those involved in the caregiving process should also have options; they are more likely to be willing and useful when they have been included in treatment planning rather than when they are suddenly faced with demands they cannot or will not fulfill.

In addressing a combination of medical, psychological, and social problems, the psychiatrist must establish treatment priorities. The mobilization of family and informal supports and the setting up of formal support systems when necessary may determine whether or not the beneficial effects of treatment will last. Gains made in treating depressed patients may depend on their compliance with medications or therapy. The early treatment stages of a patient who has suffered a cerebrovascular accident or myocardial infarction may be successful, but without continued monitoring, encouragement, and supervision, the patient may regress. If family members take on more responsibilities than they can handle over an extended period, a respite from care for the patient or help from other caregivers may be necessary.

All psychiatric treatment modalities are useful for elderly patients. Therapists must match their skills with their patients' needs and minimize the importance of chronological age as a determining factor. Treatment possibilities are limited more often by therapists' preconceptions than by patients' age. Thus decisions to use psychotherapy, electroconvulsive therapy, medications, counseling, and other approaches should be made collaboratively with patients, families, and therapists.

Psychotropic Drugs and Electroconvulsive Therapy

Psychotropic medications may help to alleviate emotional or behavioral symptoms. Attention to dosage and side effects is important, as is caution concerning a drug's potential interaction with other medications being prescribed.

Generally, one should begin treating elderly patients with small doses of drugs. Desired effects may be achieved with haloperidol, 0.5 mg to 2 mg by mouth two or three times a day, a chlorpromazine and thioridazine 10 mg each by mouth three or four times a day. If necessary, one should try larger doses before deciding that a medication is ineffective. Loxapine and thiothixene are also effective in controlling tension and agitation in the elderly. No tranquilizer is completely free of side effects, nor is any one medication far superior to any others. Psychiatrists knowledgeable about the potential risks and benefits of the available drugs must choose among them and then monitor the effects carefully and often in order to avoid difficulties. Despite the potential problems of medications, the benefits should be made available to disturbed patients and their caregivers.

The treatment of depressed patients rests on careful diagnostic appraisal (see Chapter 6, "Diagnosis and Treatment of the Depressed Patient"). Elderly people reacting with depression to the realities of their health status or social problems rarely respond to antidepressants. Those with typical vegetative signs and symptoms of a major depressive disorder, however, will often respond to antidepressants. The age of the patient and even the presence of dementia should not preclude a trial of an antidepressant drug. The guiding principles for tranquilizer use apply equally to antidepressants. A personal choice may be made among such antidepressants as imipramine, amitriptyline, maprotiline, amoxapine, and trazodone; one may start with small doses and increase them as need and tolerance are observed. Lithium is sometimes effective in manic states, but it requires special attention to the patient's physical health status, especially decreased renal clearance.

Electroconvulsive therapy should not be ruled out for elderly patients who have severe depressive disorders (see Chapter 23, "Electroconvulsive Therapy in Consultation Psychiatry"). Some experts consider this treatment safer than antidepressant medications that have serious side effects. For elderly patients who may be suicidal, electroconvulsive therapy can be lifesaving. Patients' age is not the critical issue when deciding on the use of electroconvulsive therapy.

A Final Word

The attitudes of elderly patients and their caregivers bear heavily on what treatment is prescribed, accepted, and implemented. The likelihood that an illness is multidetermined demands a comprehensive approach to evaluation and treatment. Certain characteristics associated with aging, especially the multiple etiology of disorder and the likelihood of increasing dependency, call for collaboration with family members, relatives, and community agencies as surrogates in order to achieve the highest level of functioning and satisfaction for elderly patients.

Often, an emotional crisis can be avoided or at least diminished in intensity if the psychiatrist gives attention to some of the problems' antecedents. Establishing or maintaining continuity of care with a physician, for example, can be very supportive. Family members and the staff of an interested institution or social agency have a heightened sense of security when they know arrangements for consultation and assistance are in place to deal with emergency situations. Anticipating problems and their resolution diminishes fear and anxiety in both individuals and families. Discussions about "what to do if . . ." help everyone involved to develop a sense of mastery and control. Together, caregivers and patients should discuss both the antecedents of a crisis and the factors in future adjustment. Treatment should not end when the urgent problem has been resolved; patients treated successfully for a depression deserve an evaluation for other problems that may arise. Without appearing to be condescending or overprotective, in collaboration with patients and families, caregivers should continue to investigate stresses that can be anticipated and means of coping with them more effectively, thus avoiding other crises and emergencies.

Suggested Readings

Busse, E.W., and Blazer, D.G. (eds.) (1980). *Handbook of Geriatric Psychiatry.* New York: Van Nostrand Reinhold.

Gaitz, C.M. (1974). Barriers to the delivery of psychiatric services to the elderly. *Gerontologist* 14:210–214.

Gaitz, C.M. (1984). Psychiatric emergencies of older persons. In *Phenomenology and Treatment of Psychiatric Emergencies*, ed. B.S. Comstock, W.E. Fann, A.D. Pokorny, and R.L. Williams, pp. 179–198. New York: Spectrum.

Gaitz, C.M. (1982). Some psychophysiological problems of the elderly. In *Phenomenology and Treatment of Psychophysiological Disorders*, ed. W.E. Fann, pp. 191–202. New York: Spectrum.

Glickman, L.S. (ed.) (1980). *Psychiatric Consultation in the General Hospital.* New York: Marcel Dekker.

Gorton, J.G., and Partridge, R. (eds.) (1982). *Practice and Management of Psychiatric Emergency Care.* St. Louis, Mo.: C.V. Mosby.

Tardiff, K., (1982). Violence in geriatric patients (editorial). *Journal of the American Medical Association* 248:471.

CHAPTER 8

The Rape Victim

MALKAH T. NOTMAN, M.D.
CAROL C. NADELSON, M.D.

Rape is a crime of violence expressed as a sexual act. It is one of the fastest-growing violent crimes. A recent urban confidential survey estimated that over a lifetime, nearly half of all women experience a rape or attempted rape.

Rape victims can be divided into three groups, related to the circumstances of rape: (1) victims of forcible completed or attempted rape, (2) victims who were "accessories" because of their inability to consent; and (3) victims of sexually stressful situations in which the encounter went beyond the women's expectations and abilities to exercise control. Despite the different circumstances, the intrapsychic experiences of all rape victims have much in common.

Many rape victims are young women who are assaulted in their own homes. The likelihood of rape varies with demographic factors and life style, and rape of the very young and very old does occur. Male and homosexual rape are reported less frequently, and the actual incidence is not known. The stigma associated with male rape may deter many victims from reporting this crime. It is estimated that at least half of all rapes are never reported. From 30 to 50 percent of female rape victims know their assailants, and this knowledge probably inhibits reporting and leads to underrepresentation in the number of cases appearing for prosecution.

The Victim in the General Hospital

In addition to the emotional effects of rape, many victims also suffer both genital and nongenital physical injury. More than 25 percent of rape victims sustain extragenital injuries, and nearly 5 percent report venereal disease as a consequence of the rape.

Psychiatrists working in general hospitals need to understand the responses of victims and of those participating in victims' care. Encounters with rape victims raise a great deal of anxiety, which caregivers handle in a variety of ways. Although some caregivers provide empathy and support, many respond to the victim with disbelief and negative humor directed against the victim, or with detachment or reluctance to be involved.

Professionals have been slow to acknowledge the legitimacy of rape as a psychiatric issue. They tend to believe it only happens to "marginal" people or that victims invite rape. Many rape victims are also seen as acting out unconscious fantasies and are therefore not "true" victims. Often women who have been raped do not receive the empathy and understanding usually extended to other people in crisis. The belief that many accusations of rape are false is still common, though this belief has been found to be without grounds in populations studied. Even women who are raped by someone they know do not invite the sexual assault that follows a social encounter. Other determinants of professionals' reluctance to respond to rape victims are the need for self-protection from feelings of guilt or responsibility and the sense of anger at what one cannot prevent. Contact with the rape victim or knowledge that the rape has taken place nearby can destroy professional helpers' feelings of invulnerability and safety and create a sense of helplessness or rage.

Many rape victims are so traumatized by their experience that they do not want to expose themselves further by going to a hospital or other health care facility. However, it is important that they go to such a facility to establish the extent of physical trauma and obtain necessary care. Nevertheless, their attitudes toward the professionals they encounter will be affected by their traumatic experience and may be a mixture of strongly positive and negative feelings.

Rape victims who do go to hospitals or to the police must tell a story that involves a fresh exposure of a degrading, frightening experience. The following vignettes illustrate some of these experiences.

> Miss O., a 20-year-old college junior, was alone in her room when a man entered through the window, held a knife to her throat, and insisted that she have sexual intercourse with him. She had been half asleep and was terrified at this sudden confrontation in which she felt she might be killed. She acceded to the rapist's demands, even to his insistence that she praise his sexual performance. When he left, she was still shaking with fear but was able to call a friend, who took her to the college health service. There, because she was so frightened, she could barely recount her story and had to be persuaded to undergo physical examination. She was not physically injured, but for weeks afterward was afraid to leave her room or to remain there alone. Friends took turns staying with her around the clock. She went to a rape counseling center where she received

minor tranquilizers and emotional support, but she remained phobic and could not return to her classes for weeks. She was a scholarship student from a relatively poor family and needed to work in order to remain in school. Convinced that she would be criticized, she could not bring herself to tell anyone at her evening job what had happened. After missing two weeks of work, she was fired.

The loss of income and missed classes made it necessary for her to leave school, which meant moving out of the dormitory. She also lost her scholarship. Although she felt stranded, her value system did not permit her to seek psychiatric help. Her friends tried to help, but they felt depleted after the initial weeks following the incident. It took months of support and other help from friends to enable her to fully return to work. She was forced to miss a year of school, however, because of the time she had lost.

Ms. P., a 28-year-old secretary, lived in an apartment with a roommate who was away for the night. She went out to visit her boyfriend and, while walking home, had a feeling that "something was wrong." Before she realized what was happening, a man emerged from a car nearby, threatened to kill her, and forced her into the car. After driving around for several hours, he raped her several times and forced her to perform fellatio. He also insulted and humiliated her. He finally released her in the middle of an unknown neighborhood. She managed to return to her apartment and called her boyfriend, who was distant and unsupportive. Although he was upset that she had been raped, he was unable to master his own feelings enough to reach out to her. She called her parents in another city for support, but when they wanted to come and bring her home, she insisted that she could manage on her own. Her father recognized her need to maintain control, but he also perceived her anxiety and insisted on visiting the next day. She was very glad to see him but still wanted to remain where she was and try to cope. For three or four weeks afterward, she could not go to work regularly. Her roommate, who returned the next day, was also frightened. They moved into another apartment and gradually settled down. About eight months later, when Ms. P. went to visit her gynecologist for a routine checkup and to obtain contraceptives, she broke down, started to sob, and tearfully recounted the story of the rape as if it were the first time she was allowing herself to fully describe the experience.

Miss Q. met a colleague on her way home from work. As they were waiting for the bus, he suggested that they have a drink together. Afterward, he walked her home. When they reached her apartment, she invited him in for a brief visit. He insisted on having intercourse, though she protested and struggled. He had interpreted her invitation to visit as an invitation for a sexual encounter. She felt guilty at having "led him on," and for some weeks she was reluctant to discuss her experience with anyone and suffered acute discomfort when she encountered the colleague at work. She was certain that she would not be believed if she told anyone about her experience and her distress.

As these cases show, the experiences we call *rape* range from surprise attacks with threats of death or mutilation to insistence on sexual intercourse in a social encounter where sexual contact is unexpected or not agreed upon. Consent is crucial to the definition of rape. The importance of mutual consent is often overlooked and misinterpreted; many people assume that certain social communications imply a willingness to have a sexual relationship.

Rape is a violent crime, not a sexual experience. The victim usually feels terrified, helpless, and deprived of control. If, as in the third vignette, the victim knows or is involved socially with the rapist, she is likely to feel particularly responsible, guilty, and ashamed. However, even women who are victims of forcible rape by a stranger are vulnerable to feelings of guilt and shame. Some worry that other types of behavior might have spared them, or they become concerned about any expression of their sexuality or about other aspects of their lives about which they may feel some guilt.

Although few rapes are "victim precipitated," guilt and self-blame are nevertheless experienced by a large number of victims. Nearly 75 percent of victims blame themselves for their specific behavior ("I should not have walked down that street alone"), and about 20 percent blame themselves for personality attributes such as naivete or being too trusting.

Rape produces an acute stress reaction that is resolved only much later on. The intentional cruelty of rape often involving physical injury, arouses feelings of being trapped and helpless. Rape challenges and overwhelms a woman's ability to maintain her defenses and thus arouses feelings of guilt, anxiety, and inadequacy. The resultant posttraumatic stress disorder observed in rape victims has been attributed to the sudden nature of the rape experience and the inability to develop adequate defenses.

As indicated earlier, certain acute reactions appear almost universally. Some of the consequences of rape include disruption of the normal biological functions of eating and sleeping (even in the absence of psychological symptoms), decreased attention span and ability to concentrate, increased dependency and emotional lability, and general diminution in ability to function in ordinary situations.

Rape Trauma Syndrome

The phases of response to rape constitute a rape trauma syndrome, with an acute phase and a long-term phase. Two general responses have been described in the acute phase: an "expressed style," in which victims are emotional and visibly upset, and a contrasting "controlled style," in which victims exhibit guilt and self-blame or apparent mastery of their emotions. The expressed style may be characterized by signs of intense distress, which include shock, disbelief, emotional breakdown, and disruptions in normal patterns of behavior and function. In this acute period, the victims are often unable to talk about what has happened and may have difficulty telling family and friends or reporting to the hospital or police. Many of those who do come to hospital emergency facilities are likely to be in this state. If their style is controlled, guilt may be prominent, with fears that poor judgment may have precipitated the rape. During the initial phase, victims must decide whether to report the crime and tell others about it. They are often worried about publicity and about the possibility of pregnancy or venereal disease. The decision to speak out can be made at many later points as well. A victim who tells no one initially may later have reactions evoked by another event and then want to talk about a past rape.

A period of apparent outward adjustment usually begins within several days to a few weeks after the rape, when the immediate anxiety-provoking issues seem to temporarily resolve. Returning to their usual life patterns, victims try to behave as if all is well. They try to reassure both themselves and those close to them, bringing an end to the acute phase.

Later, victims experience a phase of integration and resolution, and at that time they may want to talk about what happened in order to help reestablish their self-image and to resolve their feelings about the rape and the rapist. An earlier attitude of apparent tolerance may be replaced by anger toward the rapist. The victims often continue to feel guilty about the thought that they may have colluded in some way. In spite of the apparent resolution of many aspects of the disturbance, symptoms such as anxiety and phobias may persist. In this integration–resolution phase, or even long after the rape, an apparently unrelated experience may precipitate symptoms related to a revival of feelings about the rape.

The acute phase may last from a few days to weeks before it gradually merges into the long-term reorganization process. During the acute period, changes in life style are prominent, with impaired functioning at work, home and school. Some women move to another residence. Others are afraid to leave their homes at all, and some give up their autonomy and return to their families. Sleep disruptions can continue, with vivid dreams and nightmares that reenact the rape. Phobias that seem specifically determined by the nature of the rape experience may appear, with fears of crowds or of being at home or outside, depending on the location of the assault. Sexual fears are common, with a decline of general interest in sex as well as withdrawal from a sexual partner.

The existence of psychological problems or maladaptive behavior patterns prior to the rape increases the likelihood of maladaptive coping patterns following the rape. Serious medical or psychiatric problems prior to or resulting from the rape may also affect the long-term outcome.

However, even women without major preexisting problems may experience long-lasting effects. Symptoms may persist for as long as four to six years after the rape. Changes in eating and sleeping patterns, increased fear of being alone on the streets, negative feelings toward men, decreased social activities, and decreased sexual functioning are among the common symptoms. A woman's individual response is determined by the circumstances of the rape, her personality, her adaptive and defensive structures, and also her stage of life.

Life-Stage Considerations

Single young women between the ages of 17 and 24 are likely to be relatively inexperienced sexually and socially, and their emotional relationships may have been limited to family and close friends. Their lack of sophistication leaves them psychologically more vulnerable to a violent, intrusive encounter. Rape victims in this age group often have some prior acquaintance with the man who forces a sexual relationship. This prior acquaintance with the rapist may contribute to the women's refusal to prosecute. Rape victims of all ages reproach themselves because they feel they should have been more active in foreseeing and preventing the rape; they experience shame and guilt regardless of the circumstances. For young women, these feelings, together with their sense of vulnerability, may color future relationships with men. If a young woman has her first sexual experience in this context, it can result in confusion of sexuality and violence, with long-lasting effects. Counseling can be of great help in this situation.

For young women, the rape experience may stimulate or revive concerns about separation and independence. They may feel unable to care for themselves. Parents, friends, and relatives often respond by offering to take care of them again in an attempt to be supportive and reassuring. However, these well-intended offers, if accepted, can foster regression and prevent mastery of the rape.

Another problem for younger rape victims is the gynecological examination. Inexperienced or severely traumatized young women may perceive it as another rape. Thus, while they may be concerned about the well-being of their bodies, they will have difficulty with necessary procedures if these actions stimulate memories or seem to reproduce the original rape experience in any way.

Women with children must deal with the problems of what, how, and when to tell them. If the rape incident is known in the community, there are implications for the victim and her family. A mother must be concerned about the trauma she may be inflicting on her children, as well as about their perception of her. If she is married, she may be concerned about whether her husband will continue to find her sexually attractive. She may have un-expected negative feelings toward her husband if she feels he is not under-standing or supportive enough. Some relationships break up as a conse-quence of this stress.

Divorced or separated women are in a particularly difficult position. They may feel that their reputations and credibility are already in question because of their life style, and they may experience the rape as a confirma-tion of their feelings of inadequacy. They are especially likely to feel guilty and may fail to obtain aid or report the crime. Their ability to function independently has apparently been challenged. If they have children, they may also worry about their ability to protect and care for them.

Middle-aged women are often in a period of reassessment of their lives, particularly in view of changed relationships with adolescent or adult children. Their husbands may be experiencing their own mid-life reassess-ment and stress and thus may be less responsive to and supportive of their wives' sexual and emotional needs. At this point, the overwhelming experi-ence of rape is particularly damaging. The myth that women who are past their period of greatest sexual activity have less to lose than younger women is very much in error. Self-devaluation and feelings of worthlessness and shame may be especially prominent in women who are concerned about their sexual adequacy.

Therapeutic Intervention

Psychiatrists who are called in to see rape victims must know how to help and be able to provide an empathic understanding of the victims' experiences. In order to do this, they must be aware of and able to deal with the feelings evoked in them by these situations.

Because the effects of a rape vary for women at different stages of the life cycle and in different social and family circumstances, the meaning of the event must be understood in the context of the victim's life, and it must be kept in mind that positive adaptation is possible to the extent that the external world provides validation and support. The specific nature of the rape experience is also an important factor. For example, the betrayal by someone who was trusted or the impact of a particularly violent or de-grading experience is likely to have unique repercussions. Similarly, the circumstances of events immediately after the rape, including the attitudes and behaviors of those with whom the victim comes into contact, have important future implications. Here the attitudes of health care providers, police, friends, sexual partners, and families are particularly important.

Disapproval, skepticism, or any behavior that may be experienced as critical can intensify guilt and adaptation difficulties.

In the immediate aftermath of rape, issues of personal safety and control are of primary concern to victims. The presence of empathic, supportive medical personnel is extremely important. Accurate and clear information about medical and legal procedures must be provided so that victims can make informed decisions. While those caring for the victims may have opinions on what they ought to do about reporting, coercion has no place in the management of rape victims.

Psychological treatment of a rape victim after the immediate emergency usually involves a short-term, issue-oriented crisis approach, with the goal of restoring the victim to her previous level of functioning as quickly as possible. Although the goal of complete restoration may not be entirely realistic, treatment aims for mastery of as much of the experience as possible. Since the crisis disrupts the victim's physical, emotional, social, and sexual life styles, all these areas should receive attention. The goal is to integrate and work through as many aspects of the rape experience as possible. Attention to potential residual or late-occurring symptoms, such as sleep disturbances and sexual dysfunction, is also important.

The Psychiatrist's Role

In approaching victims, it is important for psychiatrists to be sympathetic and available without being intrusive. A doctor's physical examination helps to determine the extent of the injury and legally documents the assault. Because of the importance and possible stress of the physical examination, psychiatrists or counselors may need to support victims during such a procedure.

Obtaining a careful history includes attention to the circumstances of the rape, the victim's personal and family situation, her current mental state, and her available supports. It is also important to assess the victim's circumstances, her personal safety, her living situation, and the people available immediately, as well as her long-range adaptive potential and resources. If the victim lives alone or was raped at home, it is likely that she will fear returning home. Further, the assailant may have threatened to return. A temporary resolution may involve identifying friends with whom the victim can stay and helping her consider the options available for the future. The presence of empathic and supportive people will enhance the victim's sense of safety. Since her self-esteem has been threatened by the loss of control, as part of the counseling approach, she should be supported in regaining and maintaining control where appropriate.

In considering the assault, psychiatrists need to know the circumstances, the relationship of victim to assailant, the existence of physical and verbal threats, details of the assailant's behavior, the amount and nature of resistance, the use of alcohol or drugs by the victim or the assailant, the victim's immediate emotional and sexual reactions, and the victim's coping strategies before and during the assault.

The mental status of victims should be assessed. If there is a history of previous mental illness or some uncertainty about the nature of response, the consultant may want to make a further psychiatric referral or follow the victim's behavior closely. A history of previous stress responses and adaptive resources is an important indicator of responses to the rape.

It is important that victims be prepared for the range of reactions that are likely to occur, so that they have some awareness that the inevitable disruptions in life style are not pathological. They may experience mistrust of men or begin making very considerable demands on the men in their lives and find themselves sensitive to disappointment if the men do not meet their needs. Counseling for relevant family members or those close to rape victims can be very helpful, including preparing these individuals for possible later reactions that are part of "normal stress responses." Among these are a variety of sexual disturbances and phobic reactions, as well as anxiety and depression. All these reactions can be precipitated by stimuli reminiscent of the original trauma.

The memories of and reactions to the rape may be revived not only by major incidents but also by minor ones. For example, one woman who had been attacked by someone approaching from behind was frightened whenever anyone unfamiliar was behind her or moved outside her field of vision. When stopped for a traffic violation, she reacted with intense fear and anger at the policeman who approached from the rear of the car.

Victims may make decisions regarding prosecution at the time of the emergency room contact, but since victims who initially decline to prosecute may change their minds at a later date, it is important to gather enough information to corroborate details of the assault. It is not the physician's responsibility to decide whether a rape occurred. That can be decided in court if the victim does prosecute. The immediate task of the professional who sees the victim first is to support her and to gather evidence that can be used later.

Victims should be encouraged to talk with supportive personnel, to express their feelings, and to accept reassurance and validation of their responses. If they do not wish to talk at first contact, they can be encouraged to talk at another time. Coercion and insistence repeat the loss-of-control experience in the rape.

In working with victims of sexual abuse, one of the most important and difficult issues is avoiding infantilizing the victims or turning them into "sick" patients or defendants. This can be damaging and can interfere with their efforts to regain their self-esteem and sense of self-worth. Reassurance about how they handled their experience can be enormously helpful. The support and respect demonstrated in a sensitive interaction can turn these painful and tragic events into experiences that may lead to emotional growth. Support is extremely important in restoring the victim to her previous level of functioning and adaptation.

The prognosis will depend on the nature of the experience, the degree of violence and trauma, victims' personal histories and adaptive resources, and the amount and extent of support and validation available.

Suggested Readings

Atkeson, B., and Calhoun, K. (1982). Victims of rape: repeated assessment of depressive symptoms. *Journal of Consulting and Clinical Psychology* 50:96–102.

Becker, J., Skinner, L., Abel, G., and Treacy, E. (1982). Incidence and types of sexual dysfunctions in rape and incest victims. *Journal of Sex and Marital Therapy* 8:65–74.

Burgess, A., and Holmstrom, L. (1974). Rape trauma syndrome. *American Journal of Psychiatry* 131:981–986.

Hilberman, E. (1976). *The Rape Victim.* New York: Basic Books.

Kilpatrick, D., Veronen, L., and Resnick, P. (1979). The aftermath of rape: recent empirical findings. *American Journal of Orthopsychiatry* 49:658–669.

Martin, C., Warfield, M., and Braen, G. (1983). Physician's management of the psychological aspects of rape. *Journal of the American Medical Association* 249:501–503.

McCombie, S. (ed.) (1980). *The Rape Crisis Intervention Handbook.* New York: Plenum Press.

Nadelson, C., Notman, M., Zackson, H., and Gornick, J. (1982). A follow-up study of rape victims. *American Journal of Psychiatry* 139:1266–1270.

Notman, M., and Nadelson, C. (1976). The rape victim: psychodynamic considerations. *American Journal of Psychiatry* 133:408–413.

Sutherland, S., and Scherl, D. (1970). Patterns of response among victims of rape. *American Journal of Orthopsychiatry* 40:503–511.

CHAPTER 9

Emergency Assessment and Care of the Chronic Mentally Ill

JOHN A. TALBOTT, M.D.

Leona Bachrach, M.D., the foremost authority on deinstitutionalization in this country, describes the chronically ill as those individuals who are or have been on the rolls of long-term mental institutions and hospitals—and those who, but for the deinstitutionalization movement, might be on those rolls. Her definition is useful because it covers all the chronic mentally ill, whether or not they are affected by such state mental health policies as transinstitutionalization and blockage of admissions.

Bachrach's definition includes those suffering from schizophrenia, recurrent or episodic affective illnesses, and severe and chronic characterological disorders. It does not include individuals in long-term psychotherapy without attendant disability. The issue of disability in addition to disease is important because the disability, as much as the disease, occupies the thinking and actions of emergency room psychiatrists.

Principles

The principles of assessment, treatment, and care of the chronic mentally ill in the emergency room stem directly from historical developments and Bachrach's definition. These are people whose needs at one time were, or could have been, cared for under the single umbrella of the state hospital. Their removal from under that umbrella in no way diminishes the importance of these needs.

As Figure 1 shows, among the needs of the chronic mentally ill are housing, food, medical care, psychiatric care, and vocational and social rehabilitation. A move from a state hospital to any less restrictive setting requires individuals to meet one or more of these needs themselves. As a result, emergency room physicians must ascertain where individual patients reside. Treatment plans for those in nursing homes, board-and-care facilities, and independent apartments will be quite different.

The second overarching issue is disability. If we, as psychiatrists, were dealing only with acute illness and could be assured that with adequate treatment patients would return to their previous home lives or jobs, our thinking would be quite different than if we suspect that the patients, no matter how well the acute episode resolved, would be left with residual difficulty in everyday living.

With these two general issues in mind, the psychiatrist should consider the following principles when encountering a chronic mentally ill person in the emergency room.

1. The needs of the chronic mentally ill person often far exceed those of someone suffering from either a chronic nonpsychotic illness or an acute psychotic disorder. Therefore, a host of services, settings, and disciplines will have to be considered.

2. The social context of presenting symptoms will weigh heavily in the assessment, intervention, and treatment planning. Therefore, collateral information, previous medical records, and an accurate understanding of the precipitating event(s) are critical to treatment.

3. The presenting illness episode or emergency event is but one small moment in the patient's lifetime of illness or illness-vulnerability. Therefore, as much as the psychiatrist is preoccupied with solving the particular problem that brought this person into the emergency room, he or she must look at what has been tried before and what will come after.

4. If hospitalization is required, the chronically ill respond best to brief stays and prompt return to family or community, once stabilization and re-equilibration on medication have been achieved. Therefore, it is critical to think of the inpatient hospital ward not as the center for treatment (as is done far too often) but as one small part of the entire treatment approach.

5. Despite the fact that short-term admissions, with prompt return to family or community, are optimal, the alienation of many chronically ill patients from their families, combined with the inadequate quantity and quality of community settings and services for the chronic mentally ill, makes necessary the overutilization of both hospitals and other suboptimal settings, such as nursing homes.

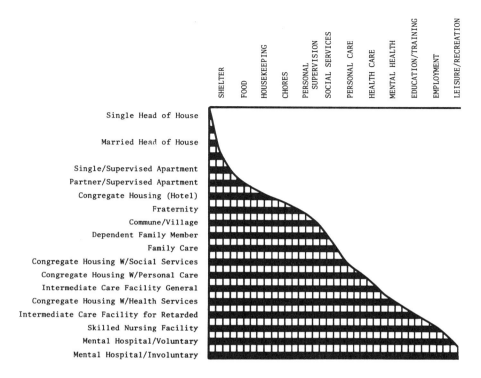

FIGURE 1.
An ideal system provides a stepwise progression of housing from the most to the least restrictive, which meets the decreasing number of needs of the chronic mentally ill. (Reprinted by permission of the author, Elizabeth Boggs, Ph.D.)

Case Histories

Miss R., a 55-year-old unemployed woman, was first hospitalized for schizophrenia at the age of 20. She stayed several months in a general hospital and was then transferred to a state hospital, where she remained until she was 35 years of age. At that point, she still talked to herself, dressed sloppily, and could work only a few hours a day folding clothing in the hospital laundry, but she was without hallucinations and delusions and seemed moderately well controlled on chlorpromazine.

Since being released after 15 years of illness, she has had eight brief admissions for reappearance of acute psychosis (presenting with auditory hallucinations, delusions of being controlled, and a thinking disorder). She has lived in many settings, including halfway houses, adult homes, single-room occupancy hotels, board-and-care homes, and foster homes, but she prefers to live alone in a one-room apartment. She can travel daily to a low-intensity "lounge program," has worked for brief periods in sheltered workshops, and spends most of her time walking the streets of the local ex-patient ghetto area of her city. She now receives intramuscular injections of fluphenazine enanthate.

She was brought to the emergency room at 10 p.m. by the police, who were called to her "welfare hotel" by the manager because she was attempting to cook some food over an open fire set on her window sill. All were concerned by her lack of judgment and by the fact that she was almost nude and had covered herself with lipstick and nail polish.

The psychiatrist who interviewed the patient found her apparently oblivious to the seriousness of her act and quite proud of her bizarre appearance. The hotel manager was called, but he provided no further information except the home telephone number of the social worker from the lounge program. The social worker revealed that the patient had stopped coming several days earlier, following a fight with another program member over who would be chief cook and who would be the cook's helper for the noon meal.

Mr. S., a 22-year-old single unemployed man who had never been hospitalized, has intermittently visited various emergency rooms, outpatient clinics, and community mental health centers for over five years. He dropped out of school five years ago because he found it boring, started work in a filling station, and occupied his evenings drinking and taking drugs with a group of friends down by the waterfront.

He has worked sporadically in more and more menial jobs for shorter and shorter periods of time. Ejected from his home because he would neither contribute financially nor help with household chores, he has been living in shabby skid-row hotels. He insists that he has no mental illness and that his contact with psychiatrists and mental health services comes only at the request of others such as the police who pick him up for "nuisance offenses," hotel managers who complain of his life style, and family members who pressure him into seeking help after he has violent outbursts with them.

He was brought to the emergency room one afternoon by his mother, who insisted that the psychiatrist do something to stop his steady social and vocational deterioration. She felt he should be on medication, get a job, and go out with a "nice girl" instead of hanging around the waterfront, drinking and smoking.

The patient looked furious but cowed by his mother. He disputed her contentions and snorted when she spelled out her ideas about a treatment plan. When interviewed alone, however, he admitted that things were not going right for him and that he hadn't yet "gotten his act together"; he claimed that all he needed was more time to get motivated. He insisted he was "no nut case" and, when verbally pushed by the psychiatrist, threatened him in a way that was frightening.

Case Discussions

Assessment, immediate intervention, and long-term treatment planning are all important components of treating the chronically ill patient. These first two components apply to all patients seen in the emergency room, but the last is particularly applicable to the chronically ill.

It is important to see the emergency room event as an opportunity to assess and reassess the chronic patient's diagnosis, current situation, and treatment plan. Several generalizations may be of help.

1. The reason that the patient is in the emergency room is frequently more important than the diagnosis.
2. Prior diagnoses may be incorrect. Once made in public facilities, diagnoses tend to stick and may point to treatable illnesses that should now be ruled out.
3. Be sure to differentiate among symptoms caused by disease, institutional or community isolation, and the aging process. Withdrawal, lack of spontaneity, and depression are common to all three. Understanding the cause will often lead to a positive intervention.

The case examples illustrate the two large groups of chronic patients commonly seen in the emergency room. Miss R. represents the older, deinstitutionalized mentally ill person, with a clear diagnosis of schizophrenia. She has led a desultory life since her 15-year hospitalization and can be seen either as shuttling helplessly between settings and services or as utilizing them as needed. The term *"revolving door"* is frequently used perjoratively, but it would be hard to argue that eight 20-day hospitalizations, over a 20-year period, which have allowed her to spend most of her time in a fashion that she considers enjoyable, are worse than one 20-year stay.

Immediately upon seeing Miss R., the interviewer must question why she is in the emergency room tonight, what went wrong in her environment, what needs to be done to restabilize it, and whether her long-term treatment plan can be improved. It is apparent initially that her presentation is different from the times when she was psychotic and necessitated inpatient hospitalization. She has no delusions, hallucinations, or thought disorder. In addition, collateral sources reveal the reason for her current presentation.

Immediate attention should be paid primarily to the precipitant of this episode, and whether therapy is accomplished in the emergency room or through a brief crisis stay in the hospital, the psychiatrist should assume that the patient will be able to return quickly to her premorbid environment. After all, she does have a home, a daily activity, and caring people involved with her medication and treatment. The circumstances of the fight with her coworker at the lounge program seem amenable to psychotherapeutic intervention, once some distance and perspective are gained.

In terms of the longer-range plan, one must measure her current treatment plan against both ideal and optimal ones. She is not in an ideal situation. One must always be careful to allow the chronically disabled person the opportunity to progress toward returning to mainstream life while not applying too great a pressure, which may result paradoxically in symptomatic or functional regression. On the other hand, her current treatment plan does not seem optimal, and perhaps some work could be done to increase her social network so that the fragility of her small interpersonal network at the lounge program does not threaten her psychiatric state.

Mr. S. represents the young or new never-institutionalized patient. Young chronic patients tend to be 20 to 35 years old and present a mixed diagnostic picture with strong characterological and affective components. They may wander the streets, abuse drugs and alcohol, get arrested for minor offenses, commit violent impulsive acts, and be high users of services, although most are noncompliant with treatment.

The psychiatrist must be sure to assess Mr. S.'s suicidal potential because he is at high risk for suicide. In addition, the psychiatrist needs to find out why his mother is so fed up with him this particular day that she brings him to the emergency room. Her involvement with him bespeaks both her possible involvement in a mutually destructive pattern and a potential solution to some of his difficulties.

In the short term, the psychiatrist must consider both people's desires— the mother's desire to stop her son's deterioration and the son's desire to get his mother off his back and yet straighten out his life. Interventions aimed at satisfying both these ends always have the highest chance of success. At this point, however, obtaining everyone's agreement to a longer-term plan is the most feasible action.

That longer-term plan should address the stated wishes of both mother and son and should perhaps involve family treatment, as well as socialization and vocational assessment and training for the son and psychoeducationally oriented counseling for the mother. A major problem for new or young chronic patients is their lack of social and vocational skills. With them, the primary task may be habilitation instead of rehabilitation.

Specific Interventions with Chronic Patients

Psychopharmacological Approaches

Many chronically ill patients appear in the emergency room because they have neglected their medication, because their illness has "broken through" their medication, because their medication requires adjustment up or down, or because the side effects of their medication have become too troublesome. Re-equilibration of their medication may be all that is necessary. Often, an adjustment is feasible on an outpatient basis, but brief hospitalization is sometimes necessary. In addition, the chronically ill may use the emergency room physician as a consultant, particularly about therapeutic or side effects of the medication.

Psychotherapeutic Approaches

Because many chronic patients appear in the emergency room in reaction to their environment, applicable interventions are often psychosocial rather than psychopharmacological. While all psychotherapeutic interventions can be utilized with the chronically ill, it is most likely that the psychiatrist will use support, clarification, problem solving, and advice giving instead of interpretation or abreaction. Often the simplest of techniques—listening, asking the reasons for the emergency room visit, and attempting to solve reality-based problems—will ameliorate the situation.

Other Psychosocial Approaches

The most common issue facing the emergency room psychiatrist when dealing with environmental problems encountered by chronic patients is housing. As was illustrated in Figure 1, an ideal system provides a step-wise progression of housing from the most to the least restrictive, including short-term and long-term hospitalization, quarterway and halfway houses, foster or group homes, board-and-care homes, crisis hostels, and independent group and individual apartments. Unfortunately, such a system is rare in this country, and we lack appropriate facilities of high quality. Therefore, the psychiatrist must often dig for whatever can be found for such patients, often settling for an inappropriate nursing home, board-and-care facility, or welfare hotel setting, instead of a more appropriate halfway house or foster home.

Social Rehabilitation

While not an emergency intervention, social rehabilitation will frequently figure into the psychiatrist's discussion with chronic patients, because it is one of their primary needs. Social contacts, socialization, and the expansion of social networks are vital to chronic patients' well-being, but these concepts have only recently been explored in such a manner that the psychiatrist can fashion the intervention to fit the need.

Vocational Rehabilitation

Although very distant from an emergency intervention, vocational assessment, vocational training, sheltered workshop settings, and competitive employment opportunities may be critical to the design of a good long-term treatment plan for the chronically ill. All these efforts are needed in programs serving the chronically ill.

Making Interventions Work

Unfortunately, knowing that a chronic patient needs medication, psychotherapy, housing, and social and vocational rehabilitation is not enough. There are usually inadequate community resources in all areas. Where available, they are rarely integrated. Such services and systems for the chronically ill have been fragmented since the state hospital ceased to be the primary locus of care.

For this population, continuity of care is more critical than whatever actual treatment interventions are offered. To achieve true continuity, each program must provide all the services needed by such people, or all programs must have a closely linked treatment system. To accomplish continuity, most programs have trained people to function as resource managers (previously called case managers) to help the chronically ill gain access to needed services of all sorts.

In addition, there is now a series of descriptions of model programs for the chronic mentally ill ranging from inpatient programs that teach patients how to survive in the community; through classical psychosocial rehabilitation programs, such as Fountain House, which provide housing, social and vocational rehabilitation, and access to medical and psychiatric care; to innovative programs that are alternatives to hospitalization and provide aggressive community care for the chronically ill.

Prognosis

The short-term emergent problems of the chronically ill are frequently resolvable through alleviating precipitating stress factors, psychotherapeutic intervention, psychopharmacological adjustment, environmental manipulation, and the design of the longer-term treatment plan. The prognosis for the underlying illness in such individuals is often not so favorable. Although we can control, ameliorate, and temper the positive symptoms of schizophrenia and we can dampen, if not prevent, many recurrences of primary affective disorders, we are at a loss to cure the major psychoses or, often, even reduce the severity of characterological disorders.

But the model programs mentioned earlier do lead us to be somewhat more optimistic than the above situation suggests. Paul and Lentz had a readmission rate under 10 percent in a group they treated, whereas the readmission rate for those receiving milieu treatment was 30 percent; those receiving traditional state hospital treatment were readmitted at a rate of over 50 percent, which approximates the national average. In addition, Fountain House residents returned to the hospital at half the rate of the control group (17 percent and 37 percent, respectively) in the first six months. Finally, the patients in Stein and Test's program demonstrated fewer symptoms, less time in hospital, and more time with friends than the control group.

A Final Word

Emergency intervention with the chronically ill is a complex, challenging, and potentially rewarding task. It offers a chance for a significantly greater quality of life to people who were previously removed from the community and deprived of the personal choices that all of us value highly. The steps in the crisis treatment of the chronic mentally ill are the same as the steps in treating a person with a less serious or chronic condition—searching for the precipitant of this episode, finding a workable and acceptable short-term intervention, and examining the feasibility of a better long-term intervention. These steps often require the psychiatrist to interact with professionals in other disciplines and with various people in the ill person's environment; in order to operate effectively, therefore, the psychiatrist needs to cultivate a broad base of professional and community support.

Suggested Readings

Bachrach, L.L. (1976). *Deinstitutionalization: An Analytic Review and Sociological Perspective.* Rockville, Md.: National Institute of Mental Health.

Bassuk, E.L., and Gerson, S. (1980). Chronic crisis patients: a discrete clinical group. *American Journal of Psychiatrty* 137:1513–1517.

Bassuk, E.L., and Schoonover, S.C. (1981). The private general hospital's psychiatric emergency service in a decade of transition. *Hospital and Community Psychiatry* 32:181–185.

Glick, R.A., Meyerson, A.T., Robbins, E., and Talbott, J.A. (1976). *Psychiatric Emergencies.* New York: Grune & Stratton.

Lamb, H.R., et al. (1976). *Community Survival for Long-Term Patients.* San Francisco: Jossey-Bass.

Paul, G.L., and Lentz, R.J. (1977). *Psychosocial Treatment of Chronic Mental Patients: Milieu Versus Social-Learning Programs.* Cambridge, Mass.: Harvard University Press.

Pepper, B. (ed.) (1982). *The Young Adult Chronic Patient.* San Francisco: Jossey-Bass.

Stein, L.I., and Test, M.A. (1980). Alternative to mental hospital treatment, I. Conceptual model, treatment program, and clinical evaluation. *Archives of General Psychiatry* 137:392–397.

Talbott, J.A. (1982). *The Chronic Mentally Ill: Treatment, Programs, Systems.* New York: Human Sciences Press.

Talbott, J.A. (1983). *The Chronic Mentally Ill: Five Years Later.* New York: Grune & Stratton.

CHAPTER 10

Commonly Missed Medical Diagnoses

MILTON K. ERMAN, M.D.

Numerous medications and medical diseases can lead to symptoms suggestive of major psychiatric disorders. And as many as 24 percent of individuals diagnosed as suffering from psychoneurotic disorders develop a significant medical disease within eight months of their initial psychiatric evaluation.

Missed diagnoses harm patients in a number of ways. Delayed diagnosis often postpones treatment and prolongs hospitalization. With many illnesses, progression of disease before appropriate treatment is begun may lead to residual symptomatology, long-term disability, or death.

Among the most obvious causes of missed medical diagnoses is the failure of many psychiatrists to physically examine their patients. In one emergency setting, 66 percent of staff psychiatrists did not perform physical examinations, nor did 59 percent of psychiatric residents.

For patients who are to be admitted to a psychiatric service from an emergency room, assessing psychiatrists must function as a "court of last resort." In an emergency room, hematological, radiological, and other diagnostic procedures are readily available and easily performed. Once patients leave the medical setting of the emergency room for the psychiatric setting of an inpatient ward, these procedures are less easily obtained and utilized and less likely to even be considered.

Medical Illnesses with Psychiatric Symptoms

Withdrawal states from addicting drugs and alcohol, seen frequently in emergency rooms, present with features that may lead unwary physicians to make a primary psychiatric diagnosis. In mild withdrawal states, the presentation and complaints may suggest an anxiety disorder. Delirious states associated with withdrawal from alcohol, barbiturates, or similarly acting sedative or hypnotic drugs may present as acute psychotic episodes, as the following case demonstrates.

> Mr. T., a 64-year-old retired fireman, was brought into the emergency room in an agitated state. He had called for an ambulance, reporting that his house had been set on fire and he had been burned. The ambulance crew arrived to find him huddled in a corner of his kitchen and brought him to the hospital. The psychiatrist on call was alerted to his arrival for psychiatric evaluation.
>
> The patient, who showed no evidence of physical injury, reported that his burns had occurred when a group of black males, who were strangers to him, had broken into his house, tied him up, poured gasoline over him, and set him on fire. He was disoriented to place and time, had impaired attention and immediate recall, and was experiencing auditory and visual illusions and hallucinations. He was tremulous and agitated and complained of anxiety. His pulse was 108 and regular; his oral temperature was 100.4 degrees; his blood pressure was 132/98; and he was hyperreflexic. Although he did not volunteer information about his drinking pattern, he did admit to long-standing regular alcohol intake of 1½ pints of whiskey per day, and reported that he had stopped drinking three days prior to evaluation.

Of interest from a dynamic perspective is the content of this patient's hallucinations and delusions. He lived in a white neighborhood that had been thrown into turmoil by the busing in of black students to a local high school. Violence had erupted, with people stoning the buses carrying the students. There was considerable fear of reprisals in the neighborhood. The patient's delusional content reflected the fears rampant in his neighborhood at the time, along with a theme that was understandable in the context of his work history, the fear of being trapped in a burning building.

The psychiatrist's ability to diagnose drug and alcohol withdrawal depends partly on a history of substance abuse. Patients may not willingly report such information for fear of the legal or social consequences, but friends or relatives can often supply the needed information. When, despite the patient's denial, there is a high index of suspicion of drug or alcohol abuse, a therapeutic trial of a short-acting benzodiazepine to assess the response to treatment i.e., of possible withdrawal symptoms may be helpful (see Chapter 21).

Endocrine disturbances are frequently associated with psychiatric symptomatology. Hyperthyroidism may lead to complaints of anxiety, to confused thinking, and to behavior disturbances with increased activity suggestive of agitated schizophrenia or mania. Depression may be related in some cases to mild hypothyroidism. More significant hypothyroidism often presents with severe psychiatric symptoms; when this is the case, the diagnosis can usually be made using standard tests of thyroid function, as in this illustration.

> Ms. U., a 44-year-old divorced white woman, was transferred from the internal medicine service to the psychiatric service of a general hospital for treatment of what appeared to be a psychotic depression. She had presented to the emergency room with complaints of lethargy and depressed mood, and with reports of recent abnormal behavior. She had been arrested in another city for refusing to leave a church, having stated that she had the same right to use the church as the priests who ran it. She was released from jail after a brief stay, returned to the church, and made her way to the bell tower. She rang the church bells, proclaimed her right to run the church as she saw fit, and denounced the priests and religious hierarchy. She was taken to a local hospital for psychiatric observation, but was released after 24 hours without a formal diagnosis. On admission to the general hospital, her lethargy and myxedematous facies were briefly noted, but she was transferred to the psychiatric service prior to completion of a medical workup for treatment of her psychiatric condition.
>
> When first seen on the psychiatric ward, she was sitting on her bed, wrapped in a blanket and wearing a scarf and cap though her room was quite warm. She appeared myxedematous and spoke with a characteristic raspy voice. Her speech was slow, as was her mental activity. She was hyporeflexic, had a pulse of 46, and an oral temperature of 96.4 degrees. Her serum thyroxin level was 0.5 $\mu g/dl$ (normal range 4.5 to 12.5 $\mu g/dl$).

Had the circumstances been different and the patient been transferred to a psychiatric hospital for long-term treatment, the diagnosis of endocrine disturbance might have been missed completely or further delayed.

Other endocrine disturbances that can lead to psychiatric symptoms are Cushing's syndrome, which may be confused with depression or mania, and Addison's disease, which may be confused with depression. True hypoglycemia, seen with insulin-secreting tumors of the pancreas, may lead to intermittent symptoms of confusion, disorientation, and bizarre behavior that may be confused with brief psychotic episodes, borderline states, or fugue or amnestic disorders.

Disorders of the central nervous system can alter brain function and thereby mimic psychiatric disorders. The evaluating psychiatrist's index of suspicion must be high when ruling out potential CNS causes, because in many of these situations the risks of delayed treatment may be great.

Central nervous system infections are rarely limited to just that system. Although patients may present with predominant symptoms of encephalitis, these are rarely seen without involvement of the meninges as well. However, psychiatric symptoms associated with the encephalitides may appear before the evidence of meningeal inflammation, leading to diagnostic confusion, as seen in the next vignette.

Ms. V., a 21-year-old single white woman, was admitted to a psychiatric service after evaluation in an emergency room. She had been followed as an outpatient for six months by a psychiatrist, and she was taking lithium. Her history revealed that she had had a psychotic episode at age 19, necessitating a 1½ year inpatient stay during which she had demonstrated aggressive and hypersexual behavior, bizarre thinking, and poor impulse control. The initial working diagnosis had been schizophrenia, but she failed to respond to antipsychotic medications. Lithium was then begun and had produced a dramatic, positive response.

When seen in the emergency room, she complained of headache, nausea, dizziness, blurred vision, and impaired thinking. She also complained of a recurrent visual hallucination, reporting that she saw a wolf or a wolf's head on occasion, and that she was quite frightened by it. Some of the findings were suggestive of lithium toxicity, but her lithium level was within the normal range.

In the emergency room she was evaluated by a neurologist, who found no localizing or pathological signs. He suggested she might have a hysterical psychosis. She was admitted to the psychiatric service for further observation. There she continued to complain of impaired thought processes and visual illusions and hallucinations, but denied delusional thought content.

Her mental state deteriorated during the first week in the hospital; she became less responsive and alert and more inappropriate, and then she developed urinary incontinence. Because of the organic appearance of her behavior, an EEG was performed. It showed generalized slowing.

Neurological consultation was requested and a lumbar puncture was performed. The lumbar puncture showed 15 lymphocytes, no red blood cells, and an elevated protein level of 60 mg/dl.

A presumptive diagnosis of viral encephalitis was made, and all psychotropic medications were stopped. The patient continued to have a mild organic hallucinosis for another ten days, then had a gradual return of functioning, and was discharged from the hospital after a total of five weeks. However, she continued to complain of mental dullness and felt that she had not completely returned to her prior level of functioning even a year after discharge. The etiological basis for the initial signs and symptoms of lithium toxicity was presumed to have been a lithium effect on a brain sensitized by a viral infection.

Viral encephalitis may have a deteriorating fatal course, or it may be self-limited with less morbidity, as in this case. When such an infection is mild and presents with only psychiatric symptomatology, diagnosis of the infection is unlikely, as this requires both a high index of suspicion about the underlying organic etiology and a diagnostic lumbar puncture.

Posttraumatic disturbances of the central nervous system are frequently missed medical conditions that may present with prominent behavior changes. Behavioral disruption occurs frequently after damage to the frontal and temporal lobes, as in the next two cases.

Mr. W., a 28-year-old single computer engineer, was hospitalized with multiple fractures following a motorcycle accident. Psychiatric consultation was requested because he was uncooperative with the nursing staff. Despite a fractured pelvis and femur and being in traction, the patient refused to use a bedpan and attempted to get out of bed to walk to the bathroom.

The medical and nursing staff's prejudices toward "bikers" had led to an erroneous assumption that oppositional behavior was typical of this man.

The psychiatric consultant determined that the patient worked for a large company and had a stable work record and no prior history of inappropriate or oppositional behavior. He enjoyed riding his motorcycle to and from work and on weekends, and had no involvement with motorcycle gangs or antisocial behavior of any sort.

Integration of the neurosurgical report and laboratory data was important. The patient had experienced trauma to the occiput at the initial impact, and contrecoup damage had occurred to the frontal regions as well. This latter injury was reflected in the CT scan, which indicated edema of the frontal lobes and decreased ventricular size. The patient showed some improvement when steroids were begun. Over the course of his hospital stay, his behavior improved considerably. No residual frontal lobe damage was evident.

Mr. X., the 23-year-old single unemployed son of a prominent local lawyer, was seen in consultation after his fourth arrest for exposing himself to women. Eighteen months previously, he had been in a motor vehicle accident. He had suffered a skull fracture and had been comatose for nine days.

The patient's behavior pattern prior to his arrests was remarkably similar. On the street or in public places, he met women whom he wanted to "get to know better," and attempted to introduce himself. When they rejected his advances, he became frustrated and responded by exposing himself to them. At the time of these acts, he did not consider the consequences of his actions and made no effort to flee or avoid arrest.

Review of his medical record yielded a CT scan, performed six months after his accident, which demonstrated frontal lobe atrophy.

These two examples show the problems with impulsivity and poor judgment, which may be perceived initially as deviant life-style behavior but may actually be caused by frontal lobe disturbances. Unfortunately, psychotherapeutic work is quite difficult with patients whose frontal lobes are damaged because they are literally unable to recognize the consequences of their actions and to learn to avoid dangerous and self-destructive behavior.

Disorders causing increased intracranial pressure may also present with psychiatric symptomatology. Subdural hematomas give rise to confusion and depression. Chronic alcoholics are at particular risk for presentation with these complaints. Normal-pressure hydrocephalus may present with dementia, ataxia, and urinary incontinence, symptoms that may be misinterpreted as resulting from depression. In rare instances, the appearance of apparent psychiatric symptoms may be the first suggestion of a brain tumor, as in the following case.

> Miss Y., an 18-year-old white student, was transferred to a university psychiatric service from an outlying medical hospital with a differential diagnosis that included catatonic schizophrenia, depression, and anorexia nervosa. She had lost 40 pounds in the preceding three months, had withdrawn emotionally, and had decreased her involvement in activities that she had previously enjoyed. She was transferred to the psychiatric service after having spent 5½ weeks in the other hospital, during which time various tests, including psychological testing, multiple routine blood studies, and serum protein electrophoresis, had been performed. No persistent abnormalities were noted in the extensive array of studies that had been performed, so psychiatric diagnoses were considered likely.
>
> On the inpatient psychiatric service, the patient was first seen by a medical student, who reviewed the history and found no psychiatric abnormalities except loss of appetite and weight, which could be suggestive of depression, as could her reports of muscular weakness and loss of interest in previously pleasurable activities. However, the medical student noticed ptosis of the right eyelid, facial asymmetry with sagging mouth and jaw muscles, a lowered palate, and upper arm weakness, all on the right side. The resident confirmed these findings.
>
> The patient was transferred to the neurosurgical service. Surgery later in the week revealed a glioblastoma, which had extended into multiple areas of the brain.

Although this example is not typical, it points out the dangers inherent in relying excessively on laboratory values and not observing the patient carefully.

Autoimmune disorders can also cause psychiatric symptoms, especially systemic lupus erythematosis. Patients with lupus cerebritis frequently present with emotional lability, auditory and visual hallucinations, and even frank psychotic delusional states. Electroencephalograms are generally abnormal, and the psychiatric disturbances are presumed to be caused by brain inflammation.

Ankylosing spondylitis usually presents initially with low back pain; other symptoms are weight loss and fatigue, which may be misinterpreted as depression.

Symptoms associated with blood and bone marrow diseases may also be misinterpreted as emotional in origin, as in the next case.

> Mrs. Z., a 34-year-old married white woman, was admitted to the hospital for evaluation of complaints of increasing fatigue, lethargy, and

shortness of breath both at rest and with exertion. She denied any recent trauma or blood loss and appeared to be in good physical condition. Although she experienced a decrease in symptomatology when given oxygen, the medical house staff felt that she was depressed, hypochondriacal, or malingering. A psychiatric consultation was requested.

The psychiatric consultant could find little to suggest that these symptoms provided the patient with secondary gain, or that they were part of a repetitive behavior pattern on the patient's part. The explanation of her symptoms was provided by the hematology report, which revealed a microcytic anemia, with a hematocrit of 20 percent.

She was transfused with three units of packed red blood cells, and her psychiatric symptoms disappeared as her hematocrit returned to a normal level.

Similarly, hematological disorders such as leukemia, lymphoma, and multiple myeloma may present with complaints of weakness, malaise, and depressed mood that may be mistakenly attributed to a primary psychiatric disturbance.

Medications That Produce Psychiatric Symptoms

Various medications, including psychoactive drugs, may lead to complaints or symptoms that suggest psychiatric illness. Some individuals treated with tricyclic antidepressants may develop an acute psychotic illness. Individuals with a personal or family history of bipolar affective disorders, or a predisposition to such disorders, may become hypomanic while taking these medications. People with a prior history of or predisposition to schizophrenia may develop a psychosis with schizophrenic features when taking antidepressant medications.

Stimulant medications often produce psychotic symptomatology. When stimulants are used chronically, people with no prior psychiatric history may develop depression, perhaps caused by neurotransmitter depletion or by the repetitive process of dysphoric withdrawal from the euphoriant effects of these medications. More intensive chronic use of amphetamines or the use of large doses over a short period of time may lead to the development of a toxic psychosis with schizophreniform features.

Benzodiazepines are remarkably safe agents, especially with regard to overdosing. However, their chronic use can lead to a state of physiological dependence, and when regular use is discontinued, withdrawal symptoms that can be confused with anxiety disorders may be seen. Rarely, patients experience a disinhibition syndrome with these medications, with prominent hyperactivity and affective lability. In some patients, the use of these medications may lead to depressive symptoms as well.

Many nonpsychotropic medications cause psychiatric symptoms. Medications with anticholinergic properties can produce excitement, anxiety, disorientation, confusion, and psychosis. When such symptoms are seen in patients with prior histories of drug abuse, these medications should be considered as a possible cause.

Psychiatric symptoms—most commonly symptoms of depression—have been associated with many hypertensive agents and may be explained by the effects of these agents on CNS neurotransmitters. Compounds containing rauwolfia alkaloids, neuronal blocking agents such as guanethidine, and alpha-methyldopa have all been implicated in the etiology of depression.

The use of steroid medications may lead to psychiatric symptoms. Euphoria is probably the most common presentation, although confusional states and depression may be seen as well. Cimetidine, a potent H_2 receptor antagonist, produces confusional states, depression, and paranoid symptomatology.

The list of possible causes of psychiatric symptomatology is long, and we certainly do not yet appreciate all the causes of such symptoms that do not lie in primary psychiatric illness. Indeed, it is possible that many of the disorders that we now consider to be primarily functional in nature may in fact have a toxic or infectious etiology.

Abnormal presentations or clusterings of psychiatric symptoms, as well as the typical presentation of these symptoms in individuals without a prior history of emotional disorder or the appearance of these symptoms at an unusual age, should lead to consideration of possible organic etiologies. Such possibilities should especially be considered when visual illusions, distortions, or hallucinations are present.

Suggested Readings

Conroe, B. (1936). Follow-up studies of 100 patients diagnosed as neurotic. *Journal of Nervous Diseases* 83:679–684.

Erman, M., and Guggenheim, F. (1981). Psychiatric side effects of commonly used drugs. *Drug Therapy* November:117–126.

Hall, R., Gardner, E., and Popkin, M. (1981). Unrecognized physical illness prompting psychiatric admission: a prospective study. *American Journal of Psychiatry* 138:629–635.

Hall, R., Popkin, M., Devaul, R., Faillace, L., and Stickney, S. (1978). Physical illness presenting as psychiatric disease. *Archives of General Psychiatry* 35: 1315–1320.

Hoffman, R. (1982). Diagnostic errors in the evaluation of behavioral disorders. *Journal of the American Medical Association* 248:964–967.

Johnson, D. (1981). Drug-induced psychiatric disorders. *Drugs* 22:57–69.

Koranyi, E. (1980). Somatic illness in psychiatric patients. *Psychosomatics* 21:887–891.

McIntyre, J., and Romano, J. (1977). Is there a stethoscope in the house (and is it used)? *Archives of General Psychiatry* 34:1147–1151.

Muecke, L., and Krueger, D. (1981). Physical findings in a psychiatric outpatient clinic. *American Journal of Psychiatry* 138:1241–1242.

Winokur, A., Rickels, K., Greenblatt, D., Snyder, P., and Schatz, N. (1980). Withdrawal reactions from long-term, low dosage administration of diazepam. *Archives of General Psychiatry* 37:101–105.

CHAPTER 11

Legal Issues

PAUL S. APPELBAUM, M.D.

The psychiatrist in the emergency room faces legal obligations in three areas: the evaluation of patients, the treatment and disposition of patients, and patients' relationships with people outside the immediate clinical setting. Although the clinician may be tempted to deal with these obligations by denying their existence or by elevating them to primacy in the decision-making process, such temptations should be resisted on both legal and clinical grounds. The goal of the psychiatrist in the emergency setting, as elsewhere, should be to integrate legal considerations into an appropriate plan of clinical care.

Standards of Emergency Care

Several peculiarities of the emergency situation complicate the psychiatrist's task. Frequently, the evaluator and the patient have not seen each other before. Although it is likely that their mutual unfamiliarity will be taken into account by the legal system in the event of an untoward outcome, the clinician's burden is increased nonetheless. Another problem is that often the patient does not give the psychiatrist sufficient information on which to base an assessment. Reasonable attempts should be made to contact a patient's primary clinician, prior caretakers, or family members to confirm the patient's account and to clear up remaining areas of uncertainty. The evaluator is also expected to act more cautiously in reaching conclusions, especially if those conclusions result in releasing potentially dangerous patients, than will a clinician who is familiar with a particular patient.

The psychiatrist's lack of a previous relationship with emergency room patients may also raise the question of whether he or she is obligated to perform any assessment at all. In urban locales, which are usually divided into multiple catchment areas, it is not uncommon for patients to appear in crisis at other than their assigned facilities. Similarly, indigent patients without insurance coverage may present at private hospital emergency rooms.

Busy staff members or psychiatrists may be tempted to refer such patients to their usual sites of care without taking the time to evaluate them first. This course of action is always a mistake. Ethical strictures, reinforced by the law, against turning away patients in crisis should dissuade the clinician from that course. The existence of a doctor-patient relationship requires that the psychiatrist evaluate and treat patients in a reasonable fashion. And in a facility claiming to provide emergency care, this relationship is presumed to exist as soon as patients request assistance. This is not to say that all people, including people seeking shelter from the cold, are entitled to complete psychiatric examinations. It is clear, however, that every patient must be evaluated carefully enough that the appropriate disposition— whether admission, outpatient referral, referral to another facility, or even a refusal to provide care—can be made with the confidence that the patient's safety will not be endangered.

Many large emergency room services utilize nonmedical personnel to screen walk-in patients. Such a practice is acceptable as long as the evaluation is supervised by a physician. Supervision means that the psychiatrist is involved enough with the evaluation to ensure its accuracy and the appropriateness of the disposition. There may be some circumstances in which it is possible for the clinician to reach that degree of certainty without actually seeing a patient—but such circumstances are much rarer than current practice would suggest. As a rule, the supervising psychiatrist should see every patient who presents to a psychiatric emergency service. In the event of a mistake and a consequent mishap, the psychiatrist may be held responsible under the legal doctrine of *respondeat superior* for subordinates' errors. The same is true for attending psychiatrists who supervise emergency room evaluations by residents—although, as physicians, the residents can more safely be accorded a degree of discretion commensurate with their clinical experience.

Clinicians have long been told that there is no legal liability for a simple error in judgment. According to this line of thought, as long as the proper procedures have been followed, no one will hold a doctor liable for a mistaken conclusion. If that cliché was true at one time, it certainly is not today. Error in judgment, seen in retrospect by a jury that has just heard of the harm caused by that error, may be indistinguishable from the most clear-cut negligence. In the current legal climate, an evaluation must not merely be commendable—it must be correct. Still, there are steps that a clinician can take to avoid being found negligent, even in the event of a bad outcome.

Foremost among them is consultation with another experienced clinician. Consultation not only increases the likelihood of a correct outcome, but also serves as persuasive evidence that the clinician has prudently followed the standard of care. What, after all, is a professional standard but the course of action that other members of the profession would take in similar cases? The most useful maxim in this area is *when in doubt, obtain a second opinion.*

When psychiatrists fulfill their clinical responsibilities in the course of an emergency room evaluation, they are, in the process, substantially meeting their legal obligations as well. Nothing more is required than that clinicians perform an assessment that conforms to the standards of the psychiatric profession. Failure to live up to professional standards—for example, failure to inquire of all depressed patients about the possibility of suicidal ideation— opens a psychiatrist to the possibility of a suit for malpractice should harm occur.

General Principles of Legal Responsibility

Psychiatrists' legal obligations have three sources: statutes, regulations, and judicial decisions.

All states have statutes governing the operation of their hospital and mental health facilities. For historical reasons, however, the rules controlling treatment in medical hospitals are often embodied in different (and less rigid) statutes than are those regulating mental hospital operations. Thus, the location of the emergency assessment may affect its legal context.

Statutes typically address the issues of which patients can be detained or committed, how voluntary and involuntary admission procedures should be structured, and what rights patients possess in the evaluation and admission process. The diversity of statutes from state to state makes firsthand acquaintance with applicable laws in a given jurisdiction mandatory for all clinicians. There is no reason for psychiatrists not to have read the mental health statute in their states; remaining questions should be answered by a competent lawyer. This procedure is eminently preferable to the usual reliance on clinical lore or notes taken long ago at a seminar.

Regulations are typically generated under legislative authority by administrative agencies such as the Department of Mental Health. Although their ostensible purpose is to concretize statutory mandates, regulation writers often modify the original legislative intent. In any event, regulations have the status of law and may provide penalties for violations. Regulations dealing with emergency mental health care may address such subjects as confidentiality of patient communications and may elaborate on statutory requirements for commitment. As with statutory law, all clinicians should possess a copy of the regulations that govern their work.

The final body of law concerning clinicians is case law—the accumulated legal wisdom resulting from centuries of litigation. In most instances, the decision as to whether a psychiatrist is guilty of malpractice will be based on the tradition of common law rather than on a particular statute. Malpractice occurs when a clinician with a duty to care for a patient negligently departs from the profession's usual standard of care, with resulting harm to the patient. Although failure to adhere to statutory and regulatory requirements may provide supporting evidence of a deviation from the standard of care, it does not always constitute malpractice.

Case law may also be the controlling factor in allegations of improper confinement, breach of privacy, wrongful actions leading to a patient's death, and other civil wrongs (called *torts*). Case law differs from jurisdiction to jurisdiction, but its general principles tend to be the same from state to state.

Legal Responsibilities in Treatment and Disposition

The major areas of responsibility where legal questions coincide with care issues in the emergency room are informed consent, competence to make decisions, involuntary commitment, and confidentiality. At times, clinicians will find themselves faced with patient, family members, and community members making contradictory demands, each excitedly demanding his or her "rights." At other times, it is difficult to determine what rights patients or their families have. The following case illustrates some of these difficulties.

> Mrs. A., a chronic schizophrenic woman who was well known to the hospital, appeared at the emergency room with her schizophrenic husband in tow. She reported that his condition had deteriorated during the previous week to the point where he was pacing about the house day and night and responding in a loud voice to auditory hallucinations. He had not eaten for several days.
>
> The wife herself appeared distraught, giving evidence of moderate thought disorder and making frequent bizarre statements. Close questioning revealed that neither patient had taken prescribed antipsychotic medication for nearly two weeks. The examining psychiatrist believed both patients could avoid admission if they could be stabilized in the emergency room. The wife agreed to receive an injection of a long-acting antipsychotic medication, but her agitated husband refused to respond to any questions, including a query about his willingness to receive several injections of haloperidol over the next few hours. The wife offered to consent on her husband's behalf; the psychiatrist, however,

was uncertain about both the legality of such a consent and the wife's competency to make a decision.

The legality of such a consent and the wife's competency to make a decision in the above case would be different in different jurisdictions.

When the assessment is completed and a plan of action is formulated, statutory and regulatory law join case law as important sources of psychiatric responsibility. Nowhere is that responsibility better exemplified than in the question of emergency treatment, as in the preceding example. During the last quarter century, the judiciary has developed and refined the doctrine of informed consent. More recently, statutes and regulations have expanded its scope, especially in psychiatric care.

The doctrine of informed consent reflects the law's desire to protect the autonomous decision-making power of every individual. The judiciary has pursued that goal by expanding earlier common-law notions of consent to require that all patients be provided with sufficient information about the proposed treatment to make an informed and uncoerced decision. Relevant information is usually conceived to include the nature of the proposed treatment, its most noteworthy risks and benefits (by virtue of frequency or severity), and possible alternatives, including the alternative of no treatment and its associated risks and benefits. Many states' statutes and regulations have further elaborated these requirements.

It is important to stress that apart from the narrow set of exceptions to be discussed, this requirement for informed consent applies in the psychiatric emergency room just as in any other medical setting. Whether it applies when patients have been admitted involuntarily to a facility—that is, whether committed patients have a right to refuse treatment—is currently being decided in the courts. But the assumption in the emergency room should be that patients have the right to be informed about all interventions and to refuse them. Treatment, even with patients' consent, without adequate information to permit an informed decision to be made, may constitute malpractice if harm occurs. Treatment without consent or over patients' objections may constitute battery.

The exceptions to this mandate for informed consent are not as broad as is commonly assumed. Treatment may proceed without consent in an emergency, but only when the delay involved in obtaining consent would place the patient in substantial danger. A patient can also be treated without consent to protect the safety of others in the emergency room who would be endangered by the failure to act. Interventions without consent are thus permitted for imminently dangerous, out-of-control patients.

The situation for patients who are not competent to give a consent is less clear. The consent of a guardian is required for patients who have been adjudicated incompetent. In the absence of a formal adjudication, the consent of an adult family member is probably acceptable. If no adult family member is available, the situation becomes complex indeed. The standard practice in most facilities is to treat incompetent patients even without their consent, in effect permitting the doctor to make a substituted decision on the patient's behalf. Although that practice is often desirable from the clinical point of view, its legal basis is tenuous. Certainly, such treatment should be limited to what is absolutely necessary to help resolve the situation that provoked the emergency room visit. A second opinion as to the need for treatment would also be advisable. Psychiatrists can, in addition, encourage legislatures to clarify their rights and responsibilities in such situations.

As indicated, psychiatrists have a common-law obligation to live up to the standard of care in deciding on dispositions for emergency evaluations. In most cases, the crucial issues will be whether the patients are clinically appropriate for admission and, if patients refuse admission, whether involuntary commitment is indicated. With regard to the decision to admit a person or to treat the person as an outpatient, the most important forensic issue is whether harm is likely to occur to either patient or others if admission is foregone. Given the uncertain nature of much psychiatric treatment, where there is no physical harm, a decision to admit or to release is not likely to be challenged simply on the basis that it contribute to less than optimal care.

Nontreatment and Release from Care

Something should be said about the release of patients from the emergency room. Experienced clinicians know that not every episode labeled an emergency actually requires immediate intervention. In retrospect, however, it may seem odd to a jury that a patient who requested urgent care was turned away, only to suffer or inflict subsequent harm. Release decisions call for careful documentation in the patient's record of the assessment, the reasons why hospitalization was not indicated, and the alternative plan of care developed.

> Mr. B., a 35-year-old single handyman, came to the emergency room complaining of an imminent fear of losing control. He requested hospitalization to prevent him from harming someone, although he had no particular victim in mind. On examination, there was no evidence of psychosis, but the patient was obviously anxious. He admitted to having a past criminal record, to being on probation, and to having a court hearing scheduled in three days, but he refused permission for the emergency room staff to contact his probation officer. The staff were suspicious that the patient's request for hospitalization might have been designed to establish a history of mental disorder in order to avoid responsibility for the pending criminal charges. On the other hand, they were concerned about his admitted potential for violence and their

possible liability in the event that a failure to admit the patient was followed by a violent assault.

As in the first case, the law varies from jurisdiction to jurisdiction and from state to state. Consultation with the hospital attorney can establish local precedents, procedures, and safeguards.

Documentation is also important in situations such as turning away borderline patients following suicidal gestures. The nuances of dealing with borderline patients, particularly the importance of avoiding regression-promoting hospitalization, often appear counterintuitive to lay people. A clear record of the decision-making process can be invaluable in defending such an action.

Paradoxically, supervisory practices are often more lax for patients who are being released to outpatient follow-up than for individuals who are being admitted as inpatients. Nonmedical mental health professionals and residents may be given the authority to release patients but not to admit them without supervisory approval. This practice makes little sense. Patients who are being released are at much greater risk of harm than are those facing admission. To minimize the possibility of liability, supervisory procedures should be made uniform without regard to ultimate disposition.

Hospitalization

If the decision is made to hospitalize a patient and if that patient is willing to enter the hospital, relatively few problems are presented. An informed consent should be obtained from the patient, who should be given some idea of the reasons hospitalization has been recommended, the likely benefits, any obvious risks, and any possible alternatives. (Of course, there may be no reasonable alternatives; if such is the case, the patient should be told so.) State statutes and regulations often prescribe additional information that must be presented to patients and may require elaborate form-signing procedures. The utility of many of these procedures is questionable, but the hospitalization may be invalid without them. State laws vary on the question of whether patients must be competent in order to sign themselves into the hospital; psychiatrists should consult laws in their states for particulars.

Involuntary admissions, of course, are fraught with legal implications. State statutes set out conditions under which commitments can take place. Because fine judgments are often required in such decisions, many state statutes provide immunity for actions that are not grossly negligent or in willful violation of the law. Commitments in defiance of statutory provisions, however, raise the possibility of suits for false imprisonment. False imprisonment need not involve force. Patients who seek to leave a facility and who are told that they will be prevented from doing so can sue for false imprisonment even if actual restraint is never employed. If the possibility of emergency commitment is being entertained in the emergency setting, it is proper to prevent patients from departing until a final decision is made.

Legal Responsibilities Involving Third Parties

Third parties typically become involved in emergency assessments as conveyors or seekers of information. They also become involved when their safety may be threatened by a patient.

Confidentiality

Patients have common-law rights to have the confidentiality of their communications protected; in many states these rights are supplemented by statutory and regulatory provisions. Generally, a patient's consent should be sought before any information is released to third parties, including the information that an evaluation is in progress. One important exception to this rule occurs when a disclosure must be made in order to obtain information that is essential to the completion of the emergency evaluation. Third parties can be contacted in such circumstances, even without the patient's consent, but information should be revealed only to the extent needed to obtain the third parties' cooperation.

Another exception to the requirement of patient consent for disclosure occurs when the patient is being transferred to another facility, such as a state hospital, for care. Failure to send along adequate clinical records to enable the receiving facility to initiate proper treatment and institute appropriate precautions, including the protection of the patient's privacy, is bad clinical practice. Any information relevant to the patient's immediate care, such as the presence of suicidal ideation or a known tendency to assault male or female staff members, must be communicated.

A more difficult problem occurs when patients are brought to the emergency room by the police. For the sake of public safety and because the police may want to pursue other measures, they should probably be told in such circumstances what disposition is planned for each patient. On the other hand, police need not be told any of the specific information that is uncovered in the course of the assessment. If a promise has been made to a court or to the police that a patient will not be released without their being contacted, it is particularly important to follow through on the promise. Facilities and clinicians have been held liable for harm caused by patients who would have been arrested had the police known that they were being released.

Protection of Third Parties

Two lines of legal reasoning have recently converged to heighten the responsibility of clinicians to prevent their patients from harming others. Although in our legal system citizens are ordinarily under no obligation to restrain others from breaking the law, an exception has long been made for circumstances in which one party exercises physical control over another, for example, when a dangerous patient escapes from a mental hospital. More recently, some state courts have defined (while others have rejected) an obligation of outpatient therapists to take measures to protect identifiable potential victims of their patients.

In practical terms, the psychiatrist in the emergency room needs to make sure that potentially dangerous patients do not escape during the evaluation or while awaiting transfer to an inpatient facility. Every emergency facility should have a security guard on duty at all times and means to close off escape routes, such as doors that can be closed and bolted by remote control. Commitment decisions about potentially dangerous patients should, of course, be made with particular care.

When patients are admitted, voluntarily or involuntarily, the need to take other measures to protect third parties is ordinarily noted. If for some reason a patient who is deemed to be potentially dangerous (as problematic as that determination may be) is not admitted, the issue of taking further measures to protect third parties arises. Court decisions such as *Tarasoff* in California may require other measures to be taken, including warning the potential victim(s) or alerting the police. Courts in other jurisdictions have rejected such an obligation on the grounds that it violates the patient's privacy.

Preferably with the advice of counsel, facilities should develop a policy on warnings before a case arises. Even in the absence of a legal obligation, a high degree of certainty that a patient intends harm to other people places an ethical burden on the clinician to act to preserve life.

A Final Word

The basic principles of law for the emergency room clinician are easily stated. The permutations of the legal responsibilities that arise in the course of everyday practice, however, are endless and complex. Of utmost use is ready access to a lawyer familiar with clinical practice or a clinician who is up to date on legal issues, and preferably both. For problems that occur when no counsel is available and an instantaneous decision must be made, the best advice is to follow one's clinical instincts. Doing what is clinically best for the patient rarely results in legal repercussions.

Suggested Readings

Appelbaum, P.S. (1982). Confidentiality in psychiatric treatment. In *Psychiatry 1982: The American Psychiatric Annual Review*, ed. L. Grinspoon, pp. 327–334. Washington, D.C.: American Psychiatric Press.

Appelbaum, P.S., Mirkin, S.A., and Bateman, A.L. (1981). Empirical assessment of competency to consent to psychiatric hospitalization. *American Journal of Psychiatry* 138:1170–1176.

Bonnie, R.J. (1982). The psychiatric patient's right to refuse medication: a survey of legal issues. In *Refusing Treatment in Mental Health Institutions—Values in Conflict*, ed. A.E. Doudera and J.P. Swazey, pp. 19–30. Ann Arbor, Mich.: AUPHA Press.

Ennis, B., and Emery, R. (1978). *The Rights of Mental Patients*. New York: Avon Books.

Fishalow, S.E. (1975). The tort liability of the psychiatrist. *Bulletin of the American Academy of Psychiatry and the Law* 3:191–230.

George, J.E. (1980). *Law and Emergency Care*. St. Louis, Mo.: C.V. Mosby.

Gutheil, T.G., and Appelbaum, P.S. (1982). *Clinical Handbook of Psychiatry and the Law*. New York: McGraw-Hill.

Meisel, A., Roth, L.H., and Lidz, C.W. (1977). Toward a model of the legal doctrine of informed consent. *American Journal of Psychiatry* 134:285–289.

Roth, L.H., and Meisel, A. (1977). Dangerousness, confidentiality, and the duty to warn. *American Journal of Psychiatry*, 134:508–511.

Slovenko, R. (1979). On the need for record-keeping in the practice of psychiatry. *Journal of Psychiatry and Law* 7:399–440.

PART II

MEDICAL/SURGICAL WARDS

Supporting Difficult Patients and Patients with Difficult Dilemmas

All patients have many psychodynamic elements in common, and illness and hospitalization have psychological consequences for all people. In this section we will discuss patient attitudes, behaviors, and situations that pose particularly complex problems of detection and resolution.

The section begins with an overview of issues that consultants should be familiar with and behaviors that occur between consultees and consultants. Anticipation of consultee needs and awareness of the consultee's countertransference enable the consultant process to function at its best. Next follows an overview of behaviors that are regularly seen in many ill, hospitalized persons. Interaction between personality variables, illness, and hospital staff may be smooth; but it may also escalate into a crisis for patient and staff alike. Special attention must be given to the somatically concerned patient; anxieties about physical concerns must be heeded, but must also be dealt with in ways that stimulate healthy coping. Difficulties in dealing with illness and hospitalization occasionally culminate in that most difficult of situations—the patient who threatens to leave against medical advice. The potential A.M.A. patient must sometimes be allowed to leave the hospital when no other alternatives are acceptable. Hopefully, kindly support and acknowledging frank differences of opinions can allow such a patient access to the hospital upon further, cooler reflection and reframing of the important issues.

The patient with anorexia nervosa is presented as an example of the combined medical-psychiatric approach to a disorder in which psychological and physical issues must receive equal attention and in which the relationship to the primary therapist may be the key to the outcome of treatment. The problems of dealing with the patient who has lost hope and the patient whose death is imminent are dealt with in the final chapters of this section. Managing these patients effectively becomes more important as we deal with increasing numbers of chronically ill people who are subjected to life-sustaining procedures that drain reservoirs of hope and lead to a breakdown of the relationship between patient and medical staff, with life-threatening demoralization. Recognizing the imminence of death is a multifaceted process involving the patient, the family, and medical caregivers. Being at the boundary between severe illness and the approach of death profoundly affects the medical staff, whose need to establish and maintain their potency as healers may outweigh the reasonable benefits of sustaining life.

M.W.

CHAPTER 12

Communicating with the Referring Physician

MICHAEL K. POPKIN, M.D.
THOMAS B. MACKENZIE, M.D.

Knowledge of typical behaviors in a consultant-consultee dyad, as well as sources of dyadic tension and potential obstacles to effective engagement and outcome, is crucial to good work. In order for consultants to implement interpersonal and pharmacological treatment, not only must there be effective contact with patients, but also some type of collaborative effort must be instituted between consultants, medical staff, and nursing staff. This chapter presents an optimal sequence of steps to guide psychiatric consultants in communications and exchanges with referring physicians. Content issues important to consultants are also discussed.

The Initial Dialogue

Most consultation sequences begin with a written request for intervention. Despite the best intentions, this request seldom conveys accurately the referring physician's agenda or dilemma. Instead, it is a limited message that must be followed by pointed, if brief, dialogue with the referring physician prior to engaging the patient. An optimal consultation sequence begins with direct dialogue with the referring physician—unless the situation is an emergency and the referring physician is not accessible. Although this discourse may be effected by phone, a face-to-face discussion is preferable—even if it is restricted to a few minutes in the nursing station. This permits the consultant to acquire valuable data and to establish the dyad in precise ways. When feasible, the consultant should review the patient's chart before speaking with the referring physician.

At the outset, the consultant needs to find out why the consultee has requested a consultation. Many consultees do not explicitly acknowledge their reasons. The simple inquiry by the consultant, "How can I be of help" often sets the stage for a more candid reply. For example, consultees are frequently embarrassed by their wish to have patients transferred to a psychiatric unit. Anticipating such a concern can be helpful, though a consultant needn't promise the impossible or implausible. The consultant can say, "I expect you may be concerned about transferring the patient. If that's the case, I'll conduct my evaluation with that in mind." Since this exchange often sets the tone for all that follows in the dyad, a positive, open, nondefensive approach is usually advisable, though it is not always easy to effect.

Determining specific consultation questions is equally important. The usefulness of a consultation is directly linked to this step. The more specific the consultation question or questions, the more likely the consultant is to be of service. A request asking only for evaluation can be honored, but the resultant data, formulations, and recommendations are unlikely to focus on the consultee's primary concerns. Accordingly, it is the consultant's responsibility in the initial dialogue to clarify or draw out what the referring physician has in mind. Does the referring physician want diagnostic assistance? practical management of troublesome behaviors? guidelines for psychotropics? a transfer or provisions for follow-up care after discharge?

Referring physicians are usually more interested in practical management of patients than in evaluation and formal diagnosis. Despite psychiatry's current fascination with nosology, consultees are indifferent to the various categories and implications of psychiatric diagnosis. They prove far more responsive to recommendations for disposition and psychotropic medication than for further diagnostic measures.

Unraveling the mysteries of consultation and consultees' actions is an ongoing process. For example, most general-hospital psychiatric consultation services see approximately 3 percent of all admissions to the medical/surgical services. The incidence of psychiatric disturbance in medical/surgical inpatient populations probably ranges from 20 percent to as much as 50 percent. The disparity between the observed rates of referral and the purported incidence of psychopathology is striking and raises a number of important questions. Why, for example, are certain patients and not others (despite diagnostic similarity) referred for psychiatric consultation? Difficulties in the physician-patient dyad are usually the key factor in deciding to consult the psychiatrist. A physician frequently finds it difficult to make a full and objective examination of patients with obvious emotional symptoms and often prematurely terminates the workup of such medical/surgical patients. A psychiatric consultant is most often called when the primary physician finds the patient too emotionally close or distant. The psychiatric consultant restores or effects a more comfortable interpersonal distance.

This construct offers a working hypothesis about referral patterns and directs the consultant's attention to what is transpiring or has already transpired between the referring physician and his or her patient. Dialogue about these issues can be extremely useful; it may permit the primary physician needed ventilation or allow him or her to get the situation back into perspective. Inquiring about the physician's experience with and sense of the patient as an individual is therefore often instructive.

Another requisite in the initial dialogue is ensuring that the consultation request has been discussed with the patient. When the patient is unprepared to see a consultant, the probability of an untoward outcome is great. Patients are prone to conclude that their physicians regard them as "crazy" or in need of rebuke or punishment, and they may be quite correct. Often, it is the physician's discomfort with broaching the discussion of the patient's emotional difficulties with the patient that prompts the request. Nevertheless, the consultant must establish that the primary physician has shared with the patient the point of concern and the interest in obtaining a psychiatric consultation. Quick assurances that patients have been apprised are not always completely reliable. Not long ago, a patient acknowledged to the consultant that he had been informed of the impending visit: "Sure, you're here to review my MMPI with me, aren't you?" he said.

Brevity is important in the initial dialogue. It is, however, helpful to explain the approach to be used and, finally, to arrange to provide the consultee with a report of findings and recommendations. The explanation of the approach need not be extensive or detailed—for example, "I'll check with nursing, conduct an initial evaluation session, and try to contact the patient's family. I'll recontact you no later than tomorrow morning with my initial impressions and recommendations." This gives the referring physician a time frame for the consultation and the elements of the assessment. Should the plan be ineffective or fail to address a specific concern, the consultee can so indicate before the sequence proceeds further.

In short, the initial dialogue establishes the contract in the physician-consultant dyad. It sets the tone and the likelihood of an effective interchange. Consultants' opportunities to maximize their skills in the interest of patients are greatest in the earlier phases of both the hospitalization and the physician-consultant dyad. A decisive, organized approach conveys working knowledge and a willingness to implement it.

The Consultation Report

The consultation report is a legal document requiring thoughtful preparation. When writing it, the consultant should bear in mind that it may be read by the patient. The written report should be accompanied and complemented by discussion with the consultee. Unfortunately, circumstances sometimes preclude such dialogue, and the report alone must suffice.

Over the past few years, our approach to the written report has been repeatedly revised and restructured in response to observations and data emerging from our Consultation–Liaison Outcome Evaluation System (CLOES). Currently, our service uses a consultation report form in which the diagnostic impressions are given first (in DSM-III format). Explicit recommendations follow in order of their priority, as judged by the consultant. Then, approximately 1½ pages are provided on the form for a synopsis of the pertinent psychiatric problem, history, and mental status examination. The body of the consultation is completed on a separate form that is not placed in the medical record but is kept instead in the consultation service office. At the top of the form is a statement indicating that the full consultation report is available on request. The paucity of such requests has convinced us that our consultees are concerned with the "punch lines" of consultations rather than the details. Accordingly, we have little more to say about the written report than suggestions concerning the consultant's recommendations and diagnoses.

Data from CLOES demonstrate that consultees are more receptive to recommendations regarding direct management of the patient and are less responsive to recommendations involving evaluative actions and to issues of psychiatric nosology. Comparison studies show that psychiatrists' recommendations for psychotropic medication fare no differently than cardiologists' recommendations for cardiac drugs. However, the diagnostic action recommendations put forth by psychiatrists achieve strikingly less concordance than do those put forth by the cardiologists. This underscores the interest of primary physicians in guidance regarding the behavioral management of the patient referred for psychiatric consultation. Consultees either have been indifferent to, or have failed to distinguish among (1) specific psychiatric diagnoses, (2) specific psychotropic drugs, and (3) specific diagnostic proposals. Studies of drug recommendations have shown that brevity, specificity, and decisiveness influence the likelihood of consultee concordance. In the last regard, consultees perceive the presentation of options as the consultants' uncertainty or ambivalence.

Collectively, such observations have led us to advise certain steps in offering and writing recommendations to consultees. Psychiatric consultants should gauge the likelihood of consultee concordance before making recommendations. They should consider known concordance rates, the influence of critical variables, and the possibility of using a novel strategy if the recommendation is likely to go unheeded. Knowing consultees in these regards is quite important to achieving desired outcomes. Established working relationships can be highly beneficial in this respect.

The form and substance of written recommendations are related to outcome. It is imperative that recommendations and diagnoses be clearly demarcated from the body of the consultation note. The most important recommendation should be placed first. Wording should be brief, and directives specific with regard to agent, dosage, timing, form of test, and so on. Conditional recommendations are to be avoided; they suggest uncertainty and are likely to get lost in the shuffle. The premium is on recommendations that can be acted on immediately. Similarly, decisiveness carries the day; consultees perceive indecisiveness as consultants' inadequate knowledge. Despite consultees' limited interest in formal psychiatric diagnoses, poor consultation outcomes signal a need for greater consistency, uniformity, and future education in diagnosis by consultants. DSM-III diagnoses are preferable to nicely couched phrases designed to obscure or not offend consultee or patient. The following vignette and the consultation report shown in Figure 2 illustrate the principles described here.

Psychiatric consultation was requested by the gynecological oncology service for Miss Y., a 32-year-old white school teacher, on the second day of her third admission. Three months earlier, she had received a diagnosis of cervical adenocarcinoma with metastases to the right kidney and colon, and underwent a nephrectomy and total colectomy. Chemotherapy was also begun. During the early part of her third hospitalization, her primary physician sought psychiatric intervention. In his written request, he noted a diagnosis of cervical carcinoma with poor prognosis and asked for suggestions regarding "appropriate antianxiety therapy and supportive counseling."

In response to the formal request, the consultant contacted the referring physician and on the oncology ward briefly discussed the consultee's specific questions, his observations of the patient, and his presentation of the prognosis to the patient. This dialogue led to a partial reformulation of the reasons for consultation (see Figure 2); the consultant understood that the patient had become increasingly anxious and despondent in the preceding weeks. With these data, the consultant specifically addressed the possibilities of anxiety and mood disorders in his clinical examination of the patient. He ascertained that the patient had been apprised of the request for psychiatric evaluation. In the first exchange with the consultee, he also promised to recontact him promptly after seeing the patient. Prior to seeing the patient, the consultant reviewed the current and old medical records and discussed the patient with a nurse who had worked with her for several days.

The patient was receptive to the consultant and related that six years earlier she had been treated successfully with doxepin (Sinequan) for a major depressive episode. She noted that four family members had histories of affective disorders. She reported a month of sleep disturbance, increasing anxiety, lack of enjoyment of previously pleasurable

UNIVERSITY OF MINNESOTA HOSPITALS AND CLINICS
DEPARTMENT OF PSYCHIATRY
CONSULTATION REPORT

A more detailed report of this Consultation may be obtained by calling 3—8644.

DATE OF EXAM 12/4/82	PATIENT IDENTIFICATION PLATE

REASON FOR CONSULTATION
Patient with complaints of anxiety and depression,
evaluate and recommend therapy.

HOSPITAL NO.

PATIENT NAME
O.Y.

DIAGNOSTIC IMPRESSION
1. Major depressive episode

RECOMMENDATIONS
1. Sinequan 50 mg po qhs x3d, then increase to 100 mg po qhs x4d
2. Follow-up with me in Psychiatry Outpatient Dept. on 12/28/82 at 11:00 a.m.

PERTINENT HISTORY/BEHAVIOR   _32 year old single white female with Stage 3 adenocar-_
cinoma of the cervix with metastases to the right kidney and colon (s/p nephrectomy
and colectomy) admitted 12/3/82 for second course of chemotherapy.

The patient gives a 1 month history of depressed mood with increased sleep
(except intermittent insomnia), decreased appetite, 5 pound weight loss, decreased
energy, decreased ability to concentrate, anhedonia, and feelings of helplessness
with decreased self-esteem. The patient denies hopelessness or suicidal ideation.
She does note episodes of crying over the past month but no diurnal variation in
mood. Patient has additional complaints of increasing anxiety over the past 2-3
weeks with increased startle response but no panic attacks.

Past history is positive for a depressive episode 6 years ago treated with
Sinequan 150 mg po qhs with improvement in mood. No prior suicidal ideation. Family
history is positive for depression in mother (2 hospitalizations), aunt, 2
uncles - all on mother's side of family.

Mental Status Exam:
Alert, cooperative white female with wig, enters good relationship

Speech: Delivered in a coherent monotone;

Psychomotor: Slowed; without abnormal movements;
Affect: Tearful, appropriate, slight constriction of range;

Mood: Depressed, anxious;

Thinking: No evidence of associative loosening; no hallucinations, delusions
paranoid ideation; no homicidal or suicidal ideation. Expresses
concern for her children ages 3 and 7 who are staying with her
mother.

Insight: Fair (little knowledge re malignancy);

Judgment: Not impaired;

Intellectual: Oriented x3; recalls 3/3 items at 5 minutes; recalls 6 digits
forward and 4 reverse; fair fund of general information; abstracts
well.

M. Popkin, M.D.

P S Y C H I A T R Y   C O N S U L T A T I O N

FIGURE 2.
Sample of the author's format for consultation reports. Note that the diagnostic
impressions and recommendations are given first.

activities, crying spells, decreased energy, and feelings of being overwhelmed by her illness and her situation. In his mental status examination, the consultant observed features consistent with an affective disturbance. Corroborative history was obtained from the patient's mother. Despite confounding factors, including the malignancy, surgery, and chemotherapy, the consultant diagnosed a major depressive disorder. In his subsequent discussion with the consultee, he explained that the anxiety, which had been the physician's original concern, was a feature of the mood disturbance. He proposed a trial of doxepin, the antidepressant to which the patient had responded six years earlier; an explicit protocol for the drug was provided. In addition, the consultant indicated his plan to meet regularly with the patient through the remainder of her hospitalization and beyond to explore her responses to and her coping with her illness. Finally, the consultant reviewed the consultee's approach to the patient in terms of the prognosis and encouraged the physician to create additional opportunities for the patient to ask questions about further therapies, complications, and prognosis. These recommendations were endorsed by the physician; the antidepressant medication was instituted the next day. The consultant met with the patient five times during her hospitalization to monitor the antidepressant and to explore the patient's responses to her illness. He advised the consultee of the patient's ability to tolerate the medication and of her difficulty in discussing her illness.

Following discharge, the patient evidenced steady improvement in mood. At her first clinic visit three weeks after the original consultation, the patient's sleep pattern had normalized, her anxiety had diminished, and her crying spells had ceased.

Subsequent Dialogue and Monitoring

Ongoing dialogue with the consultee should complement each step of the consultation process. Once the initial evaluation is effected, the findings and recommendations are best discussed in advance of the written note. Such discussion is more important if the observations or directives depart from what is routine or perhaps anticipated. Given the limitations of consultees' grasp of psychiatric diagnoses and distinctions among psychotropic drugs, these exchanges can ensure that a consultant's rationale for a course of action is appreciated. When a particular diagnosis has been ruled out or a consultant advises against an antidepressant, clarifying criteria for diagnosis of a major depressive disorder, which would warrant prescription of an antidepressant, can be very helpful and can forestall the consultee's anger at not getting the hoped-for recommendation from the consultant. When a specific course of treatment has been proposed, discussion can reduce problems in sequential administration, as with increasing the dosage of a psychotropic medication.

Consultants need to monitor the outcomes of their recommendations. If a suggestion has been implemented, the consultant needs to ascertain the clinical results. When a consultee does not follow the consultant's advice there may in discourse be an opportunity for the consultant to learn from the consultee's failure to follow the advice rather than be offended by it.

At the end of an optimal consultation sequence, the consultant should have a final conversation with the referring physician, checking on the outcomes and on the physician's perceptions of the intercession. This and other important closure steps are the ones most frequently omitted by consultants.

Obstacles

A number of factors interfere with consultants' interaction with primary physicians. Principal among these are fundamental tensions operative in the dyad.

Despite the common bond of medical training, referring physicians and psychiatric consultants are not always likely to enjoy similar constructs regarding medicine and, in particular, the issue of emotional disorders in the medically ill. This small degree of shared conceptual framework is among the greatest problems faced by consultation psychiatry. Though consultants quickly glean something of these conceptual differences, most consultants cannot or will not readily bring up the belief systems of consultees for discussion.

There is often tension over what consultees want or expect and what consultants wish to provide. For example, consultees seek active management of what they presume are mood disorders in patients undergoing chemotherapy. Consultants, keen on organic mental disorders and on ruling out psychiatric symptoms secondary to physical illness, dismiss or downplay the issue of mood disturbance and seek further evaluation of a possible organic mental disorder. Though the consultants are being thorough and are diagnostically accurate, consultees are likely to be upset. Not only has their diagnostic assumption been found wanting, but an entirely unanticipated course of action has been suggested. Such conflicts, invariably unspoken, color much of consultation. In some cases, consultants may use too narrow an approach, repeatedly proposing those steps with which they are most intrigued, skilled, and comfortable.

Another fundamental source of tension in the consultant-consultee dyad is referring physicians' view of psychiatry. Psychiatric consultants are often viewed as intruders with vague and alien concepts. Many physicians perceive psychiatry as a nonmedical entity. It appears that a sizable number of consultees are psychologically minded and receptive, but many regard psychiatry as anathema. The majority are in the middle, capable of being influenced by their ongoing experience. By the same token, psychiatrists' biases and preconceptions about consultees may be equally detrimental to the functioning of the dyad.

Finally, for those engaged in consultation work, there is often an unspoken conflict between what best serves referring physicians and what helps patients. The clinical task of consulting psychiatrists is to facilitate the best possible care and outcome for the patient. Consultants can best accomplish this by giving thoughtful and careful attention to engaging referring physicians and communicating with them in the context of the individual case.

Suggested Readings

Coles, R.B., and Bridges, H. (1969). The consultant and his roles. *British Journal of Medical Psychology* 42:231–241.

Hackett, T.P., and Weisman, A.D. (1960). Psychiatric management of operative syndromes. I. The therapeutic consultation and the effect of noninterpretive intervention. *Psychosomatic Medicine* 22:267–282.

Karasu, T.B., Plutchik, R., and Conte, H. (1977). What do physicians want from a psychiatric consultation service? *Comprehensive Psychiatry* 18:73–81.

Lipowski, Z.J. (1967). Review of consultation psychiatry and psychosomatic medicine. I. General principles. *Psychosomatic Medicine* 29:153–171.

Lipowski, Z.J. (1971). Consultation-liaison psychiatry in the general hospital. *Comprehensive Psychiatry* 12:461–465.

Mackenzie, T.B., Popkin, M.K., Callies, A.L., and Kroll, J. (1983). Consultation outcomes: the psychiatrist as consultee. *Archives of General Psychiatry* 40: 1211–1214.

Meyer, E., and Mendelson, M. (1961). Psychiatric consultations with patients on medical and surgical wards: patterns and processes. *Psychiatry* 24:197–220.

Popkin, M.K., Mackenzie, T.B., and Callies, A.L. (1981). Improving the effectiveness of psychiatric consultation. *Psychosomatics* 22:559–563.

Popkin, M.K., Mackenzie, T.B., and Callies, A.L. (1983). Consultation-liaison outcome evaluation system (CLOES). I. Consultant-consultee interaction. *Archives of General Psychiatry* 40:215–219.

Popkin, M.K., Mackenzie, T.B., Callies, A.L., and Cohn, J.N. (1981). Interdisciplinary comparison of consultation outcomes. *Archives of General Psychiatry* 38:821–825.

CHAPTER 13

Coping Styles and Behaviors of Medical/Surgical Patients

MYRON F. WEINER, M.D.

Certain behaviors or coping mechanisms are commonly seen in general-hospital medical and surgical patients:

- Regression
- Clinging and demanding behavior
- Overindependence
- Overdramatization
- Long-suffering attitude
- Suspicious quarrelsomeness
- Haughty entitlement
- Emotional and physical withdrawal
- Passive aggressiveness

The interaction of these patient behaviors as well as other coping styles with the value systems and personalities of hospital personnel often lead to staff-patient interactions that culminate in hostile behavior by the staff toward patients or in the staff's neglecting patients' emotional and physical needs.

Before considering these behaviors, it must be stated that the aspects of a person's personality exaggerated by illness and hospitalization may not be that person's predominant behavior or coping style under other circumstances. Illness and the hospital environment often trigger maladaptive behavior in people who otherwise cope successfully. Therefore, a diagnosis of a personality *disorder* should be made only when the patient's in-hospital behavior fits with a long history of similar behavior in daily life and is consistent with DSM-III criteria. In fact, the consulting psychiatrist would do well to avoid making a diagnosis of a personality disorder without strong corroborating evidence from outside informants, because illness and the hospital environment may place a significant strain on a particular person and may call forth unique behaviors. Finally, the clinician must be aware that a patient's behavior in the hospital results from a complex interaction between the patient, the personalities of the caregivers, an alien hospital culture, and the physical environment of the hospital. For example, a person who values physical activity highly may be uncomfortable in an intensive care unit, in which physical inactivity is demanded. On the other hand, a person who has long been physically inactive because of illness or injury may find the activity level of a rehabilitation unit frightening and overwhelming.

Regression

Psychological regression, the reappearance of primitive, poorly organized patterns of thinking and behavior, is a usual accompaniment of severe illness. Severely ill people do not perceive their environment clearly and do not organize their responses well. The effect of the normal regressive process depends on the patient's personality structure and the nature of the illness. Clinging and demanding behavior may be a direct acting out of normal regression; overindependent behavior is a frequent reaction against regression. Regression in the form of diminished physical activity or self-care may be readily accepted by a person with a painful injury but may be poorly tolerated when strict bedrest is required in a relatively pain free illness such as hepatitis. In addition, the patient's ability to regress in terms of self-care and the patient's style of regression have a profound impact on medical caregivers, as will be seen in the discussion of some of the regression-stimulated behaviors that ill people develop.

Clinging and Demanding Behavior

The clinging and demanding pattern of behavior frequently begins with the patient eagerly trying to please the staff as a way of obtaining emotional nurturance. After experiencing this for some time, physicians and nurses begin to feel emotionally drained and angry because their emotional nurturance of the patient seems insufficient. Staff members try to protect themselves by turning off their emotional spigots, thereby intensifying the patient's clinging. This type of coping style is best dealt with by kind, firm limit setting in which the patient is told what can be had, what can be expected, and when. For example, the nurse can tell a patient whose medical condition is stable that she will check every two hours but will not respond to the emergency buzzer. The doctor can tell the patient what time to expect daily rounds. Knowing that attention will be regular, the patient will be less inclined to fear an arbitrary cutoff of emotional supplies. The psychiatrist's interpretive comment that the patient needs to be seen as a needy person is less valuable than finding ways to help patient and staff meet those needs. For example, the medical staff's praising the patient for appropriate self-care can provide emotional nurturance through rewarding self-sufficiency instead of through the staff's performing chores, such as bringing p.r.n. medications or straightening sheets.

Overindependence

Overindependent behavior is common in people who pride themselves on their ability to manage their own lives without help from others, and who fear dependence on others. Many of these people belong to Friedman and Rosenman's Type A personality classification. They cause great consternation on a medical intensive care unit when, following a severe myocardial infarction or cardiac arrhythmia, they insist that nothing is wrong and that they must leave the hospital to tend to business. In these cases, there is often an element of illness denial, but it usually cannot be addressed directly. Instead, the best way to deal with this type of behavior is through negotiation: giving these patients some control of their own activities in exchange for their allowing themselves to be monitored and kept to a reasonable amount of bedrest or restricted activity. A certain number of telephone calls per day, for example can be exchanged for a certain number of hours of bedrest. Patients with this type of behavior respond poorly to the staff's expressions of concern about their physical well-being. It is better if the staff members tell a patient that *they* become anxious in dealing with heart attacks and arrhythmias and that the patient can help relieve their anxiety by staying in bed. The following vignette illustrates the principles of dealing with overindependent behavior.

> Miss D., a 33-year-old truck driver, was hospitalized for a recurrence of pulmonary embolism secondary to deep venous thrombosis. She had previously been treated with subcutaneous heparin but had discontinued that medication two weeks earlier when her prescription for syringes ran out.
> Psychiatric consultation was requested because she refused to stay in bed, insisted on walking to the end of the hall to smoke, and was pressing strongly to leave the hospital.
> The patient had been abandoned by her parents when she was 11 months old. She was raised by her grandmother until she was 12 years

old, when her grandmother died. She lived briefly in several foster homes and then left, as she put it, "to make it on my own." She became a truck driver at age 18 and thoroughly enjoyed her work. She resented the house staff attempting, as she saw it, to boss her around.

The psychiatric consultant indicated to the medical staff that this woman's primary means of maintaining her self-esteem was doing for herself and that threats to her autonomy resulted in prompt and intense negative responses. The consultant suggested a course of negotiation, making concessions in return for partial cooperation. She also suggested that the staff frame their suggestions in terms of the patient's taking care of herself, and encouraged the staff to put aside their needs to be in charge of the patient.

Overdramatization

Overdramatizing is often a thinly disguised bid for attention. Doctors and nurses who feel guilty about meeting their own dependency needs directly (instead of vicariously, through caring for others) react to their envy of the patient's easy conscience by getting angry and chastising the patient for histrionics or by attempting to ignore the patient, which only makes matters worse. Small doses of admiration for the histrionic patient's good grooming and efforts at self-care are frequently helpful in settling everyone down. Angry confrontation plays into dramatization. The consultant should advise staff members that finding something they genuinely admire and respect about the patient is far more helpful than criticizing the patient's behavior. Pairing a positive comment about the patient with a request for something from the patient usually gets better results.

Long Suffering Attitude

Medical staffs are made uncomfortable by the hostility underlying the behavior of patients who seem long-suffering and self-sacrificing. Often they induce angry behavior in the staff by refusing offered help and by responding negatively to encouragement. Staff members feel they are being needled, but they don't know exactly what is going on or why. The psychiatric consultant points out an ironic piece of patient behavior: While apologizing profusely for complaining, long-suffering patients are still complaining. The patients are saying, without accepting responsibility for doing so, that they are being badly treated but are tolerating it as long as possible. Another perplexing thing about these patients is that they worsen if complimented—feeling that if they're doing well, they shouldn't be in the hospital. Short, businesslike replies to these patients' complaints are more effective than avoidance or trying to get everything just right to stop the complaining. It is appropriate to agree with patients that many aspects of their care are unsatisfactory and to attempt amelioration; however, the psychiatrist also points out that certain aspects of hospital life cannot be changed because of necessary hospital policies or staff shortages.

Suspicious Quarrelsomeness

Suspicious quarrelsomeness rightly raises the staff's concern about potential legal action and makes the staff reluctant to be firm. Nevertheless, quarrelsome patients can be told firmly that they have a choice of staying in this hospital, going to another hospital, or going home, but if they choose to stay in this hospital certain ground rules need to be followed by them and other rules will be followed by the hospital staff. The hospital staff will explain each procedure that needs to be done but will not engage in argument. In exchange for staff members' explaining what they are doing, these patients are asked to cooperate with the diagnostic or treatment measures that are deemed necessary and important by the medical staff.

Haughtiness and Entitlement

Haughtiness and entitlement, typical of narcissistic individuals, are difficult for hospital personnel to tolerate. Some staff members are intimidated, but most resent being treated like servants. Some of the staff's anger can be eased by pointing out that haughtiness and entitlement are often means to bolster shaky self-esteem. Viewing patients' behavior as a defense against insecurity often allows the staff to feel less demeaned and more potent. Limit setting is also appropriate, indicating to the patient that staff members must divide their time among all patients, who are accorded staff time and effort in relation to their physical needs.

Emotional and Physical Withdrawal

Emotional and physical withdrawal arouses concern instead of anger on the part of the medical staff, who may call the psychiatrist and raise the question of an emotional disorder. The withdrawn, unresponsive patient needs to be scrutinized closely by the psychiatric consultant from both a psychiatric and a medical standpoint. The patient may be experiencing a significant depression. But the patient may also be more seriously ill than hospital staff suspect, or the patient may have a metabolic imbalance, mental retardation, a conservation-withdrawal response, or an organic brain disorder caused by intracranial or systemic factors. At times, calling in the psychiatrist to evaluate a withdrawn patient is part of the staff's denying (1) the severity of illness, (2) the patient's failure to respond to treatment, or (3) the adverse effects of medical treatment.

Passive-Aggressive Behavior

Passive-aggressive behavior is probably the most common type of covert uncooperativeness seen in hospitalized medical/surgical patients. Ill people who are angry with the physicians in whose hands they have placed their lives, or with the nursing staff responsible for their day-to-day care, will often have difficulty expressing their anger directly to the hospital staff. They also have trouble acknowledging their anger when it is noticed by the staff.

Causing difficulty by not giving urine specimens on time or by being off the ward when the doctor makes rounds may be indicative of a personality disorder, but it may also be a patient's effort at self-assertion while feeling impotent in the face of illness or authority figures and fearful of standing up to the staff. The first task of the psychiatrist is to see whether there is a significant conflict between the patient and the staff. Often, the passive-aggressive person has failed to live up to staff expectations. Staff punish the patient by being less responsive to his or her needs. The patient then responds with less attention to staff needs. In this situation, the psychiatric consultant serves as a go-between, indicating to the warring parties that there is more to lose by fighting than by cooperating, and encouraging both sides to heed the other's demands. Occasionally, a passive-aggressive person will need to be offered the option of leaving the hospital.

Passive aggression may be suspected in many situations in which patients fail to cooperate adequately. But patients may often be uncooperative because they do not understand where they are or what is required of them. People with mental illnesses, mental retardation, or personality disorders can be uncooperative. The psychiatric consultant frequently finds that the uncooperative patient is delirious or demented, or that the staff explained a procedure inadequately and the patient became terrified. In the following case, a delirium, not a passive-aggressive personality, contributed to the patient's lack of cooperation.

> Mr. E., a 36-year-old married black man who had received a kidney transplant six months previously, had rejected his transplanted kidney, and plans had been made to remove the nonfunctioning organ. On the day of surgery, his doctors told him surgery had to be delayed because another emergency had arisen. They rescheduled the procedure for

several days later, but the patient refused to sign the consent form, stating that he had already undergone the surgery. The doctors were unable to convince him otherwise. When they appealed to his wife, she also refused, saying that she would wait until his parents came in. With the support of his wife and his parents, he realized that the surgery had not been done and consented to the operation the following day while his entire family was at the hospital. This man's belief that his surgery had already been performed was partly due to severe clouding of consciousness from uremia, but the specific trigger was psychological—his wish to have had the surgery over with.

Mental illness and mental retardation are usually detected on mental status examination. People with antisocial and borderline personalities often disrupt hospital routines and fail to cooperate with trivial demands made by the hospital staff. The mentally ill can be appropriately medicated; the borderline retarded can be educated to cooperate (or subjected to less complex demands), but people with severe personality disorders may not be treatable in a hospital and may have to be discharged to their own care instead of further demoralizing the hospital staff. Attempting to coerce or physically restrain people with personality disorders is to everyone's disadvantage in the long run. It reinforces these patients' view of themselves as victims and intensifies their struggle against their persecutors or tormentors.

A Systems Approach

Throughout all of this material runs the thread mentioned earlier: that the patient's behavior in the hospital does not arise solely from internal factors. The consulting psychiatrist must therefore pay attention to the hospital environment and to the people who are concerned about or disturbed by the patient. Each area of the hospital makes its own unique demands on patients. In the coronary care unit, during renal dialysis, and during convalescence from a fracture, quiet bedrest is required. On a chronic pain unit or a diabetes control unit, self-care and ambulation are the rule. Patients need to be educated to the demands of the hospital environment and to changes in the staff's expectations when they are transferred from one part of the hospital to another. When staff fail to do this, they often find themselves at odds with patients who are transferred from an intensive care unit in which they rightly played a highly regressed, dependent role to a room in which they are expected to meet some of their own needs. "Good" patients in one setting often become "bad" patients in another setting— through no fault of their own.

Inevitably, there are personality or attitudinal differences between patients and staff that cause difficulties. For this reason, it is important to interview both the staff members who have difficulty with a particular patient and the ones who do not. Interns with great therapeutic expectations are disappointed because their patients respond slowly or not at all; surgeons find it difficult to understand that maintaining autonomy by saying no to a potentially life-prolonging procedure can be more important to some people than prolonging life.

The psychiatric consultant should be cautious in communicating an evaluation of the patient's coping style to the medical staff. Assigning a personality diagnosis may accelerate or set in motion a process of scapegoating and lead to the medical staff's discounting the patient's problems, as illustrated here.

> A psychiatric consultant was called in to advise on the management of Ms. F., a very emotional 25-year-old nurse with multiple sclerosis. When the psychiatric resident diagnosed her as a histrionic personality, the medical staff became suspicious that her inability to empty her bladder or rectum was functional. As the consultation/liaison attending later observed, the problem in this case was not that the woman's personality was interfering with her treatment, but that staff members were extremely frustrated by her worsening condition. They wished to see her worsening as caused by her emotional state instead of having to face the fact that medical treatment was not slowing the progress of the disease.

It is useful for a psychiatrist to make a personality diagnosis to help in the formulation of a plan of psychological management for a patient. But the psychiatrist may need to leave that diagnosis unrevealed and instead point out the significant stressors for a patient, indicate the patient's characteristic means of reacting to certain stresses, and make concrete suggestions for patient management.

Closing Thoughts

The psychiatric consultant called on to evaluate a patient must consider the multiple factors that impinge on the patient and help create the behavior with which the hospital staff must deal. Included in this evaluation are the patient's illness, the hospital milieu, and the staff. The three cases presented in this chapter point up the need for the consultant to pay careful attention to the patient's medical status. Histories obtained from people who know the patient well in everyday life are extremely important, as is thorough medical and psychiatric history taking by the psychiatrist, paying attention to cultural and religious factors as well as intrapsychic and socioeconomic factors. Generally speaking, it is unwise for the psychiatric consultant to assign a personality disorder diagnosis to a patient unless so labeling the patient helps staff maintain their equilibrium. Otherwise, it is best for the psychiatrist to simply describe the patient's behavior in the hospital and to make concrete suggestions for its amelioration. The psychiatrist often serves as go-between, interpreting for staff and patient alike until effective communication begins or is restored. If the situation between medical staff and patient reaches an irreversible impasse, the psychiatrist may have to help both sides disengage and allow the patient to move to another setting so that negotiations do not engender a trapped feeling on the part of patient or staff.

Suggested Readings

Friedman, M., and Rosenman, R.H. (1974). *Type A Behavior and Your Heart*. New York: Knopf.

Goodwin, J., Goodwin, J., and Kellner, R. (1979). Psychiatric symptoms in disliked medical patients. *Journal of the American Medical Association* 241:1117–1120.

Grouse, L.D. (1982). Dirtball. *Journal of the American Medical Association* 247: 3059–3060.

Groves, J.E. (1978). Taking care of the hateful patient. *New England Journal of Medicine* 298:883–887.

Hackett, T.P. (1978). Disruptive states. In *Massachusetts General Hospital Handbook of General Hospital Psychiatry*, ed. T.P. Hackett and N.H. Cassem, pp. 234–235. St. Louis, Mo.: C.V. Mosby.

Kahana, R.J., and Bibring, G.L. (1965). Personality types in medical management. In *Psychiatry and Medical Practice in a General Hospital*, ed. N. Zinberg, pp. 108–123. New York: International Universities Press.

Myint, S., and Weiner, M.F. (1981). Management of a borderline patient in a surgical setting. *Psychosomatics* 22:71–72.

Peabody, F.W. (1927). The care of the patient. *Journal of the American Medical Association* 88:887–892.

Weiner, M.F. (1983). Conservation withdrawal and mental retardation in medical/surgical patients. *Psychosomatics* 24:41–43.

CHAPTER 14

The Somatically Concerned Patient

DOUGLAS A. DROSSMAN, M.D.

Medical and surgical patients have obvious concerns about their bodies. Their physicians respond psychologically to those concerns through explanation, reassurance, and personal availability. However, some patients become preoccupied with bodily concerns, cannot be reassured, and display illness behaviors disproportionate to their medical problems.

The psychiatrist who evaluates such patients attempts to understand the reasons for their need to be symptomatic, identify specific behavioral patterns, and consider the needs and expectations of the referring physician before establishing a treatment plan.

The Patient

Somatically concerned patients are a heterogeneous group. Identified by their behavior within the health care system, they are called problem patients, hateful patients, crocks, turkeys, or other pejorative names because they elicit strong negative reactions from their physicians. They may have no diagnosable medical disease, or their somatic preoccupation may exaggerate and distort their experience of illness and their reporting of symptoms. The prevalence of these patients in medical settings is not known, but patients with major psychosocial difficulties comprise over half of those presenting to outpatient medical clinics and at least a third of medical inpatients.

The reasons why some individuals deal with psychosocial difficulties by excessive concern about their bodies are multiple and complex. Society, family, and personality shape attitudes, expectations, and behaviors related to illness throughout life. This learning influences how the person experiences, reports symptoms, copes, uses medical facilities, and complies with treatment.

Cultural factors greatly influence the experiencing, attribution, and reporting of symptoms (see Chapter 28). For example, mental illness is highly stigmatized in China, and patients with even minor psychological problems present to physicians with physical complaints. Ethnic differences can influence a patient's behavior in reaction to physical symptoms. Among medical inpatients in a New York City hospital, it was observed that first and second generations of immigrant Jews and Italians had more dramatic responses to pain, while the Irish tended to deny their symptoms, and "old Americans" were even more stoic. Cultural mores can play a role in sex differences in seeking health care. In Western society, women predominate among patients with irritable bowel syndromes, perhaps reflecting the tendency for men to be more stoic about relatively minor health complaints. However, in India, where men more often seek medical attention, the sex ratio among patients with this condition is reversed.

Once a person assumes the status of patient, certain benefits accrue from the sick role. These benefits may include exemption from work or family obligations, avoidance of stressful situations, and gratification of other needs through socially acceptable dependence on friends and family. Therefore, chronic disease itself, regardless of cause, can reinforce illness behaviors.

Diagnosis

Several identifiable patterns of cognition and behavior are associated with somatic preoccupation and increased seeking of health care (see also Chapter 28). By identifying these patterns, the consulting psychiatrist makes the patient more understandable to the primary physician and helps in the development of specific treatment strategies. At times, it is difficult to make a specific psychiatric diagnosis because a patient with these behaviors may have one or more medical or psychiatric disorders, or none at all. The patient's bodily complaints and concerns may result from genetically determined traits, learned maladaptive forms of social communication, expiation of guilt through suffering, or gratification of basic needs through a dependent relationship with a physician. The DSM-III psychiatric disorders that are most commonly accompanied by physical complaints are psychological factors affecting physical condition, somatization disorder, conversion disorder, psychogenic pain disorder, hypochondriasis, depression, and schizophrenia.

Psychological Factors Affecting Physical Condition

Psychological factors including anxiety, depression, and interpersonal conflict commonly contribute to the initiation or exacerbation of medical disorders. The frequency of such an association often depends on the clinician's interest and skill in identifying such influences. In some cases, it is not only the patient's physical condition that intensifies, but also the patient's preoccupation with the disorder and the sick-role behavior. Patients with chronic, recurring, or debilitating medical disorders (e.g., rheumatoid arthritis, inflammatory bowel disease, neurological disorders) are particularly vulnerable. These patients may be referred to the psychiatric consultant when they seem noncompliant with treatment strategies, when their poor handling of stress exacerbates their underlying disease, or when their complaints appear out of proportion to the assessed extent or activity of the medical condition, as in the following vignette.

> Ms. G., a 29-year-old single woman, had a 15-year history of Crohn's disease complicated by frequent hospitalization for enterocutaneous and rectovaginal fistulas and perianal abscesses. Her latest admission was for new symptoms of epigastric pain, nausea, and vomiting. She feared that her condition would worsen and that she might require surgery, or die.
>
> Radiological evaluation showed involvement of the jejunum, ileum, and colon, but no evidence of disease progression or complications such as intestinal obstruction or infection. Her condition improved slightly with increased doses of prednisone and sulfasalazine. When told that she could leave the hospital, her symptoms worsened and psychiatric consultation was obtained.
>
> The patient reported to the psychiatrist that her father had died of cirrhosis one year earlier (with symptoms of pain, nausea, and vomiting). She harbored ambivalent feelings about his death. An earlier good relationship with her father had deteriorated when his progressive alcohol consumption led to frequent episodes of verbal and physical abuse. Two weeks prior to admission (on the one-year anniversary of his death), she began having recurrent dreams of him, and her symptoms began soon thereafter.
>
> She was seen as a psychiatric outpatient six times over a two-month period. The issues of her unresolved grief were explored, and her symptoms abated.

Somatization Disorder

Patients with this disorder, also called Briquet's syndrome, present with a long-standing history of numerous chronic or recurrent vague physical complaints. This behavior begins in adolescence, is much more prevalent in women, has a strong familial predisposition, and may lead to multiple surgical procedures.

Identification of this disorder can help to minimize unneeded laboratory studies and procedures. In the face of diagnostic uncertainty, it is easy for the physician to pursue evasive medical disorders (e.g., systemic lupus erythematosus, multiple sclerosis, occult carcinoma) by the "shotgun" ordering of procedures. It is important to evaluate new somatic symptoms, of course, but treatment and invasive diagnostic decisions should be based on signs of disease, not symptoms.

Conversion Disorders

Conversion disorders result from unconscious adaptive processes in which unconscious conflict is dealt with through symbolic physical complaints or symptoms. Conversion disorders involve the sensory organs, producing symptoms such as blindness, or the voluntary motor system, resulting in various types of paralysis that do not conform to the actual innervation of the affected limb or limbs. A diagnosis of conversion disorder should not be made in the presence of physical findings that might otherwise explain the patient's symptoms.

Some patients with conversion disorders may respond to brief insight therapy, but most respond best to nonconfrontive supportive medical care and an explanation that the symptoms will ameliorate with conservative medical treatment. A man with a functional leg paralysis, for example, can be encouraged to gradually bear weight on the limb, with the assurance that its strength will return. Meanwhile, attempts are made to strengthen environmental supports and reduce secondary gain.

Psychogenic Pain Disorder

The pain-prone patient has an affinity for pain and pain-producing situations. Pain-proneness can be conceptualized as a type of conversion disorder. This pain-prone patient is seen more often in medical than psychiatric settings and presents with a history of multiple physical traumas, operations, and pain episodes. Patients with symptoms of more than two year's duration are not likely to ameliorate. Some patients improve their functional capacity over time, but many do not, as indicated in the next case.

Mr. H., a 28-year-old married native American with three children, developed abdominal pain at age 16. He recalled his gym teacher's stepping on his abdomen at the time. One month later he was expelled from school for pulling a knife on his classmate. Over the years, he had

had five hospitalizations to evaluate his pain. An appendectomy and a cholecystectomy were performed; his appendix and gallbladder were found to be normal.

He had had multiple injuries that included a truck rolling over his legs, a tree falling on him, three bales of tobacco dropping on him, and two major car accidents in which he sustained multiple fractures. He was illiterate and had had difficulty keeping a job. He enjoyed hunting and fishing by himself. His father had back trouble and peptic ulcer disease, his mother had back pain, and two uncles had stomach pain. In the last year, he had also experienced leg, hip, and neck pain and severe headaches. Continuing care by internists, orthopedists, psychiatrists, neurologists, surgeons, and social workers had been unable to alleviate his symptoms or return him to work.

Pain-proneness may derive from feelings of guilt established early in childhood in reaction to an overbearing, abusive environment. A family history of alcoholism and broken marriages is common. Throughout life, pain or demeaning situations serve as means of atonement for established feelings of self-devaluation and guilt. These patients have a need to fail and to suffer. By making the physician aware of this character style, the consultant can help the physician recognize that heroic attempts to cure are unlikely to succeed. The physician can thereby minimize personal frustration by resetting the treatment goals to helping the patient live with the pain instead of aiming to cure it. (This is further discussed in Chapter 24.)

Hypochondriasis

Hypochondriasis is a behavior pattern characterized by preoccupation with bodily function and a search for a physical illness that justifies that preoccupation. Hypochondriacs interpret ordinary physical sensations as abnormal, maintain a persistent fear of harboring serious disease, and are preoccupied with a variety of vague and shifting complaints. Many of these patients have limited social relationships outside the health care system, and their complaints maintain their self-esteem and provide a means of social communication.

Recommendations to the referring physician begin with accepting the patient's need to complain. New diagnostic evaluations should be based on objective changes in the patient's clinical status such as fever or abnormal blood chemistries, not simply on the patient's complaints. Invasive procedures should be avoided if possible. Patient visits should be brief but scheduled regularly to avoid the increasing physical complaints that occur when potential abandonment is suggested by the physician's refusal to meet the patient's psychological need to be a patient.

Depression

Somatic preoccupation also occurs as a symptom in other functional psychiatric disorders. Patients with a major depressive disorder, for example, may focus primarily on their somatic symptoms. An internist focusing on physical complaints might overlook a clinically significant depression (see Chapters 6, 10, and 22 for further discussion). The patient who attributes sadness, sleep disturbance, loss of appetite, and weight loss to a chronic physical disorder may also misdirect the physician. This is particularly true if the physician fails to explore the clinical signs of depression. The consultant can recommend an antidepressant, can help the referring physician reevaluate the need for continued medical diagnostic exploration, and can refocus the clinical approach toward counseling, home health care, or other methods of psychosocial support.

Schizophrenia

Although a relatively uncommon occurrence in the general-hospital medical setting, patients with schizophrenia may present with physical complaints ("My intestines are rotting"; "There's something moving inside me") that are somatic delusions. The peculiar quality of the complaints is a clue to their delusional nature. Treatment of the developing psychotic disorder (see Chapters 5 and 20) often resolves the somatic symptoms along with the psychosis.

The Physician

Somatically overconcerned patients have varied impacts on their physicians. The physician's uncertainty about diagnosis can lead to a feeling of being ineffective, particularly if the patient insists urgently that something be done. The adaptive value of the illness in patients with somatoform disorders is not always recognized by the physician, who may set an unrealistic goal of freeing the patient from symptoms and complaints. The physician's resultant frustration can then cause anger, which results in poor medical care. Physicians often believe that the care of these patients is out of their area of responsibility and expertise and may refer them for psychiatric care. However, these patients see themselves as medical patients and are reluctant to obtain psychiatric evaluation and treatment, although some may eventually require psychiatric hospitalization.

The insistent behaviors exhibited by patients with somatoform disorders can impair the physician's clinical decision making. Ordering unneeded and potentially harmful studies and treatment plans (*furor medicus*) often occurs when physicians care for demanding, somatically overconcerned patients. Test ordering tends to reinforce patients' sense that they are ill and frequently debilitates them even more.

The Psychiatric Consultant

The following general approach is useful for the consulting psychiatrist in dealing with a somatically concerned patient.

ENCOURAGE A BIOPSYCHOSOCIAL APPROACH TO ILLNESS. The psychiatrist is skilled in obtaining psychosocial data. However, the major role with the somatically concerned patient is to obtain and communicate information that enhances the referring physician's understanding of the illness and identifies psychological determinants that can be applied in specific treatment strategies. For example, the psychiatrist attempts to establish the feasibility of changing the patient's behavior. The primary physician is also helped by knowing whether the patient's current somatic preoccupation is part of a long-standing characterological pattern or results from more recent stresses such as the recent death of a loved one. The consultant determines whether the patient has a psychiatric disorder amenable to specific treatment such as antidepressant medication. The essential aim is to help the primary physician establish certain behavioral strategies, such as accepting the complaints and paying more attention to other issues, or encouraging greater patient participation in treatment. The consultant also determines whether the patient is a good candidate for psychiatric treatment or the physician's request belies other concerns (e.g., "Am I capable of managing this problem?").

HELP RESET TREATMENT GOALS. For a variety of reasons, the somatically concerned patient with long-standing symptoms benefits from feeling ill. The patient must be informed that it is unrealistic to expect rapid and complete relief when the condition has existed for so long, but that with sufficient commitment, real benefits can be expected. Similarly, the physician should be informed that removal of the symptom is not the goal of treatment. Instead, a reasonable goal may be the patient's achieving a higher level of functioning (e.g., return to work, participation in church activities) despite symptoms. Some patients, such as those who are pain-prone, may continue to be symptomatic. When this occurs, the physician's efforts are better directed toward minimizing unneeded and potentially harmful diagnostic studies and addicting medication. The consultant may need to emphasize that the physician should not construe failure to cure the patient as a sign of clinical incompetence.

Long-Term Treatment Strategies

In many cases, the patient can benefit from brief, regular visits to the primary care physician or other health care provider, such as a nurse practitioner. During these visits, the physician can listen without feeling compelled to respond to each complaint. When the patient recounts misfortunes and continued discomfort, the physician can communicate understanding of the difficulty in coping with such distress. When doing well, the patient should be praised for good effort but cautioned not to overextend himself or herself.

The physician should recognize and avoid behaviors that reinforce the patient's sick role. Examples include paying exclusive attention to the patient's symptoms and ignoring other issues, responding to each complaint by ordering diagnostic studies or prescribing medication, and assuming total responsibility for the patient's well-being. Instead, efforts should be made to minimize the benefits of the patient's somatic preoccupation and encourage the patient to take more personal responsibility. The patient can be given the option to choose among several medications (or to choose no medication) after being apprised of their benefits and potential side effects. The physician thus relinquishes some control in an effort to foster the patient's independence. In addition, the physician can focus strongly on positive aspects of the patient's life and limit attention to the patient's symptom recital to what is needed to satisfy medical considerations. This technique of differential attention is a form of operant conditioning that reinforces acceptable forms of social communication.

When new or different complaints arise, they should be assessed from biological, psychological, and social standpoints. Both medical and psychological causes should be considered. The physician must avoid becoming complacent, labeling each complaint as functional, but at the same time should not feel compelled to respond to each complaint with another round of diagnostic studies.

Once a trusting relationship is established, the patient may begin to focus on more significant concerns involving thoughts and feelings that might not have been expressed previously. If the physician continues to provide a nonjudgmental environment conducive to the expression of those concerns, the patient's symptoms may begin to lose their adaptive value. As these issues become more apparent, the physician can assess the extent of the psychological disturbance. If psychiatric referral seems indicated, the patient, being more trusting and more cognizant of his or her emotional concerns, may now accept the recommendation.

At times, symptoms may worsen and urgent requests may be made for the doctor to "do something." Late-night calls or emergency visits by patients may be needed during times of stress. If the physician can provide calm reassurance, the patient's anxieties will be reduced and excessive diagnostic and treatment procedures avoided. Once a positive relationship has been established, the physician should continue periodic contact with the patient instead of terminating the relationship when the patient's symptoms disappear or seem under control. It is better for the physician to gradually decrease the frequency of visits to once or twice a year than to stop them completely. The patient is thereby assured of the physician's ongoing recognition of the illness and the continued open door to care.

A Final Word

The medical or surgical patient who is referred because of seeming somatic overconcern requires careful consideration. The consultant must seek to understand the patient within the context of the sociocultural setting and to identify specific psychological determinants or psychiatric disorders for which there are specific treatment strategies. The consultant must also appreciate the referring physician's feelings and reactions to these patients who challenge his or her professional potency.

Suggested Readings

DeVaul, R.A., Faillace, L.A. (1978). Persistent pain and illness insistence. *American Journal of Surgery* 135:828–833.

Drossman, D.A. (1978). The problem patient: evaluation and care of medical patients with psychosocial disturbances. *Annals of Internal Medicine* 88:366–372.

Drossman, D.A. (1982). Patients with psychogenic abdominal pain: six years' observation in the medical setting. *American Journal of Psychiatry* 139:1549–1557.

Drossman, D.A. (1983). The physician and the patient: review of the psychosocial gastrointestinal literature with an integrated approach to the patient. In *Gastrointestinal Disease: Pathophysiology, Diagnosis, Management*, ed. M.H. Sleisenger and J.S. Fordtran, 3rd ed., pp. 3–20. Philadelphia: W.B. Saunders.

Engel, G.L. (1959). Psychogenic pain and the pain-prone patient. *American Journal of Medicine* 26:899–918.

Groves, J.E. (1978). Taking care of the hateful patient. *New England Journal of Medicine* 298:883–887.

Lazare, A. (1978). Hysteria. In *Massachusetts General Hospital Handbook of General Psychiatry*, ed. T.P. Hackett and N.H. Cassem, pp. 117–140. St. Louis, Mo.: C.V. Mosby.

Lipsitt, D.R. (1970). Medical and psychological characteristics of "crocks." *Psychiatry in Medicine* 1:15–25.

Tseng, W.S. (1975). The nature of somatic complaints among psychiatric patients: the Chinese case. *Comprehensive Psychiatry* 16:237–245.

Zborowski, M. (1952). Cultural responses to pain. *Journal of Social Issues* 8:16–30.

CHAPTER 15

The Patient Who Leaves the Hospital Against Medical Advice

WALTER F. BAILE, JR., M.D.

A patient's threat to leave the hospital against medical advice often reveals a serious psychological disturbance and causes considerable dismay in the attending physician and ward staff. On entering the ward, the consultant who has been asked to evaluate such a situation may find an angry or insistent patient "packed and ready to go," an atmosphere of tension, and feelings of helplessness on the part of the staff. This situation is especially uncomfortable when the patient is actually quite ill and departure from the hospital might be seriously health-endangering. The referring physician is concerned about keeping the patient in the hospital and about the patient's ability to make a rational decision regarding the need for treatment; in addition to these concerns, the psychiatrist wants to know how such a crisis developed.

The Patient Who Leaves

In most instances, the psychiatrist is not consulted when a patient leaves the hospital against medical advice. In dealing with patients threatening to leave A.M.A., it is therefore important to distinguish between those for whom consultation is requested and those for whom premature hospital discharge is mutually agreed upon by the physician and the patient. Retrospective reviews of patients' charts show that about 1 percent of all general-hospital discharges are against medical advice.

Patients who leave against medical advice are frequently young, of black or Hispanic background, and from a lower socioeconomic class. There is often a history of multiple A.M.A. discharges. Most sign-outs occur within the first five days of hospitalization. Patients who sign out A.M.A. tend to be anxious or agitated. Psychosis, organic brain syndrome, and addiction to alcohol and drugs are frequent in these patients.

When 29 patients (1.2 percent of admissions) who left a city hospital coronary care unit A.M.A. were compared to a matched control group, A.M.A. sign-outs were younger and, unlike the control group, did not have acute cardiac disease. Twenty-five percent of the A.M.A. patients and none of the controls had histories of previous A.M.A. behavior, and about half of the A.M.A. patients had a history of psychiatric problems (mostly anxiety, depression, or alcohol abuse). Although the average length of stay was brief (under 3 days), chart review revealed clear-cut evidence of emotional and behavioral disturbance prior to discharge in over 75 percent of A.M.A. patients.

Patients addicted to narcotics and alcohol frequently enter the hospital system for treatment of illness (such as cellulitis or gastrointestinal bleeding) resulting from their habits. These patients often present difficulties for, and are disliked by, the ward staff. They may be uncooperative and ungrateful for treatment. They evoke strong feelings in staff members who focus on the indulgent and self-destructive aspects of their behavior, and the patients often become scapegoats for staff frustrations and tensions. Because of the conflict between these patients and staff, it is not surprising that A.M.A. discharges are disproportionally large. Thus the "irregular discharge" often occurs in disruptive patients who are not seriously ill. The discharge is an acceptable alternative both to the patients, who do not consider themselves sick and are unhappy with ward regulations and routine, and to the physician, who is glad to be rid of problem patients.

Having the patient sign an A.M.A. form is one way to relieve the physician of both medicolegal responsibility and guilt feelings about rejecting the patient. It is important to note in these cases, however, that the physician may view drug and alcohol abuse as a moral instead of a medical issue and may fail to allow or encourage drug or alcoholism service consultation for the patient.

To prevent premature discharge of these patients, consultation-liaison programs dealing specifically with the drug addict and the alcoholic in the general hospital have been implemented. (See Chapter 21 for a discussion of the alcoholic patient.) Crucial in the management of the patients has been intensive education and support of ward staff and the use of drug abuse and alcoholism counselors. Patients with substance abuse problems perceive these counselors as allies, as do the ward staff.

The Patient Who Threatens to Leave

The patient who threatens to leave the hospital prematurely is often seriously ill, and the physician may feel a strong responsibility to continue care.

Many of the same principles used to understand other acute psychological disturbances on the medical and surgical wards—agitation, refusal of procedures, noncompliant behavior—can be applied to the symptoms of the A.M.A. patient. Many times, these problems will precede the sign-out threat by several days. It is the dramatic expression of the disturbance and the features of the intervention in such circumstances that make a psychiatric consultation unique. The patient is threatening to fire the doctor, and strong feelings have been evoked in both the patient and the staff. The consulting physician is often aware of the tension and the pressure to act. However, the consultant needs to avoid immediate overreaction, because these disturbances are not usually sudden, capricious, totally unexpected acts of the patient. They result from crises of trust and communication that have been brewing for some time.

Conceptual Framework

The hospital is a system in dynamic interaction with the tasks of treating disease and alleviating suffering. The protagonists—doctor, patient, and nursing staff—have complementary roles that facilitate treatment. Traditionally, doctors diagnose disease and prescribe treatment. Patients submit to examination, procedures, and therapy in the interest of their own health. The nurses attend to specialized patient needs. Other factors, however, enter into the interaction. These include the patient's personality and background and the extent to which they color the illness experience; the stresses of illness and the needs created in the patient; the style and sensitivity of the physician, including the physician's values and attitudes about sickness and the ill; and the entire ward milieu, which may heighten or mollify the discomfort, uncertainty, and frustration of the patient's hospital experience. The interaction of these factors, and the way in which they may affect staff-patient relationships, sometimes result in a patient's leaving or threatening to leave the hospital.

Patients, physicians, and staff are part of a social system in which membership is constrained. That is, the members of the group interact for their own advantage and personal liking does not play a primary role. It is advantageous for patients to get well, for the house staff to learn and fulfill professional training requirements, and for the attending physicians and staff to earn a living and see patients get well. Because of these and other factors, the group interaction is task-oriented, with high emphasis on efficiency. This orientation is particularly evident in teaching hospitals, where most of the care is provided by overworked house staff who feel a continual pressure to reduce their patient load by turning over patients quickly. As a result, strong norms for behavior emerge, and roles are often rigidly defined. Physicians are the authority, patients are expected to be dependent and submissive, and communication is often minimal. Moreover, communication tends to be instrumental and focused far more on problem solving than on feelings, with the physician asking, "Where does it hurt?" rather than saying, "You look upset."

A part of this system is the patient—worried, fearful, in pain and distress, uncertain of the future, and presenting unique personality characteristics. Each patient usually has a half-formed set of notions about the nature of the illness, which may or may not coincide with the notions of the staff. The patient's distress often arouses a state of heightened suggestibility, in which somewhat distorted cognitive processing increases the likelihood of the patient's reacting to the environment with increased emotionality.

Specific Problems in the A.M.A. Situation

Certain problems that emerge from the interaction of the various personalities in the context of the hospital system may cause a breakdown in the doctor-patient relationship. These problems include:

1. Distorted perception of the actions of others, as in the case of the patient with an ulcer who, assuming a conversation about a cancer patient held in the hallway outside his door refers to him, becomes panicky and distrustful of his physicians.
2. Issues of dependency and helplessness that result in disturbances such as severe denial of illness, as in the patient with recent myocardial infarction who, in response to restriction of her mobility, claims she has "never felt better in my life" and demands to go home.
3. Issues of control, which arise when a patient's demand for more activity is taken as a challenge to the physician's authority.
4. Diffusion of care, when the patient is managed by a multispecialty team and receives several conflicting messages about diagnosis, treatment, or prognosis.
5. Displacement of staff conflicts onto the patient, which often involve disagreements over treatment but which can also include personality differences that are acted out in communicating with the patient. An

example of this is the physician who, because of irritation with the staff, comments to a patient on a specific nurse's inexperience.

6. Delirium and psychosis that go undetected or ignored until patient-staff tension becomes intolerable.

In many cases, personality factors act as catalysts in escalating anxiety resulting from any of the problems just described, and finally a noticeable disturbance develops. A patient who is made anxious by misperceptions, by diffusion of care, and so forth, may show behavioral manifestations that reflect characteristic personality structure: for example, the dependent patient will make more demands, the paranoid patient will become angry and distrustful. (For further discussion of personality traits in a medical setting, see Chapter 13.) Staff's tendency to attribute the patient's behavior to illness and to avoid the patient's feelings results in their ignoring the patient's behavior at first. As disruptive behavior continues and worsens, it ultimately affects ward routine and causes frustration, anger, and uncertainty in staff members, who may begin to avoid the patient or to treat him or her differently. Soon, a crisis of mistrust and mutual hostility develops that escalates into an A.M.A. threat.

Evaluation of the Problem

By conceptualizing the sign-out threat as a problem that arises from a crisis of trust and communication in the operational group—including patient, family, physician, and ward staff—the consultant can begin to take steps to defuse the situation. First, the referring physician should be contacted and the case discussed, in order to shed more light on the nature of the patient's illness, the way the hospitalization has been handled, the patient's psychosocial background, and the referring physician's emotional reaction to the patient. The discussion can be followed by gathering more data from the nursing staff and, if possible, from the patient's family. As the consultant collects information, the therapeutic effects of ventilating and clarifying feelings will often begin to lower staff tensions. Careful chart review will allow the consultant to obtain an understanding of the patient's illness and a longitudinal perspective on the problem. Often the progress notes will enable the consultant to characterize the onset and nature of the problem and to correlate it with medical procedures, changes in the patient's medical condition, and so on. By the time these tasks are completed, the consultant should be able to answer the following questions.

1. What is the patient's medical condition?
2. Has there been a series of behavioral disturbances leading up to the

current crisis, and if so, how have staff members dealt with these disturbances?

3. Have there been recent changes in the patient's environment—distressing information, scheduling of unexpected procedures, worsening of medical condition, new house staff, family crisis?

4. Has medical care been uniform?

5. What is the patient's premorbid personality? Is there a history of psychiatric disorders?

Evaluation of the Patient

The consulting psychiatrist often meets angry, defensive patients who feel that he or she is there to label them crazy. The consultant can best deal with such situations as a concerned physician eager to understand what would make a person leave the hospital when ill—not as an emissary of other caregivers, trying to control the patient's behavior. By allowing ventilation of the patient's own version of the problem, the psychiatrist can begin to assess:

1. The patient's understanding of the illness and perception or misperception of hospital routine.

2. Problems in communication.

3. The patient's view of events leading up to the crisis.

4. The presence of overt psychiatric disorders such as severe depression, schizophrenia, or delirium.

5. The patient's personality and the use of defense mechanisms such as denial or acting out.

Intervention

On completion of the assessment, the consulting psychiatrist often develops a dynamic formulation of the case. Along the way, the consultant may take the opportunity to correct some of the patient's misperceptions. Empathizing with each party about the difficulties each has experienced is helpful as long as the consultant resists taking sides. Impartial empathy often reduces anger and soothes hurt feelings. Focal issues, such as patient misperceptions and diffusion of care, and their impact on the patient can be presented to the staff so as to make the patient's behavior understandable. This initial understanding often increases effective communication between patient and staff and allows reconciliation.

Despite the best efforts of the consultant, a patient sometimes does decide to leave the hospital. If this does occur, the strategy outlined here may still allow a reduction in mutual hostility. House staff, in accepting a dynamic interpretation of a patient's behavior, may feel less guilty, be less rejecting of the patient, and be encouraged to provide a follow-up appointment for the patient.

When the factor of competency arises, detaining patients against their will becomes a significant issue. Because hospital administrative policy and state laws differ considerably in this area, each consultant should be familiar with the legal and technical aspects of this problem. (Competency is discussed more fully in Chapter 11.)

The psychiatric consultant has done well in dealing with patients threatening to leave against medical advice if staff and patient accept that each has a different point of view that is valid in its own way. Even if reconciliation is not possible, each party can still maintain self-respect and avoid angry recriminations toward the other.

Suggested Readings

Albert, H.D., and Kornfeld, D.S. (1973). The threat to sign out against medical advice. *Annals of Internal Medicine* 79:889–891.

Baile, W.F., Brinker, J.A., Wachspress, J.D. and Engel, B.T. (1979). Sign-outs against medical advice from a coronary care unit. *Journal of Behavioral Medicine* 2:85–92.

Galanter, M., Karasu, T.B., and Wilder, J.F. (1976). Alcohol and drug abuse consultation in the general hospital: a systems approach. *American Journal of Psychiatry* 233(8):930–934.

Goldberg, R.J. (1980). The social system as a factor in medical treatment. In *Strategies in Psychiatry for the Primary Physician*, ed. R.J. Goldberg, pp. 23–30. Darien, Conn.: Patient Care Publications.

Iverson, L. (1972). Discharge from hospital against medical advice: a documentary investigation from a medical department. *Ugeskrift for Laeger* (Copenhagen) 134:1057–1061.

Janowski, C.B., and Drum, D.E. (1977). Diagnostic correlates of discharge against medical advice. *Archives of General Psychiatry* 34:153–155.

Meyer, E. (1956). Acute psychologic disturbance in the course of hospitalization of patients with chronic illness. *Journal of Chronic Disease* 3:111–121.

Meyer, E., and Mendelson, M. (1961). Psychiatric consultation with patients on medical and surgical wards: patterns and processes. *Psychiatry* 24:197–220.

Schulauch, R. W., Reich, P., and Kelly, M.J. (1979). Leaving the hospital against medical advice. *New England Journal of Medicine* 300:22–24.

Wise, T.P. (1974). Psychiatric management of patients who threaten to sign out against medical advice. *International Journal of Psychiatry in Medicine* 5:153–160.

CHAPTER 16

The Patient with Anorexia Nervosa

DAVID A. WALLER, M.D.

Patients with anorexia nervosa confront the consulting psychiatrist with a number of difficult tasks. Confirming the diagnosis according to specific criteria is one primary concern; it is also crucial to rule out other medical and psychiatric disorders. Patients' psychological and physical status must be carefully assessed, and a treatment plan defined that addresses biological and psychosocial issues. An attempt must be made to ally with patients and their families, and consultation should be provided to other medical and nursing staff who are caring for the patients. Medical complications must be recognized quickly. Although no two cases of anorexia nervosa are exactly the same, these patients do have much in common with one another. As a result, specific guidelines can be outlined for the tasks described here.

Diagnosis

Anorexia nervosa stems from a relentless, irrational fear of overweight and a pursuit of thinness in the face of severe emaciation. The term *anorexia*—loss of appetite—is misleading. Appetite is denied rather than absent. Like other people who are starving, patients with anorexia nervosa think about food much of the time, but because of their fears of obesity, food-related thinking is apparently redirected. Many women with the disorder are waitresses or attend cooking school. One young anorectic girl, for example, had her father construct her own personal kitchen.

Recent controlled studies cast doubt on the common assertion that patients with the disorder exaggerate their fatness more than people without the disorder. Feeling fat despite emaciation may not be a disturbance of body image. On the other hand the *fear* of overweight helps in understanding much of the patient's behavior. Dieting, exercising, self-induced vomiting, purging with laxatives and diuretics, and deceiving those who encourage eating all serve the purpose of pursuing thinness as the result of a "fat phobia."

Ninety-five percent of anorectics are female. Typical patients are middle- to upper-class white adolescent girls. The vulnerability of this particular population to the disorder is not understood. In recent years the incidence of the condition has apparently increased, with serious cases reported in 0.5 to 1.0 percent of girls in private schools. As the overall number of cases has increased, there has been a growing number of reports of the disorder occurring among nonwhites and lower socioeconomic classes.

The predominant physical finding of weight loss is easily overlooked, given society's current tendency to view extreme thinness as attractive. By the time help is sought, usually by patients' families, patients have generally lost 20 to 30 percent of their weight. The extent of emaciation may be concealed by extra layers of clothing, worn partly in response to patients' increased sensitivity to cold.

Amenorrhea invariably occurs in women who are anorectic, sometimes before much weight has been lost. Reproductive system hormone patterns shift to an immature, prepubescent configuration, but the secondary sexual characteristics are not lost. Men experience an analogous decrease in sexual interest. Body temperature, pulse, and blood pressure are reduced, apparently to conserve energy in the presence of starvation, and even the increase in soft body hair (lanugo) may relate to conserving heat.

To make the diagnosis, the characteristic abnormal attitudes toward food and physical findings should be present. Patients may be asked whether they feel fat or thin and whether they are more frightened of gaining weight (the anorectic stance) or of losing more weight (the more realistic concern shared by those caring for the patients). Garner and Garfinkel's Eating Attitudes Test may be useful to quantify the abnormality of attitude.

Differential Diagnosis

If the criteria just described are used, it should not be difficult to distinguish anorexia nervosa from other types of weight loss in which psychological factors play an important role. An example is an individual with schizophrenia whose delusions about food make it difficult for the person to eat. Pituitary disease can cause weight loss and amenorrhea, but here secondary sex characteristics are lost, and one does not find the characteristic weight phobia and relentless pursuit of thinness. In pituitary failure, patients are inactive and lethargic. Anorectics have a drive to activity that may originate in food-searching behavior prompted by starvation.

A more complex diagnostic issue is the possible presence of concomitant medical illness. The exclusion of other medical illness in the DSM-III diagnosis of anorexia nervosa violates the spirit of the multiaxial classification system and is an unfortunate reversion to either-or thinking. The anorexia nervosa syndrome has been reported with hypothalamic tumors, regional enteritis, seizure disorders, and gonadal dysgenesis. In such cases it would seem appropriate to list Anorexia Nervosa as the Axis I diagnosis, and the associated medical disorder on Axis III. Although the precise relationships between these medical disorders and anorexia nervosa have yet to be defined, their association appears to be more than chance, and there are obvious critical implications for treatment.

Treatment

Although numerous biological and psychosocial hypotheses concerning anorexia are under investigation, the etiology of the disorder remains unknown. The disease may be a final common pathway of many physical and mental factors. In the future, a biological breakthrough may explain how the disorder "takes hold" of patients and keeps them in its grip. Such an explanation may lead to a more specific treatment than is currently available. In the meantime, much useful clinical experience has accumulated regarding the management of the characteristic physical and psychological findings.

It is clear that patients must be helped to gain weight, but it is equally clear that weight gain per se does not alleviate the fundamental weight phobia. In fact, a weight-restoration program undertaken without due consideration of psychological factors may intensify patients' distress, and suicides have been reported. The dilemma is in figuring out how to address both the physical and the psychological distortions in the disease. In practice, the best results may be achieved when a psychiatrist and an internist or a pediatrician work together closely, one taking responsibility for the mental aspect, the other for the physical aspect. For purposes of discussion, these two areas will be discussed separately, beginning with management of patients' physical condition.

Physical Assessment and Management

In confronting this disorder, it is important to recognize the occasional patient whose physical status has deteriorated to a life-threatening level. Useful criteria are a drop of more than 35 to 40 percent in patients' usual body weight, or a drop of 25 to 30 percent occurring in less than three months; the presence of cardiac arrhythmias in the absence of electrolyte imbalance; progression to the stage of listlessness; significant metabolic stress such as infection; and failure of adequate trials of other methods. Any of these situations is a medical emergency and may warrant a period of parenteral alimentation. Death may occur quite suddenly, and the exact cause of death may be difficult to determine.

Much more typical are patients whose weight losses have been more gradual and have not reached quite such extreme proportions. Such patients can sometimes be literally nursed back to health by experienced nurses who provide firm, gentle support and supervision at eating time. Patients can be assured that they will not be allowed either to become too fat or to starve to death. Moreover, the goal is to allow them to take full charge of their eating as soon as it is safe for them to do so, as demonstrated by the establishment of a pattern of slow but definite weight gain.

Patients often appear so habituated to their habits of food aversion, dieting, and exercising that a behavior modification program must be implemented in a hospital setting. In general, these programs make activity and other privileges contingent on fulfilling a contract for a specific amount of daily weight gain, such as a half-pound per day. It is essential that patients' weighings be supervised and that care be taken regarding patients' state of dress and water intake prior to weighing. Heavy shoes, for example, can be deceiving, as are lead weights in underwear. If patients do not gain the amount of weight contracted for, they are confined to their rooms or to bed, to conserve energy and weight. Behavioral programs can be very effective, but they should be entered into collaboratively. The contingency contract offers patients a means whereby *they* can gain control over their eating behavior. Other helpful suggestions are conceptualizing food as medicine or as fuel, and using high caloric nutriments, such as Ensure, before placing the patient on a full food regimen. If these programs fail, tube feedings may have to be used. Many times, fear of the tube, not of physicians' veiled threats, motivates patients to continue the difficult, dreaded task of increasing caloric intake. Tube feedings are a safe, effective means of delivering calories, but it is easy for such a situation to deteriorate into one in which patients quite properly feel attacked.

Although attempts to promote weight gain with medication have generally not been successful, there has recently been a great deal of interest in the potential role of antidepressants. An increased incidence of affective illness has been reported in the families of anorectic patients, as well as in the patients themselves, following remission of the "weight phobia." Abnormalities of dexamethasone suppression, urinary MHPG (3-methoxy-4 hydroxyphenyl glycol), and thyrotropin-releasing-hormone–induced thyroid-stimulating hormone response have also been found but may be secondary effects of starvation. In a recent double-blind trial, Halmi and associates found cyproheptadine to be more effective than amitriptyline or placebo. They hypothesize that the antidepressant effects of cyproheptadine are mediated through its serotonin antagonist action. However, other investigations have not found cyproheptadine to work better than placebo. Until further studies clarify this situation, it would seem appropriate to search for evidence of affective illness in these patients, and to consider a trial of antidepressant medication when such evidence is found.

Another intriguing biochemical finding has been the recent demonstration by Kaye and associates of increased cerebrospinal fluid opioid activity in patients with anorexia nervosa. It is interesting to speculate that these patients' "addictlike" behavior may be perpetuated by endorphins.

To summarize, there is as yet no definitive medication or other somatic treatment that will correct anorexia nervosa. Reports of successes with new agents must be put into perspective. The disorder has a highly variable natural history and outcome, and dramatic treatment successes and failures have been reported with almost every imaginable form of intervention.

Psychiatric Treatment

The situation with regard to behavioral therapy and medications has been described in the preceding section. Given the current incomplete state of knowledge regarding anorexia nervosa, it is extremely important that the consulting psychiatrist have a thorough grasp of the typical kinds of psychological conflicts these patients are experiencing. First is the issue of control. Patients' histories often reveal that as children they were quite compliant with the wishes of others, apparently failing to develop a sense of their own feelings and ideas. They have grown up with feelings of pervasive ineffectiveness. The onset of the disorder seems to be a last-ditch attempt to be in control of something—every morsel of food, every calorie, every ounce of weight—and to excel in dieting, if nothing else. One patient is reported to have announced proudly that she had already had her breakfast: She had licked a postage stamp.

Patients and their families often seem to be engaged in a bitter struggle for control that extends beyond food and eating. It has been suggested that the parents' behavior is understandable as a reaction to their child's inability to take adequate care of herself or himself. At times, however, parents who are bright and well-meaning seem blind to their difficulty in truly allowing their child to individuate. During one family therapy session, the psychiatrist suggested that it might be helpful for the patient to reach her own decision about a certain matter. The father replied, "That was exactly what I kept telling her to do." Possibly he was merely expressing the frustration of dealing with a person who could not make up her mind. But when the decision was later made to hospitalize the patient, her mother commented that it was difficult to relinquish control of her daughter's mind to strangers.

Whatever its origins, the dilemma remains: How does one turn control over to individuals who seem bent on starving to death? One answer is that there is generally a great deal of room for exploring and respecting these patients' feelings and attitudes without putting their lives in jeopardy. For example, if patients prefer an outpatient program, there may be an advantage to temporarily pursuing outpatient care in order to foster an alliance with them, provided that weight is physician-monitored and that there is a clear agreement that below a certain weight, hospitalization will be mandatory.

The guiding principle in working with these patients is to care for them without controlling them. One hopes that through the psychotherapy relationship patients will come to know their own minds and feelings and develop a sense of self that will allow them to cope more effectively with the newly encountered stresses of adolescence. However, as discussed earlier, it is imperative not to lose sight of patients' physical condition in the course of psychotherapy. A starving brain is probably incapable of functioning at a level that permits meaningful psychotherapy to take place.

The following case illustrates a psychodynamic approach to the treatment of anorexia nervosa.

Miss I., a 15-year-old ninth-grader, was referred for consultation by her family physician because of weight loss. She was 5'5", but weighed only 95 pounds, having lost 25 pounds during the previous year. The process had begun as a fairly reasonable diet, undertaken after some friends at school commented that she appeared to be getting fat. At the time of consultation, the patient was unable to eat more than a bite or two of food and could not stop her vigorous exercise program because she feared that if she were to "indulge" herself in a regular meal, she would lose all control and quickly become obese. She was aware that others thought she looked ill and malnourished, but she did not see herself that way and thought she looked trim. The family physician had found no physical disease responsible for her weight loss and referred her for consultation with the presumptive diagnosis of anorexia nervosa.

The patient had recently entered the freshman year at an exclusive girls' school. Her father was an extremely wealthy, successful business-man who was highly obsessive-compulsive and very ill at ease expressing feelings. Her mother had a long history of depression and alcoholism. The parents described their daughter as a "perfect child" while she was growing up. She had always complied with their wishes. She was their only child, and they found her current behavior totally inexplicable— surely she could eat if she would simply make up her mind to.

She and her family preferred an outpatient treatment plan, and it was decided that she would be followed simultaneously in an adolescent medicine clinic and in outpatient psychotherapy. Together with the patient, the consulting dietitian in the adolescent medicine clinic worked out a diet consisting of small meals supplemented with a high-calorie liquid nutrition drink, which was designed to provide a slow but steady weight gain. The patient was assured that she would not be allowed to become fat. She would be weighed weekly at the medicine clinic, and after the weighing she would see her medical physician briefly. If her weight dropped to 90 pounds, she was to be hospitalized in the psychiatric unit.

Outpatient psychiatric treatment focused on helping the patient gain some sense of who she was, how she felt about things, and what she wanted for herself from her life. At the outset, much of her existence revolved around playing certain roles dictated by family dynamics. She was her mother's "little girl" and closest ally, because of the mother's empty marital relationship and the social isolation imposed by her drinking problem. The mother referred to her daughter's activities with plural pronouns, as in "We've been having some trouble at school lately." Her father longed to see his daughter follow in his footsteps and achieve success at an Ivy League college, though her grades and intelligence were average. It appeared that without a reasonable "growing up" option, she was instead embarked on a course that would lead to her disappearance altogether.

Progress was slow. For a while the patient's weight appeared to stabilize, but then it began to slip down to 91 pounds. The possibility of hospitalization began to loom larger. The patient was actually more agreeable to hospitalization than were her parents. The turning point occurred when the parents gave in and agreed to hospitalization if the patient lost the final pound to 90. At that juncture, they acknowledged her need to exist as a separate person, whatever that entailed, and the patient began a process of steady weight gain.

Medical Complications

Most of the physical changes in anorexia nervosa appear to be starvation-related and to reverse with weight gain. Amenorrhea, however, may precede weight loss, and may even persist in some patients who are "weight recovered" but still have anorectic thinking. Sometimes, anorectic patients initially present with a complication related to starvation, such as infections or growth failure of apparently unknown cause, and the underlying disorder goes temporarily undiagnosed.

Vomiting is often self-induced. Persistent vomiting can result in a loss of tooth enamel. Vomiting can also result from a superior mesenteric artery syndrome in patients who have lost a great deal of weight, and from acute gastric dilatation in patients who are refed too rapidly. This last condition may be a life-threatening emergency, as are the profound electrolyte disturbances that can be caused by vomiting. More insidious is the wasting of myocardium that takes place in cases of profound starvation, which may account for some instances of heart failure during refeeding, and which may be associated with sudden death in severe cases. Estimates of mortality rate for the disease vary, but 5 percent is probably a conservative figure for serious cases that come to medical attention.

Consultation with Ward Staff

Anorectic patients can be extremely upsetting to ward staff. On one occasion, a new student nurse was reduced to tears at the end of a shift that had consisted of grappling with a patient's endless manipulations. The final straw came when the patient's dinner was found concealed under her pillow. Frequent ward staff meetings are essential to provide mutual support and to coordinate care plans. In these meetings staff members are reminded that these patients may perceive hospital staff as the "manipulators" and may then respond accordingly to what they experience as misguided attempts to help. There is no substitute for good sense of humor in this situation, provided staff realize that the patient is suffering truly desperate fears of fatness and of losing control in general.

Prognosis

Most patients recover. However, as many as a third may go on to a chronic and, in some instances, fatal course. There is no sadder sight than chronically wasted treatment-resistant patients who have had the disorder for many years and have long since withdrawn from all meaningful interaction with other people. Conversely, the emergence of vibrant human beings where once there had been only gaunt, robotlike creatures is one of the most gratifying treatment successes in medicine.

Predicting outcomes for individual patients is difficult. It was formerly stated that an early age of onset (11 to 15 years) was associated with a better outcome, but a recent critical review casts doubt on the dictum. Halmi and associates have divided patients into bulimic anorectics, who engage in binge eating and vomiting, and exclusive dieters. The bulimics seemed to be a more chaotic group, with personality disorders, habitual lying, "psychotic tendencies," and stressful interpersonal relationships. The exclusive dieters were more depressed during pretreatment and at the one-year follow-up. There was no significant difference between the groups in terms of mean weight at the time of follow-up.

We are left with more questions than answers for this enigmatic disorder. A recent patient commented about her dieting and exercising, "If I don't do this, what am I?" We must seek to fill that psychological void while we search for a biological breakthrough.

Suggested Readings

Bruch, H. (1978). *The Golden Cage.* Cambridge, Mass.: Harvard University Press.

Drossman, D.A., Ontjes, D.A., and Heizer, W.D. (1979). Anorexia nervosa. *Gastroenterology* 77:1115–1131.

Garfinkel, P.E., and Garner, D.M. (1982). *Anorexia Nervosa.* New York: Brunner/Mazel.

Gerner, R.H., and Gwirtsman, H.E. (1981). Abnormalities of dexamethasone suppression test and urinary MHPG in anorexia nervosa. *American Journal of Psychiatry* 138:650–653.

Halmi, K.A., Eckert, E., and Falk, J.R. (1982). A study of outcome discriminators in exclusive dieters and bulimics. *Journal of the American Academy of Child Psychiatry* 21:369–375.

Hsu, L. K. G. (1982). Is there a disturbance in body image in anorexia nervosa? *Journal of Nervous and Mental Disease* 170:305–307.

Kaye, W.H., Pickar, D., Naber, D., and Ebert, M.H. (1982). Cerebrospinal fluid opioid activity in anorexia nervosa. *American Journal of Psychiatry* 139:643–645.

Kron, L., Katz, J.L., Gorzynski, G., and Weiner, H. (1977). Anorexia nervosa and gonadal dysgenesis. *Archives of General Psychiatry* 34:332–335.

Powers, P.S. (1982). Heart failure during treatment of anorexia nervosa. *American Journal of Psychiatry* 139:1167–1170.

Rollins, N., and Piazza, E. (1981). Anorexia nervosa: a quantitative approach to follow-up. *Journal of the American Academy of Child Psychiatry* 20:167–183.

Swift, W.J. (1982). The long-term outcome of early onset anorexia nervosa. *Journal of the American Academy of Child Psychiatry* 21:38–46.

Vigersky, R.A. (1977). *Anorexia Nervosa.* New York: Raven Press.

Waller, D.A. (1979). A clinician's guide to the psychologic and medical diagnosis and treatment of anorexia nervosa. In *Psychiatric Medicine Update,* ed. T.C. Manschreck, pp. 109–123. New York: Elsevier.

Weller, R.A., and Weller, E.B. (1982). Anorexia nervosa in a patient with an infiltrating tumor of the hypothalamus. *American Journal of Psychiatry* 139:824–825.

CHAPTER 17

Complications of Pregnancy

MICHAEL C. FITZPATRICK, M.D.

Psychiatrists are often called in to make difficult decisions regarding prophylaxis or treatment of emotional symptoms and syndromes that may profoundly affect the mother-child unit. This chapter examines the clinical psychiatric syndromes associated with pregnancy and childbirth and suggests rational pharmacological and psychotherapeutic approaches to them.

Pregnancy and childbirth are major life events; a woman's emotional stability is an important requisite for developing a positive mother-child relationship. The physical and psychological changes of the puerperium may also enhance psychological vulnerability and trigger psychiatric symptomatology. Major psychiatric syndromes, schizophrenia, and affective illnesses, as well as mild or incapacitating adjustment disorders, may arise during this period. Women with puerperal psychosis comprise up to 8 percent of female psychiatric admissions, and most pregnant women report at least some disturbing mood changes.

Hyperemesis Gravidarum

Most women experience nausea and vomiting in the first trimester of pregnancy. If severe vomiting continues into the second trimester, dehydration and electrolyte imbalance may require hospital treatment.

Hyperemesis gravidarum can best be conceptualized as a somatization disorder whose organic and psychological features become most prominent after the 12th week of pregnancy. It often afflicts women with immature personality styles, borderline object relations, or low intelligence—women in whom somatization is common. From a psychological standpoint, women with hyperemesis may be responding to feelings of inadequate emotional support. Many women also feel ambivalent about their pregnancies and respond with heightened dependency and regression. Hyperemesis may therefore be a response to psychosocial stress or a reaction to unconscious conflict.

Pregnant women often feel trapped between the need to please those on whom they depend and the need to sort out their own confusing feelings. Husbands frequently focus their attention and interest on the expected child. They fail to acknowledge their wives as individuals and are unaware of their wives' conflicted feelings. Their attitudes reinforce their wives' feelings of isolation. The more threatened many women feel, the more regressed they become.

In the ideal approach to hyperemesis gravidarum, the psychiatric consultant identifies the environmental stressors, considers means to alleviate them, explores patients' ambivalence, allows for realistic decision making, and redirects husbands' attention and support. In talking to patients, psychiatrists should pay as little overt attention as possible to the physical symptoms. If patients require hospitalization, the administration of intravenous fluids and antiemetics (prochlorperazine, 25 mg by suppository b.i.d. or 5 to 10 mg intramuscularly p.r.n. to a maximum daily intramuscular dose of 40 mg) makes it easier to focus on emotional issues rather than on nutritional needs. An active plan to minimize regression is important. When interacting with the psychiatrist, the patient is encouraged to sit up. The psychiatrist talks face to face with the patient despite the likelihood of intermittent vomiting. Small doses of intramuscular haloperidol (1 to 2 mg b.i.d.) are often beneficial if the patient is regressed but are usually not necessary when prochlorperazine is used to control nausea. Anxiolytics are not recommended. Certainly, the most drug-free environment is best for fetal well-being. Keeping patients out of the hospital is best, but more than one admission may nevertheless be required.

Women with primary organic illnesses such as diabetes mellitus are often difficult to maintain outside a hospital. Adequate control of diabetes may be impossible with persistent vomiting. Diabetic women are frequently caught between their desire to have a child or the need to have a baby to please their spouses or to feel complete as women and their realistic fear of life-threatening diabetic complications of pregnancy. They may have been given conflicting advice by physicians about the safety of pregnancy and labor. In addition, if they have already experienced diabetic complications in this pregnancy or earlier ones, they may feel guilty over their hostility toward the fetus for putting them in such a precarious position.

Short-term psychotherapeutic intervention to help patients identify and verbalize their ambivalence is important. Once stated openly, patients' reality-based or fantasy-based fears become less intense and are more easily resolved.

Alcohol Abuse

Many pregnant women abuse alcohol, sometimes as a continuation of a habit, sometimes as a means of relieving anxiety or depression. Moderate to heavy antenatal exposure to alcohol may result in the fetal alcohol syndrome. Forty-five drinks per month classifies a woman as a heavy drinker in terms of fetal outcome studies. Characteristics of the fetal alcohol syndrome include (1) small infant size at birth, (2) delayed developmental milestones, (3) craniofacial, cardiovascular, and joint and limb abnormalities, and (4) mental retardation. Even consumption of small amounts of alcohol has been associated with partial expression of the syndrome and may lead to behavioral teratogenicity, including diminished cognitive ability and symptoms similar to minimal brain dysfunction with hyperactivity.

An aggressive approach to pregnant women who are problem drinkers is necessary. If heavy drinking is a part of a mood disturbance, early hospitalization with behavioral, pharmacological, and supportive approaches is useful. Family therapy and vigorous use of such groups as Alcoholics Anonymous and Al-Anon may also be beneficial. Their pregnant condition and the danger to the fetus from alcohol may stimulate these women to deal actively with their drinking problems and the factors that determine their drinking.

Miscarriage

About 15 percent of pregnancies result in a spontaneous abortion. Loss of a nonviable fetus is often not consciously acknowledged as a major loss by mothers. As a result, the inevitable grieving process can be impeded because of the absence of the social support that is usually forthcoming at times of loss. Health care professionals and friends may themselves deny the significance of the loss by referring to the possibility of future pregnancies. Many of these mothers harbor strong feelings of self-doubt or guilt concerning their role in the aborted pregnancy. Many feel personally responsible. It is essential that psychiatrists identify these feelings and provide reassurance about them as well as accurate information on the probable causes of the miscarriage.

To the mothers, unborn children often possess idealized qualities or symbolize a fantasized relationship felt to be essential to the mothers' own well-being. If a hysterectomy is required following a spontaneous abortion, loss of the ability to reproduce may foster resentment toward the aborted fetus. This anger in turn hinders the grief process.

It is important that physicians facilitate grieving by identifying fantasies and ambivalent feelings that may block the expression of grief. Women who have miscarried may need to be taught that such mixed feelings exist and are very understandable in these circumstances. They also need a cognitive focus around which to initiate their grief work. Providing such a focus may include bringing the fetus (if it was sufficiently developed) or photographs of the fetus to the mother. A memorial service may also be helpful.

Frequently these women are regressed. Involving them in specific decisions about their immediate care and about their future helps them regain control. There may be a concomitant insomnia related to anxiety surrounding the loss. Short-term use of anxiolytics such as alprazolam, 0.25 mg at bedtime, is beneficial.

Postpartum Psychosis

Pregnancy produces tremendous alterations in maternal physiology and requires significant intrapsychic reorganization in the expectant mother to accept responsibility for the care and protection of an infant. Accordingly, pregnancy can be a major precipitating factor in psychotic disorders. The incidence of postpartum psychosis ranges between 1.0 and 2.5 per 1,000 deliveries, with a markedly higher rate of morbidity after delivery if there has been an earlier psychotic episode. In addition, primiparas have a higher risk than multiparas for new onset of functional psychosis. In the puerperium, the two major psychiatric diagnoses of psychotic patients without prior psychiatric morbidity are schizophreniform disorder and major affective disorder, although other brief reactive psychoses may occur.

Schizophreniform illness following delivery is usually acute and begins sometime after the third postpartum day. Prodromal symptoms of insomnia and agitation are frequent. Initial diagnosis may be uncertain. Symptoms of delirium, especially confusion, are common, and new mothers may exhibit considerable agitation. Delusions tend to be grandiose, religious or supernatural, or persecutory. The mood-congruent affect and guilt seen in affective illness tend to be absent. A potent neuroleptic such as haloperidol (in an initial dosage of 5 mg IM b.i.d. or t.i.d.—depending on the level of agitation) is usually appropriate. (See Chapter 5 for a description of rapid neuroleptization.)

Schizophrenia

For women with a history of nonpuerperal schizophrenia, the risk of recurrence during the first and subsequent pregnancies approaches 20 percent. Women with a first-degree relative with schizophrenia are at high risk for postpartum schizophrenia. The likelihood of an episode may range from 5 to 10 percent.

Although, in general, the less medication during pregnancy the better, schizophrenic women who need maintenance antipsychotic medication should be allowed to continue taking their medication throughout the puerperium. Phenothiazines have not been shown to increase the chance of fetal anomalies, and follow-up studies have shown no effects on perinatal mortality, birth weight, or intelligence. Chlorpromazine in dosages greater than 500 mg daily and equivalent dosages of other antipsychotics have occasionally been associated with the "floppy infant" syndrome and with newborn respiratory distress at delivery. However, these problems do not seem to be major. Phenothiazines and butyrophenones are secreted in breast milk, but no significant difficulties have been encountered with the babies of lactating mothers.

Depression

Nowhere is the biopsychosocial model more useful than in understanding and treating depressed pregnant women. About half of all women who develop postpartum psychiatric morbidity have experienced antenatal psychological symptoms, especially anxiety, feelings of despondency, and somatic complaints. The puerperium requires an intrapsychic reorganization on the part of the mother to accept her new role and a period of family adjustment to accommodate the new family member. Successful adaptation to these anxiety-producing changes requires considerable maturity. Positive change can usually occur when a woman feels emotionally secure. Therefore, when the relationship between spouses is disturbed, when emotional support is lacking, or when the patient is psychologically immature, the likelihood of antenatal psychological symptoms increases, and such women should be regarded as being at risk for postpartum psychiatric complications.

Psychiatric consultation early in the antenatal period is strongly suggested if psychological symptoms are expressed by the patient or observed by the primary physician. The correction of misinformation and the provision of support with family assistance if possible generally assuage patients' fears. If a pregnant woman develops a major depressive disorder, treatment with tricyclic antidepressants is indicated. As with neuroleptics, there is no evidence of teratogenicity. Tricyclics can be used safely and effectively. By contrast, monoamine oxidase inhibitors should be avoided. They require dietary restrictions, produce hypotension and have been shown to cause fetal resorption in some animal studies.

Anxiolytics should be avoided in the first and third trimesters. Diazepam has been associated with cleft palate when used during the critical differentiation period of fetal development. Accumulation may occur in fetal tissues if anxiolytics are used frequently or in high doses and may lead to the "floppy infant" syndrome. A newborn's efficiency in metabolizing and excreting antianxiety drugs is compromised because of its immature glucuronyl transferase system. If benzodiazepines are unquestionably indicated, oxazepam is preferred because of its short half-life and its lack of active metabolites.

In the 48 hours immediately following the delivery, nearly 80 percent of women develop a syndrome of emotional lability and oversensitiveness associated with feelings of being let down. Presumably, these postpartum "blues" are concomitants of precipitous changes in hormonal levels. Self-limited (lasting 48 to 72 hours), these blues require only psychological support.

There is a danger, however, that symptoms of true depressive illness may be misdiagnosed by medical staff or attributed to a mere prolongation of these third-day blues. Moreover, patients may avoid telling physicians their affective symptoms, which typically are indicative of depression; or they may present with hypochondriacal symptoms masking their illness. The onset of a true depressive disorder may occur while the mother is still on the obstetrics floor or up to six months after she has returned home. A mother suffering from an untreated postpartum depression will be highly dysfunctional and may have a protracted illness.

From a psychosocial standpoint, factors predictive of postpartum depression include:

1. An undesired or unplanned pregnancy.
2. Marital discord or feeling unloved.
3. A history of violence in the family.
4. Pregnancy without a mate.
5. Older age.
6. Previous history of depression.

The thought content in postpartum depression generally centers around recurrent themes of self-doubt concerning mothering ability. Mothers may feel incapable of loving adequately or may express uncertainty about their love for their children. They may have disturbing thoughts of injuring the newborn child. Unconscious conflicts seen in these depressed women often include feelings of sibling rivalry with their infants, discomfort with their own sexuality, hostility toward their mothers for providing inadequate mothering, and threatened loss of dependency as they become required to be caregivers rather than care receivers.

If women meet DSM-III criteria for major depressive disorder, a two-step plan of somatic and psychological treatment is appropriate. Tricyclics in therapeutic doses or electroconvulsive therapy can diminish the troubling vegetative symptoms. Psychotherapy is indicated for conflict resolution and exploration of feelings of inadequacy. A psychotic depression requires hospitalization, family involvement, and direct encouragement of daily mother-child interaction. At the other end of the spectrum of symptoms, there are many reactive states with less severe, intermittent symptoms. Psychotherapy is the treatment modality of choice in such situations.

Bipolar Affective Disorder

Special problems arise in managing pregnant women with manic-depressive illness, as they require careful monitoring throughout the puerperium. Women with a history of bipolar affective disorder have a 30 to 40 percent chance for exacerbation of their illness following delivery. After one episode of postpartum psychosis, the risk of an episode after subsequent deliveries approaches 50 percent.

Discontinuing maintenance lithium during pregnancy has been related to postpartum mania. Unfortunately, lithium readily crosses the placental membrane and can result in fetal dysmorphogenesis. Cardiovascular malformations including Ebstein's anomaly, thyroid dysfunction with fetal goiter, and muscular hypotonia have been reported.

It is preferable for patients with a history of bipolar affective disorder to plan their pregnancies. If possible, they should be withdrawn from lithium prior to conception. If no troublesome symptoms develop and there is no change in mood, patients can remain lithium-free until the third postpartum day, when lithium should be reinstituted. Hypomania after the first trimester of pregnancy can be controlled with haloperidol, but if the symptoms are severe, lithium can be safely restarted in the second trimester. If, in a woman taking lithium, the pregnancy is not known until after the 12th week, there is no need for her to stop taking the lithium.

Other problems with lithium include obstetrical complications, such as eclampsia, and the need for salt and fluid restrictions. At parturition, there may be a change in the body's distribution of lithium. Since tight control over the distribution is impossible to achieve, the lithium can be discontinued at this time and reinstituted on the third postpartum day. Women taking lithium should not breastfeed.

First onsets of bipolar affective disorders may be difficult to distinguish from schizophreniform illnesses. Hallucinations and delusions are common in manic episodes, but the themes are less bizarre than in those found in schizophrenia. A prolonged hospital course is required, and total family involvement is usually beneficial. If bipolar patients have thoughts of injuring their children, the children should be considered at risk until the illness is controlled. The prognosis and outcome are the same as for non-puerperal affective disorders.

This chaper concludes with an illustration of the management of a pregnant woman with an affective disorder.

Mrs. J., a 35-year-old white woman who was 20 weeks pregnant with her first child, was brought by her husband to the hospital emergency room with complaints of insomnia and "nervousness." The physician reassured the patient that her baby was fine and gave her triazolam to help her sleep.

The patient returned alone two days later with similar symptoms and became quite agitated when she was told the same physician was not on duty. A psychiatric consultation was obtained.

The consultant found that the patient was working as a legal secretary and studying for a master's degree in business administration at night. She had returned to school after feeling her husband was "too involved in other things." When she first learned she was pregnant, she felt uncertain about her mothering ability and then impulsively purchased several cases of diapers and baby food. She had also made numerous long-distance calls to ask advice of relatives.

The patient was the older of two sisters in an upper-middle-class family. She had always excelled in order to please her father, who was vice president of a local bank. She described her mother as an alcoholic who had suffered from bouts of depression.

At age 20, while in college, the patient had seen a psychiatrist when she became acutely confused after taking phenmetrazine (Preludin) to help her study. She had felt pressured to maintain her B+ average and to continue as a cheerleader and as president of her sorority.

On examining the patient in the emergency room, the consultant found her to be well dressed, anxious, and demanding, but oriented in all spheres. Her mood was labile, with affect appropriate to mood. Her conversation was circumstantial, she was distractible, and exhibited pressured speech. There was no evidence of hallucinations, loosened associations, or loss of thought control. She did feel there was "something terribly wrong with my baby." She also asked that the mayor be called to expedite her admission to the hospital.

The patient was diagnosed as having a bipolar affective disorder with mixed features, and she was hospitalized. She was treated with haloperidol, 5 mg t.i.d. Her symptoms abated within a week. During that time, the patient and her husband acknowledged and discussed for the first time their concerns about their marriage. She was discharged ten days later on haloperidol, 5 mg at bedtime, with arrangements made for the consultant to follow her progress.

At term, the patient was admitted with moderate anxiety. Labor and delivery were uneventful. On the third postpartum day, lithium was begun (1,800 mg PO daily), and therapeutic levels were obtained on the ninth postpartum day. The patient continued to express feelings of self-doubt, but she accepted her newborn easily. She was discharged from the hospital, with arrangements made for outpatient follow-up.

Suggested Readings

Abel, E.L. (1980). Alcohol syndrome: behavioral teratology. *Psychological Bulletin* 87:29–45.

Ananth, J. (1978). Side effects in the neonate from psychotropic agents excreted through breast-feeding. *American Journal of Psychiatry* 135:801–804.

Barglow, P., Hatcher, R., Wolston, J., Phelps, R., Burns, W., and Depp, R. (1981). Psychiatric risk factors in the pregnant diabetic patient. *American Journal of Obstetrics and Gynecology* 140:46–52.

Kadrmas, A., Winokur, G., and Crowe, R. (1979). Postpartum mania. *British Journal of Psychiatry* 135:551–554.

Katon, W.J., Ries, R.K., Bokan, J.A., and Kleinman, A. (1980–1981). Hyperemesis gravidarum: a biopsychosocial perspective. *International Journal of Psychiarty in Medicine* 10:151–161.

Kendell, R.E., Rennie, D., Clarke, J.A., and Dean, C. (1981). The social and obstetric correlation of psychiatric admission in the puerperium. *Psychological Medicine* 11:341–350.

Kowalski, K. (1980). Managing perinatal loss. *Clinical Obstetrics and Gynecology* 23:1113–1123.

Nurnberg, H.G. (1980). Treatment of mania in the last six months of pregnancy. *Hospital and Community Psychiatry* 31:122–126.

Protheroe, C. (1969). Puerperal psychosis: a long-term study, 1927–1961. *British Journal of Psychiatry* 115:9–30.

Targum, S.D. (1979). Dealing with psychosis during pregnancy. *American Pharmacy* 19:18–21.

Vandenbergh, R.L. (1980). Postpartum depression. *Clinical OB-GYN* 23:1105–1111.

CHAPTER 18

The Hopeless, Suicide-Prone Medical Patient

LINDA GAY PETERSON, M.D.

Patients at high risk for becoming hopeless and suicide-prone are those with prolonged hospitalization, debilitating disease, or terminal illness accompanied by an extended period of suffering. These patients may have illnesses with uncertain prognoses or with diagnostic confusion. Other high-risk individuals are those who are emotionally troubled, have little social support, and must contend with an extended hospitalization. Certain situational factors also contribute to inducing hopelessness and suicide-proneness, especially a real or fantasized breakdown of the relationship between patients and significant caregivers, including family or members of the professional staff actively involved in treatment.

The following case illustrates the conjunction of many of these factors:

Mr. K., a 40-year-old married sales executive, was readmitted to the hospital six weeks after a motor vehicle accident. Previously in good physical and mental health, he had sustained fractures of the mandible, maxilla, and orbital floor and leaked spinal fluid from his left ear. Immediately following the accident, his jaws were wired shut to stabilize his fractures. After several days of observation, he had no further spinal fluid leakage and was sent home. His chief complaint on readmission was stiffness and swelling of his neck. Cervical spine film on admission showed a subluxation of the cervical spine at C3, C4 with osteomyelitis. The responsible organism was identified and antibiotic treatment was initiated. Shortly after admission, the patient developed a bradycardia of 20 beats per minute and became anoxic. He could not be intubated because his jaw was wired closed, so an emergency tracheostomy was performed, further limiting his ability to communicate. Afterward, he had a number of seizures and developed multifocal myoclonus and delirium. As the patient's delirium cleared, he was noted to be depressed over his mental and physical problems. On several occasions he wrote on his clipboard that he wished to die, which prompted psychiatric referral.

On examination, the patient had impaired short-term memory and fluctuating mild to moderate depression. He often did not remember that his physicians had seen him or that his wife had visited, and as a result he felt that he was receiving poor care and that his wife did not want him. His private duty nurse also noted that from the time that the patient had been in isolation because of his infection, staff and family visits had been short and infrequent. The patient felt that if his myoclonus were to be permanent, he would be better off dead, as he would not be able to support his family and would be a burden on his wife and children.

The factors that led this patient to feel hopeless and suicidal included illness, physical disability, the presence of an organic amnestic syndrome, and perceived lack of family support.

Patient-Related Factors

Many individuals suffering from prolonged illnesses or from illnesses that result in major changes in body image or function exhibit suicidal ideation or behavior. In this category are those who have recently experienced considerable life stress, disintegrative symptomatology such as loss of sight and renal function in diabetics, and chronic renal failure. Patients with collagen vascular diseases, progressive neurological diseases, and cancer and those enduring severe burns, amputations, or quadriplegia are also included in this category.

Active lethality, with hopelessness and the making of plans for suicide, may go unnoticed if it takes the form of poor compliance with medical regimens or of sudden unexplained deterioration. Cheerfulness in the face of worsening physical conditions may be due to gratification of lethality—the desire to stop living rather than endure further suffering or physical disintegration. Patients who have changes of mood or attitude out of character with their general response to illness should therefore be assessed carefully.

Aside from medical illness itself, past psychiatric illness or current psychiatric disability can induce hopelessness. Patients who become depressed while ill, whether as a response to stress, as part of a recurrent depressive or manic-depressive illness, or as a result of medications, are a significant concern. Along with psychotic patients and patients with organic mental syndromes, depressed individuals are at risk from their mental symptoms and from the tendency of medical staff to identify their mental problems or their problem behavior as uncooperativeness. Staff tend to spend less time, give less information, and provide poorer-quality care to patients perceived as having frank mental illness. Depressed patients may not ask important questions and may have a more negative view of their illness owing both to their attitude and to their lack of accurate understanding. Because of their negativism, irascibility, and uncommunicativeness, they may alienate the staff and thus further increase their feelings of hopelessness and isolation. Often, they tell their families not to visit because they feel they are a burden on them. This diminishing of their support base augments their sense of unimportance and isolation.

Treatment

Intervention necessitates treatment of the patient's depression through psychotherapy and medication, plus treatment of the staff's anxieties with a clear plan and active followup. Therapeutic agents that may exacerbate depression such as cimetidine or antihypertensive agents should be discontinued. Metabolic imbalances, infections, and neoplasms—all of which may cause depression—must be corrected if possible. (For further discussion of depression in medical patients, see Chapter 22.)

Psychotic patients may feel hopeless and suicidal because they misperceive or misinterpret reality. The staff's tendency to fear and reject them as people reduces both time spent and meaningful interaction with them. Fear and rejection are present both when the psychosis is a functional psychiatric disorder of long duration and when it is secondary to the current illness or its treatment. Psychotic individuals may behave erratically and unpredictably, resulting in moments of high suicide risk. The consultant's aim is to calm, contain, and reduce unrealistic staff fears during the crisis.

Psychotropic agents should be used to decrease patients' agitation, hallucinations, and delusions. Neuroleptics should be given regularly, not as needed, because nonpsychiatric staff may be afraid to use these medications or may keep the patient overly sedated. Careful directions should be given on the use and side effects of these agents, including a specified treatment regimen and specific instructions about appropriate p.r.n. use.

The needs of hopeless or suicidal patients with cognitive impairment, who do not understand their situation, add another dimension to the consultation. Since these patients cannot ask for help and information and cannot cooperate with treatment, they pose real problems for staff management. In the vignette presented, Mr. K., because of his impaired memory, felt he was receiving inadequate medical care. The problem was compounded by the medical staff's seeing him less often because he did not ask questions or communicate intelligibly. Other patients may pull out intravenous lines, disconnect traction, or remove Foley catheters because of confusion or misunderstanding about treatment. These behaviors result in staff frustration and anger and may further decrease communication and make patients feel rejected and disliked. Such actions may also lead the staff to restrain patients unnecessarily, increasing patients' view of themselves as abused, burdensome, and "better off dead." The staff must understand the prophylactic importance of regular visits and the need to explain repeatedly the treatment plan, even if the patient has limited understanding. Sometimes, putting *do not touch* signs on traction wires or intravenous tubing helps to prevent patients with impaired reality contact from removing them.

Social Supports

Along with the medical and psychiatric problems themselves, social support during prolonged hospitalization is an important factor for many inpatients who are trying to maintain their will to live in the face of disability and pain. In the vignette, Mr. K.'s wife was unable to see him often because they had a small baby at home. Other patients may be separated from their families by distance, transportation problems, or preexisting family discord. Such patients may perceive their suffering as pointless or even deserved because no one seems to care, and they may consequently decide that their families would be better off if they died. Patients with little religious faith seem even more prone to despair.

Staff-Related Factors

The staff may add to patients' feelings of hopelessness. A feeling that a patient discounts or actively disparages their care may lead nursing staff to spend less time with and be less responsive to that patient. There may be an individual conflict between a patient and a member of the staff, or a patient may behave in such a way that the entire staff begins to see him or her as a "bad" patient. A patient who is demanding, abusive, or manipulative may arouse and experience staff resentment. Conversely, an uncomplaining patient may feel neglected because the nurses are very busy and thus are inadvertently neglectful. Patients with chronic illness who feel responsible for exacerbations of their illness and hate to bother the nurses or to ask for family visits may as a result become quite isolated, secondarily depressed, and then suicidal.

Difficulties in communicating with physicians can also lead patients to feel abandoned and hopeless. In this era of committee medicine, problems in identifying the primary physician often arise. The presence of multiple consultants, transfers from one service to another, and the patient's physician's unavailability because of illness or vacation all may lead the patient to a sense of abandonment with ensuing hopelessness. In teaching hospitals, the changes of interns and residents may trigger fears of abandonment in some patients. The changes in treatment plan that accompany staff changes may also lead patients to lose confidence in their caretakers. Patients who are in isolation for a prolonged period often begin to receive brief "head-in-the-door" visits. These patients may also receive fewer visits from family and staff because of the inconvenience of having to dress in isolation gowns as well as the fear of contagion.

Conflict between physicians caring for patients may be frightening and lead patients to feel pessimistic about their illnesses. One patient seen in psychiatric consultation had heard her physicians arguing outside her room over her case. She stated that if her doctors couldn't decide what was wrong with her, there was no hope of her ever getting well. Conflicts between patients and physicians can cause even more distress than conflicts with nurses. Patients' relationships with their physicians assume increased importance during hospitalization because patients are often in regressed and passive states and perceive rejection by physicians as children might perceive rejection from parents. Helping identify and resolve these conflicts is often the main task of psychiatric consultants.

Patient-Staff Interaction

After performing a mental status examination of the hopeless, suicide-prone patient for depression, thought disorder, and confusion, the consultant tries to understand the medical problem and the patient's perception of it, evaluates the patient's social support network, and conceptualizes the staff-patient relationship from both the patient's and the caregiver's viewpoints. The plan of intervention follows from a careful assessment of all these interacting factors.

When patients begin to express suicidal ideas, their relationship with the nursing and medical staff often deteriorates markedly. Voicing these ideas may stimulate the caregivers to view patients as crazy, frightening, and undesirable. Because suicidal patients and patients with impaired mental function are often the most disliked by their physicians, the consultee's primary goal in obtaining a consultation may be to effect the transfer of the patient to the psychiatric unit rather than to understand the patient's dilemma and develop ways to deal with it. (For further discussion of working with the consultee, see Chapter 12.) Commonly, a psychiatric evaluation of a regressed, hopeless patient is followed by many phone calls from nurses and doctors to reaffirm what the consultant has told them verbally and in the written report, with subtle hints that the patient would still be better off on the psychiatry service. These daytime telephone calls may be followed by nighttime attempts to have the on-call psychiatric resident transfer the patient to relieve the staff's discomfort.

Dealing with the Staff

After providing information about the cause of the patient's suicidal feelings or behavior, such as depression, organic brain syndrome, psychological responses to illness, feelings of being neglected, or conflict with nursing staff or attending physician, the consultant must provide clear recommendations for the patient's treatment. Essential are instructions on the use of medications for depression or psychosis (including dose, timing, and route of administration), protective measures such as removing sharp objects from the room or searching for medication that could be used to overdose, supportive measures such as frequent nursing observation, a 24-hour sitter for patients who appear to be a high immediate suicide risk or for whom frequent nursing checks are not possible, use of nightlights for patients with organic brain syndrome, and further diagnostic procedures.

The next step is to redefine the problem for the staff. Starting with the patient's primary nurse and then moving to other nurses involved in the patient's care, the consultant should discuss findings and recommendations and allow the nurses to express their concerns about implementing these ideas. Some modifications of the strategy may be made to fit the particular needs of the primary nurse or the nursing needs of a particular floor. In pointing out that a patient has been neglected or is actively disliked, it is crucial to reward efforts made by the staff to deal with difficult patients. Empathic support for the difficulties of dealing with personality-disordered patients or with patients whose long illnesses have not responded to the available therapy helps improve nursing staff attitudes toward these patients. Recommendations can follow about the needed frequency of nursing visits. The consultant may suggest areas of productive discussion, such as the patient's hobbies or children, or other topics that stimulate a positive affective interchange with the patient that will be more rewarding for nurses and patient alike. Support for nurses and physicians helps them acknowledge the limitations of the medical treatment that they are providing. In turn, the staff's simple acknowledgment of the patient's distress will often increase the patient's trust and faith in the medical caregiving. It may also help the nursing staff out of a defensive or evasive posture.

Nurses and physicians become concerned about addicting chronically ill patients to pain medications. As a result, they may change medications and dosages frequently and demand that patients show evidence of pain in order to earn medication. The consultant can help greatly in such situations by suggesting a reasonable pain control regimen that is noncontingent on pain behavior and establishes smooth, around-the-clock pain relief; such a program will decrease both the patient's fears of being forced to suffer and the nursing staff's fears of addicting the patient.

Pain control can be achieved by prescribing a dose of pain medication greater than that currently used, to be administered every 3 to 4 hours around the clock unless the patient is asleep or refuses the medication. After the patient has been pain-free for 24 hours, the medication can be gradually decreased if indicated. In terminally ill patients or patients with chronic pain, a tricyclic antidepressant and training in biofeedback and relaxation to improve pain control may be needed before reduction of narcotics is feasible.

When a patient pits staff members against each other, it is important to assign one person on each shift as primary communicator with the patient and to develop a consistent management plan. Shifting the responsibility for getting well to the patient, maximizing patient independence and participation in self-care, and including family and friends in supporting this approach will reduce manipulation of the sick role. The psychiatrist's being easily accessible to the staff and keeping open the option of patient transfer to the psychiatric service if the plan is unsuccessful after a specified period may further diminish staff anxiety about persevering with a difficult patient.

Prophylactic Measures

After any major psychiatric disturbance in the patient has been dealt with or ruled out, the psychiatrist may need to help the patient take a fresh look at the circumstances of the illness and its treatment. If prolonged hospitalization is necessary, arranging small, regular breaks (from a few minutes to an hour or two) from the hospital environment in a wheelchair or a stretcher, sometimes with the aid of a heparin lock, can be very helpful to patients. Most patients in traction can be placed near a window for a short period each day. Patients in reverse isolation can leave their rooms, masked and gowned, when there is low traffic flow in the corridors. Intensive care unit patients on monitors can be cheered by being moved to a bed near a window, watching TV, or having a volunteer read to them or play games with them. Occupational therapy is also useful for patients with multiple medical problems who are hospitalized for a prolonged period.

Severely ill patients can be helped to express their feelings of frustration over hospitalization, changes in body image, and future expectations. These patients can also benefit from finding ways to be more active in their own treatment. Leukemic adults in reverse isolation, with prolonged in-hospital chemotherapy and suffering the pain of their illness and the physical changes caused by treatment, report improved spirits and attitude when instructed in self-care of indwelling central intravenous lines, when allowed to participate in selecting a pain medication regimen, and when permitted while gloved and gowned to instruct new patients in ward routine.

Many patients feel they cannot express negative feelings about their care and its likely outcome. Internalization of these feelings may result in feelings of hopelessness and suicidal behavior. Providing an opportunity for ventilation individually and in groups may minimize the experience of hopelessness, isolation, and depression. Groups provide an excellent means to help patients change some of the relationships or activities that frustrate them. Patients who have given up caring for themselves and have become passively suicidal are often successfully challenged by other group members to be more active in taking care of themselves.

Nurses and physicians need to be informed that after increasing the activity of patients in their care, they are likely to be confronted with increased demands and complaints from these patients as a result of their becoming more active on their own behalf. If they are not prepared for this occurrence, the staff may respond negatively to the patients' increased self-assertion. Having the staff engage in role playing can help them to cope with more independent patients while still maintaining their own view of themselves as healers. They can play the role of a patient complaining about care and threatening to leave the hospital, of a very negativistic patient who won't cooperate because of the feeling of inevitable death, and of a demanding, seductive, and noncompliant patient. These are the three most common situations in which staff-patient relationships break down and result in the patients' feeling hopeless and even becoming suicidal.

A Final Word

When confronted with a hopeless, suicide-prone patient, the important factors for the psychiatric consultant to assess are patient-related factors, including the nature of the medical illness, the presence of psychiatric disorder, the availability of social support, and situational factors that may have disrupted patient-staff relationships. The consultant should follow a careful review of these areas with a detailed written description of the factors involved in the particular case. This formal report is complemented by dialogue with the patient and the treatment team to maximize their understanding of recommendations and their ability to follow them. Patients who have given up on themselves can also be helped by participating in groups. And having the staff engage in role playing can help them to deal better with their patients and thus minimize the chances that their own unconscious reactions will lead patients to become hopeless and suicide-prone.

Suggested Readings

Benson, D., Peterson, L.G., and Bartay, J. (1983). Neuropsychiatric effects of anti-hypertensive medications. *Psychiatric Medicine* 1:205–214.

Dubovsky, S.L. (1978). Averting suicide in terminally ill patients. *Psychosomatics* 19:113–115.

Goodwin, J.M., Goodwin, J.S., and Kellner, K. (1979). Psychiatric symptoms in disliked medical patients. *Journal of the American Medical Association* 241: 1117–1120.

Karasu, T.B., Waltzman, S.A., Linden-Mayer, J.P., and Bickley, P.J. (1980). The medical case of patients with psychiatric illness. *Hospital and Community Psychiatry* 31:463–472.

Petrich, J.M., and Holmes, T.H. (1981). Recent life events and psychiatric illness. *Psychiatric Annals* 11:207–218.

Reichsman, F., and Levy, N.B. (1974). Problems in adaptation to maintenance hemodialysis. In *Living or Dying*, ed. N.B. Levy, pp. 30–39. Springfield, Ill.: Charles C Thomas.

Robins, E. (1981). *The Final Months: A Study of the Lives of 134 Persons Who Committed Suicide.* New York: Oxford University Press.

Satinover, J., Peterson, L.G., and Perl, M. (1981). Psychiatric intervention with immigrants and non-English speaking patients. Paper presented at Sixth World Congress of the International College of Psychosomatic Medicine, Montreal, September 13–18.

CHAPTER 19

Dilemmas of the Dying Patient

AVERY D. WEISMAN, M.D.

The clinical encounter with imminent death is rarely a matter of emotional indifference. It can be exalting or exhausting, and usually is instructive. However, before the consultant ventures into the field, it is advisable to be familiar with the concept of *terminality*. Terminality is the disposition to die in the very near future. Time of death cannot be imposed arbitrarily except during the last hour or two. But terminality rarely extends more than a day or two. The very word has a pessimistic implication, just as some doctors designate certain diseases, such as metastatic cancer, "terminal," regardless of the patient's physical and psychosocial status. Not all serious disease is terminal. Sickness is a subjective state; disease is a pathological entity; and much more can be envisioned for very sick patients by referring to them as having a *posttherapeutic phase* than by calling them terminal.

A moribund person is still alive, just as is someone who is confused. Terminality is a pessimistic term that should be reserved for special conditions. The psychiatric consultant should first try to place a patient along a continuum within the posttherapeutic period, differentiating between deterioration and decline, preterminality, sickness unto death, and the deathwatch itself. Then, the consultant will find it easier both to understand major areas of concern at a specified juncture and to identify points of vulnerability.

Problems and Dilemmas

Most preterminal and terminal patients are not psychiatric patients in the conventional sense. As a result, the consultant will deviate considerably from tactics, rubrics, and policies used in most psychiatric situations. Significant assessment depends on knowing a patient reasonably well, although prolonged or profound contact over a long period is seldom needed, welcomed, or feasible. To get most and to effect most, the psychiatric consultant needs to do more than ask a few perfunctory mental status questions, write a note about a patient's depression, and then, after prescribing medication, disappear.

Four factors determine which problems and dilemmas are important: (1) *site*, or location, extent, and severity of the biological disease, (2) *social support*, or psychosocial resources available, (3) *situation*, or the clinical plight that resulted in a consultation, and (4) *self* or *style*, which the patient formerly used or is now using to deal with predominant problems. The plight includes psychosocial problems of varying severity, which are not always in proportion to the extent of disease or the degree of debilitation.

Dying and preterminal patients often have fewer problems and dilemmas to contend with than do patients who are still being diagnosed or who are experiencing a recurrence or a relapse. Despite the threat of death, dying and preterminal patients may have already dealt with psychosocial disruptions. In general, however, preterminal problems have two main sources: infringement and indecision. When a patient's autonomy and social support are infringed upon by disease, symptoms, and treatment, demoralization is apt to result, along with assorted personal problems and dilemmas. When an afflicted patient cannot choose how to cope most effectively, the quandary is one of indecision and invalid options. There is no specific correlation between treatment, spread of disease, palliative measures, and the extent of infringement and indecision.

There are certain common points of vulnerability that cause distress, regardless of the primary problem or area of concern.

UNCERTAINTY, PESSIMISM, AND DISCONTENT.   Many preterminal patients waver between awareness of inexorable disease and denial of facts or implications signifying a pessimistic outlook. Uncertainty, pessimism, and discontent are interwoven in different shades and textures. The psychiatrist should accept the disparity between what a patient says and does from one session to the next, and often from one person to another. Satisfaction and acceptance at one moment may, at another, become pessimistic discontent or even false certainty about a good prognosis.

SEPARATION FROM SOCIAL SUPPORTS.   Professional caregivers are strong sources of social and emotional support during regular duties and through informal interactions with patients and families. Separation from the support given by caregivers may occur inadvertently without overt interruption of professional activities. It can be symbolic, indirect, or actual. A caregiver may carry out duties scrupulously, but with a hostile, impatient, irritated, fatigued, or indifferent attitude. The wrong kind of social support is as alienating as separation itself. Reassurance too quickly given, without hearing details of a worry, underscores a patient's feelings of helplessness and estrangement. Supportive relationships always fluctuate. Total consistency, like absolute loyalty, is hard to find. But caregivers, including the psychiatric consultant, should recognize their own incipient frustration or sense of failure.

INABILITY TO THRIVE AND USE AVAILABLE HELP.   Failure to thrive characterizes a deteriorating, debilitating, ultimately fatal disease. From the point of view of the person, failure to thrive is failure itself. Denial is difficult, confidence is shattered, and as a result, the patient refuses to cooperate, as if it were a last gesture of waning autonomy. Failure to thrive brings on disinclination to strive, which most caregivers deplore because they value "will to live" so strongly and so dislike having their own feelings of helplessness stimulated.

REPUDIATION OF AND BY SIGNIFICANT OTHERS.   Physicians are prone to underestimate the importance of significant others in the well-being and distress of their patients. Significant others are people who occupy a place of strong relevance, such that their absence, tactical withdrawal, or tacit repudiation makes a devastating difference in the patient's life. Significant others are those who cannot be easily replaced. Nurses and social workers are usually aware of who visits often, seems most concerned, and asks pertinent questions. Furthermore, even the sickest patient, at least until terminal admission, spends only a fraction of time inside the hospital. Significant others are, therefore, likely to have more undivided influence on what a patient thinks or feels than professional caregivers. Significant others in some respects are fellow sufferers along with the patient.

As fellow sufferers, significant others grieve, become fed up, irritated, uncooperative, querulous, frustrated, and even fall ill themselves. Anger mixes readily with love and compassion, if stirred long enough over a low flame, so that the combination of feeling an incipient loss and being at a loss leads to repudiation of the patient, who reciprocates the ambivalence. Hospice programs recognize ambivalence and fatigue, and so offer respite for exhausted significant others.

DEVALUATION AND DEFECTIVE SELF-ESTEEM.   Draining of confidence and competence is almost as deleterious as wasting of tissues and impairment of organ functions. It is common to find patients who ascribe their illness to a fault or flaw in themselves as people. As dependence grows, self-esteem diminishes. Patients may not often think they cause disease, but they do think that they impose a heavy burden on significant others by their disease. This judgment is only a step away from feeling guilty and evil.

ENCROACHMENT AND EROSION OF AUTONOMY.   Lack of options and reduced freedom to act undermine the staunchest spirit. Symptoms snowball. Along with this, though at a different pace, sickness unto death begins. There is a genuine but indistinct transition point when a very sick person changes to a dying person.

Impersonal death, that is, death by disease, seldom shows the extent of spiritual death, death as a person. Patients usually resist assignment to the dying role, sometimes by becoming angry at those who have been most attentive and devoted. They do not want to languish further or to impose a heavier burden. Yet autonomy would be sacrificed even more by going to a nursing home. Still another reaction to the dying role is extreme denial. "When I get better in a few weeks (there's nothing really wrong now), I'll rest a little, gradually get back my strength, eat more (my appetite's been bad, probably because of this hospital food), and think about working again (maybe only part-time)." Such disjointed optimism is likely to herald impending death.

Encroachment and erosion of autonomy have different expressions, though all are typical of deterioration and decline (see Table 3). Goals are mainly relief, comfort, and care because truce with an implacable enemy is difficult to negotiate. The dilemma now is whether the price of struggle exceeds its value.

DEMORALIZATION AND DEPRESSION.   Common mistakes in assessing pre-terminal patients come from the evaluator's externalizing his or her emotional responses and misjudging expectations. Patients are assumed to deny more than they actually do and to be more depressed than they actually are, as the following case illustrates.

> Mr. L., a 70-year-old former school principal and artist, underwent a colostomy for carcinoma of the colon. Three years later, complaints of low back pain led to discovery of disseminated cancer of the prostate, which was then treated with orchiectomy and estrogens. Although his spirits seemed high, he had no means to support himself and his blind wife.
> The staff was certain that he was deeply depressed but managing to maintain strong denial. In talking with him, the psychiatrist found that he coped by redefining his plight, saying that since his colon cancer had been controlled for three years, perhaps the outlook was equally good for the prostate cancer. He was fully aware of having metastases and knew that he had to depend on public agencies for support and housing. Naturally, despite an effort at higher spirits than he actually felt, he was very sad, but not depressed in the sense of a formal DSM-III diagnosis, and he certainly was not "neurotically" depressed or dejected. In fact, anger far exceeded sadness. He did know that there was very little he could do on his own behalf.

TABLE 3.
DETERIORATION AND DECLINE

IMPAIRMENT	Near-total
QUALITY OF LIFE	Diminished to absent
GOALS	Relief and comfort
ATTITUDE	Resigned or angry
TIME PERSPECTIVE	Closed
DENIAL	Sometimes strong
ACCEPTANCE	Usually partial
COPING	Passive strategies
SYMPTOMS	Many and confluent

This case illustrates the inappropriateness of assigning one expected mood to any patient and ignoring other kinds of distress. Mr. L. was in reasonably good spirits, though he was not, of course, very optimistic. There was partial denial, rationalization, bravado, irritability, anger, and much discouragement. He was, however, not demoralized, because he expected treatment to work.

Other patients state frankly that their morale is low, that they foresee no positive change, and that they have no confidence in being able to cope. They may or may not be depressed. The *diagnosis* of depression is different from the *mood* of depression, which can range from sadness and solemnity to self-hatred and being suicidal (for further discussion, see Chapter 22). Terminal patients are commonly more demoralized than depressed. But the diagnosis and mood of depression are more difficult to discern than demoralization. Depressed patients may be obtunded by illness and medication; morale is easier to ask about.

IMPAIRED COMMUNICATION.   Many preterminal problems can be traced to impaired or misunderstood communication between caregivers and patients. What is said to a patient or significant other may not be what the patient later recalls and reports to other caregivers. Words and phrases are changed according to wishes, fears, and grievances. As a result, patients and significant others play one person against another, so that everyone loses.

Denial and pretense are not very effective by the time a patient reaches preterminality. There is not much left to hide. Although recovery is not a prospect, and patients might properly be insulted when given gratuitous hope, survival on good and comfortable terms for an unspecified period may be within reach.

One of the most important functions of a psychiatric consultant is to clarify distorted communication. Misconceptions can be corrected by compassionate candor and comfortable repetition of responses to questions. This is a significant contribution and permits the staff to reestablish a better relationship, as this case demonstrates.

> Miss M., a 32-year-old art dealer, was referred for psychiatric evaluation because the staff had become annoyed at her vacillation about further chemotherapy. The patient was less concerned about treatment for her advanced ovarian carcinoma than she was with the idea of becoming pregnant. The psychiatrist expected to find a rather detached, superficial, somewhat unapproachable woman who would blandly talk of romantic fantasies of becoming a mother before she died, clearly the stuff of TV drama. He also anticipated much denial because the staff thought her grasp of reality was weak.
>
> He was wrong. The patient was warm, perceptive, articulate, intelligent, and completely aware of her dilemma, knowing that treatment was risky and uncertain and that delay might be deleterious. The idea of pregnancy was not a mere "bride of death" or "mother of sorrow" fantasy.
>
> Her elderly, sick parents were already middle-aged when she was born, an only child. The key to her dilemma rested in a strong family tradition. Several members of her family, over a number of generations, had owned and cared for a large estate. With her death, the estate would be sold because her parents could not manage it by themselves. Family heritage and pride in heritage caused her to want a child to replace herself, not only for her parents who would be bereft, but to prevent the estate from passing into other hands when they died. It all made sense and, for the psychiatrist, explained her procrastination about chemotherapy. Leaving an heir was more important to her than the risk of dying, with or without chemotherapy. Besides, she knew that chemotherapy might make her sterile.
>
> When this was explained to the staff who knew and cared for her, the impaired communication was patched up, and ultimately she chose chemotherapy.

Dealing with Impending Death

In theory, everyone faces death, but that is not the issue. The reality of death is significant only for those who actually hear its rustling and feel its pangs. No psychiatrist or physician, scarcely even a significant other, truly appreciates the solitude of preterminality as death looms.

Impending death has tasks for everyone: The patient is helped to reach an acceptable demise, compatible with the best standards of earlier life. Significant others begin to grieve, a process that usually goes on for months after the actual death. The staff involved bring order to their efforts, which end in death, and try to avoid emotional depletion.

The key to impending death from a psychiatrist's viewpoint is *informed collaboration*. The task is not to console, pretend, explain, offer unrealistic hope, or urge total resignation. To promote a better quality of death, the psychiatrist who follows dying patients will look for points of vulnerability, as well as for problems that have not yet been coped with.

Specific directions for psychosocial and psychological interventions are difficult to set up, because spontaneity and serendipity cannot be cultivated or anticipated. However, a few obvious warnings and suggestions might be useful as guidelines.

Do not expect the same motivation found among healthy, verbal, psychotherapy patients. Dying patients are very sick. They have urgent physical problems to deal with. Illness, fatigue, confusion, medication effects, and frequent interruptions prevent long or deep sessions. Extended interviews are seldom needed to exert a positive influence.

Sit down, make eye-to-eye contact, and avoid the unnatural power posture of looking down on a recumbent patient who already feels submissive and dependent enough. Be willing, however, to admit that sickness and disease have superior strength, compared with our limited capacities. It is better to listen well than to speak foolishly.

Do not confuse empathy with being a surrogate mourner. It is important to respect at all times the plight and courage of the dying patient. Would we do as well?

Seek information, but do not limit inquiries to fact-finding about specific times, places, treatments, and people involved. Do not ignore physical complaints, but do not repeat questions already asked by primary physicians. Try to be familiar with basic facts about the underlying disease and customary treatment.

Do not ask questions that call for a yes or no answer. Such questions lead nowhere, and simply show that the consultant is in a hurry. Communication, to be effective beyond the limits of information, must be compassionate, calm, simple, direct, and candid. False heartiness or lugubrious solemnity is not needed.

No style or line of interviewing and interceding suits everyone, but here are a few questions that can be shaped as suitable and that might lead to picking up points of vulnerability in the patient.

> What do you see as the most important problem you have to face at present, aside from getting proper treatment?
> Looking back, how have you changed during your illness?
> What about the other people close to you? Tell me about them.

If you were to remind yourself of good things that happened in the past, when you felt at your best, what would they be?

If you could, how would you change some things that happened?

What advice might you give to someone else?

Phrasing, of course, differs. The aim is to open a path to the pressing problems unique for that patient. But do not be overcome with such zeal that you aim to rectify what cannot be corrected or reversed. A little help goes a long way, unexpectedly.

How Useful Are Psychiatrists?

There is an authentic, though modest, role for psychiatric consultants in the case of dying patients. The psychiatrist dealing with impending or preterminal death assesses and alleviates misunderstanding. The psychiatrist also does as much as possible to help the patient cope and to promote a significant survival along with an appropriate, befitting demise.

The psychiatric consultant cannot be overly concerned about or distracted by anecdotes about alternative therapies. Relaxation techniques, guided imagery, and so forth are acceptable procedures and might contribute to comfort, not remission. The atmosphere should include self-respect, reflection, even repose and relaxation, with controlled, not misdirected, emotion. Consulting with the staff can be a strong contribution when these caregivers are receptive. After all, they have major responsibility, carry out onerous duties, and experience the frustration of caring for a patient who will not get well. Moreover, we seldom appreciate that staff members suffer many of the same emotional problems faced by patients and significant others. Physical complaints take another form, but the staff often lack rewards and recognition commensurate with their efforts and the demands made on them.

Summary Advice

1. Sit down and be unhurried.
2. Listen carefully, but raise questions that encourage elaboration.
3. Formulate areas of primary concern, and try to spot tendencies to slide over problems and dilemmas.
4. Look for emotional pressure points. Because they hurt, be gentle, tactful, and persistent.
5. Separate problems that can be coped with from insurmountable ones.

6. Keep your own composure, without feigning objectivity or pretending certainty you do not feel.
7. Replace pity with compassionate candor. Resist the temptation to deny or console gratuitously.
8. If you do not expect too much, optimism can be helpful to you and the patient.
9. Be neither sad nor cynical. Do not try to do too much.
10. This is the patient's only death. Try to make sure it is a reasonably good one.

Suggested Readings

Ahmed, P. (ed.) (1981). *Living and Dying with Cancer.* New York: Elsevier.

Feifel, H. (ed.) (1977). *New Meanings of Death.* New York: McGraw-Hill.

Feigenberg, L. (1980). *Terminal Care.* New York: Brunner/Mazel.

Garfield, C. (ed.) (1978). *Psychosocial Care of the Dying Patient.* New York: McGraw-Hill.

Grollman, E. (ed.) (1967). *Explaining Death to Children.* Boston: Beacon Press.

Holland, J. (1973). Psychological aspects of cancer. In *Cancer Medicine,* ed. J. Holland and E. Frei, pp. 991–1021. Philadelphia: Lea & Febiger.

Weisman, A.D. (1972). *On Dying and Denying: A Psychiatric Study of Terminality.* New York: Behavioral Publications.

Weisman, A.D. (1974). *The Realization of Death: A Guide for the Psychological Autopsy.* New York: Jason Aronson.

Weisman, A.D. (1979). *Coping with Cancer.* New York: McGraw-Hill.

Weisman, A.D. (1980). Thanatology. In *Comprehensive Textbook of Psychiatry/III,* ed. H. Kaplan, A. Freedman, and B. Sadock, pp. 1748–1759. Baltimore: Williams & Wilkins.

Somatic Interventions

Psychiatrists in general hospitals need expertise in the use of physical treatment modalities, including antipsychotic drugs, minor tranquilizers, antidepressant drugs, and electroconvulsive therapy. In addition to knowing the indications for these treatments, the psychiatrist must be aware of their limitations and dangers, especially in patients with medical illnesses or medical complications of their psychiatric illnesses. Of paramount importance in patient management is recognizing the conditions that respond to physical treatment modalities, including delirium, withdrawal syndromes, depression, and pain. Recognition and treatment of depression in the medically ill are especially complicated in that many of the signs and symptoms of depression overlap with nonspecific symptoms of illness. Accordingly, much attention is paid in this section to the diagnosis of those depressive disorders that respond to antidepressant medication and those that are more responsive to other forms of therapy, including psychological measures.

F.G.

CHAPTER 20

Acutely Psychotic and Delirious Patients

BARRY J. FENTON, M.D.

Acute psychosis in patients on medical/surgical services is the most frequent reason for emergency psychiatric consultation. Few experiences are as frightening to medical and nursing staff or as disruptive to ward routines as agitated, disoriented patients. Many hospitalized medical/surgical patients experience functional psychosis or delirium during the course of their illnesses; treatment of such patients can be difficult and dangerous. Side effects of the most useful antipsychotic drugs become great hazards, as do the interactions of neuroleptics and the drugs used to treat the patients' medical conditions. Treatment of these patients on medical/surgical services is possible if care is taken to properly diagnose and address the underlying causes of the acute psychosis.

There are five overlapping categories of medical/surgical patients to be considered: delirious patients, demented patients with complicating delirium, chronically mentally ill individuals who are hospitalized for medical/surgical problems, patients whose mental illnesses relapse during nonpsychiatric hospitalizations, and patients who develop functional psychoses for the first time.

The Delirious Patient

Delirium is an acute condition that is life-threatening, reversible, and readily diagnosable by careful clinical examination. Some surveys show that up to 30 percent of general medical patients experience delirium during their hospital stay; delirium may occur in as many as 45 percent of older patients.

Left untreated, a delirium may resolve spontaneously, progress to a non-reversible dementia, or lead to irreversible coma or death.

Delirium is primarily a disorder of cerebral insufficiency. Any systemic or intracranial disorder that causes diffuse metabolic impairment of brain function can result in delirium. Dehydration, fasting, hypoglycemia, hypothyroidism, hyperthyroidism, hypoxia, vitamin B_{12} deficiency, postictal states, alcohol, sedatives, sleep deprivation, chemical withdrawal, drug interactions, and cardiac, hepatic, and renal failure are all common causes of delirium seen in hospitalized medical/surgical patients.

Delirious patients are confused. They are awake but disoriented, most frequently to time, less frequently to place. Higher cortical functions such as memory, perception, and attention are impaired. Visual hallucinations and misperceptions occur frequently. The affects expressed most commonly are anxiety, fear, and depression. Periods of confusion may alternate with intervals of lucidity. During the lucid periods, patients may recall having been confused and frightened. It is useful to employ a graded mental status exam, such as the one devised by Folstein, Folstein, and McHugh, several times a day to obtain an accurate picture of the changing mental status. The electroencephalogram is pathognomonic of delirium. It usually shows diffuse slowing, but there may be superimposed fast activity if the patient is in a state of high arousal and agitation.

Delirium often worsens during periods of reduced or unfamiliar sensory stimuli. "Sundowning" and "ICU psychosis" are frequently caused by loss of a familiar and comforting environment and the absence of orienting stimuli such as meals or of visual cues in windowless rooms. Night lights, pictures of families, radios, clocks, and background music can often be helpful in these situations. The staff should actively orient these patients and maintain cheerful, supportive, and personal contact with them.

The treatment of delirium begins with establishing its cause. Many deliria can be treated without drugs, especially if patients are confused in a passive and quiet manner. Such patients may require only supportive environmental measures while the etiologies of their deliria are identified and corrected. When delirium is related to a closed head injury, psychotropic drugs may cloud the clinical picture and alter the level of consciousness, and it is best to use the patient's actual, unaltered level of consciousness to monitor brain function.

A drug-induced delirium can also be treated without drugs: Often, withdrawing the precipitating drug is sufficient. Cimetidine can cause delirium, as can steroids. Barbiturates and benzodiazepines frequently cause delirium in the elderly. The elderly are also sensitive to the anticholinergic side effects of many drugs such as antidepressants, antihistamines, antipsychotics, and antiarrhythmics. In certain individuals, prednisone in doses of 80 mg or more per day can precipitate symptoms of delirium or psychosis.

Delirium may also be caused by sudden withdrawal of hypnotics, sedatives, and minor tranquilizers taken chronically by patients prior to hospitalization. In these instances, the drug may need to be restarted and withdrawn slowly over a period of a week to ten days to avoid reprecipitating a delirium or provoking withdrawal seizures. The equivalent dosage is established by giving the drug in question or a short-acting barbiturate in divided doses until patients' sensoria clear or they become slightly groggy and dysarthric. Patients who are regular, but moderate, drinkers may experience subclinical delirium tremens on the second or third hospital day. This syndrome, characterized by increased pulse and blood pressure, agitation, tremor, diaphoresis, and mild disorientation can be treated with benzodiazepines (as indicated in Chapter 21, "Alcohol Withdrawal").

Many patients receive several potential delirium-causing drugs, and it may be impossible to ascertain which one(s) caused the delirium. In these cases, delirium may be caused by the combination of drugs, not by a single medication. It may be necessary to temporarily withdraw all drugs and to restart them one at a time, beginning with the drug most needed medically. This is particularly the case with drugs with cumulative anticholinergic effects.

Psychotropic drugs do not reverse cerebral insufficiency. If a person is mildly disoriented, but quiet and cooperative, there is no reason to prescribe additional medication that will only complicate the treatment regimen. Psychotropic drugs are indicated for delirium when patients are agitated, uncooperative, uncomfortable, or unable to obtain adequate rest. In these situations, a useful drug is haloperidol, 1 to 5 mg PO or IM two to four times per day. Dosage is titrated against levels of agitation. In the event of an extrapyramidal crisis, such as an acute dystonia, benztropine mesylate, 1 to 2 mg IM, is helpful. Should Parkinsonian rigidity or akathisia begin to develop, a regular dose of benztropine mesylate, 1 to 2 mg PO b.i.d., will usually be adequate to deal with the side effects.

The Demented, Delirious Patient

Patients with a previous history of dementia often undergo an acute change in mental status after admission to the hospital. Because dementia is usually an insidious deterioration of the mental faculties, patients are often able to develop compensating mechanisms that enable them to function at surprisingly high levels in their home environments. Changes in their environment can cause such individuals to decompensate; the emotional and/or physical stress of an illness and subsequent hospitalization often can precipitate an acute delirium.

A psychiatric consultant was called to see Mr. N., age 66, because of "changing mental status" since hospital admission. The patient had been admitted via the emergency room four days earlier because of shortness of breath and chest pain. He had an abnormal EKG at the time of admission, but all other clinical and laboratory findings were unremarkable. Subsequent EKGs normalized rapidly. He was kept under observation and started on nitroglycerin p.r.n. for pain. On the third hospital day, he was found disoriented to time and place; he thought his intern was his nephew. When disorientation persisted throughout the day, a psychiatric consultation was initiated.

The mental status exam revealed an alert, mildly agitated man. He said he was scared of being in the "factory" and wanted to speak to his "nephew" (the medical intern). He could not recall any objects after two minutes, could not repeat any digits, and refused to do serial threes. He could not recall anything after 1979 and thought the year was 1979. The working diagnosis was delirium. He was treated with orienting and supportive measures. The social service worker found that he lived alone, received "Meals on Wheels," and had no family. His neighbors reported him to be friendly and quiet, and "odd," but they could not say in what way. On the fifth hospital day, he was told that he had not had a heart attack and that he would be able to return home in a few days. On the sixth hospital day, he had a CT scan, which revealed marked widening of cerebral ventricles and cortical atrophy. A second mental status exam showed that he was still disoriented to time but he was no longer agitated. He knew where he was hospitalized and where he had lived and could recall two of three objects after three minutes. He was discharged to his home on the seventh day, with a visiting nurse scheduled to see him every day. The nurse reported one week later that he was doing well.

This case is an illustration of a delirium superimposed on a dementia. The most likely causes of the patient's delirium were his fear of having had a heart attack and his hospitalization. With the added psychological stress, his compromised cerebral capacity was overwhelmed, and this was probably sufficient to precipitate an acute delirium. He responded well to simplification of his environment, support, and reassurance that he had not had a heart attack. After his delirium resolved, it became clear that his mental baseline was not normal but that he would be able to return to his previous level of psychosocial functioning.

The Chronically Mentally Ill Patient

People who enter hospitals with known chronic mental illnesses are usually taking regular doses of an antipsychotic agent or of lithium. Psychiatrists see that psychotropic medications are continued in doses sufficient to keep patients' symptoms suppressed, but they make certain that these medications will have no adverse interaction with other medications to be prescribed. Antipsychotics with strong anticholinergic activity (thioridazine, chlorpromazine, fluphenazine) may need to be temporarily replaced by medications with less anticholinergic activity, such as haloperidol. Instead of having a patient continue taking a potentially cardiotoxic phenothiazine such as thioridazine, a butyrophenone such as haloperidol may need to be substituted. Antipsychotic agents should be discontinued for at least 24 hours prior to general or spinal anesthesia because of their hypotensive effects and their potentiation of anticholinergic agents. They may be restarted in small doses as soon as patients' vital signs have been stable for 24 hours, with careful attention paid to potential urinary retention. Should patients become agitated in the immediate postoperative period, haloperidol, 1 to 5 mg IM every four hours, can be used until patients' regular medication can be restarted.

Patients on lithium need to have their lithium levels monitored carefully. Lithium is reabsorbed preferentially to sodium. Patients taking sodium-wasting diuretics may therefore need to have their serum lithium levels measured daily and their lithium dose lowered. Close attention should also be paid to fluid-restricted patients; lithium should be included in osmotic calculations. Early signs of lithium toxicity—coarse tremor, nystagmus, delirium, and/or vomiting—should be detected quickly and the medication reduced or discontinued, lest convulsions or coma ensue.

When individuals with chronic mental illnesses become more disorganized, agitated, or delusional during the course of medical/surgical hospitalizations, it is not always necessary to alter their medication. As with all patients, illness and hospitalization are frightening to those with chronic mental illness; reassurance about and explanation of their medical treatment and the hospital routine may help to reduce anxiety and agitation.

Patients with chronic mental illness may also be more sensitive to disturbances of their wake-sleep cycles. Nighttime sedation with a mild hypnotic will often provide adequate sleep. Benzodiazepines are preferable to barbiturates for sedation. It may be necessary to add a bedtime dose of the antipsychotic medication patients are currently receiving.

High-potency neuroleptics should be discontinued in mentally ill individuals who become hyperthyroid because these drugs can produce fatal pseudobulbar palsy. Mentally ill people who develop muscular stiffness and fever should also be removed from high-potency neuroleptics to prevent the development of a full-blown neuroleptic malignant syndrome.

The Relapsing Mentally Ill Patient

Individuals who enter general hospitals with a history of past mental illness need not be started on prophylactic medication, although there is some evidence that lithium may be useful as a prophylaxis against recurrence of mania induced by steroid therapy. Physicians should attempt to avoid uncertainty and ambiguity when treating patients with a history of mental illness. As with the chronic mentally ill, physicians should carefully explain diagnostic procedures and the reasons for ordering them, especially when unusual machinery or invasive methods are to be used. As physical symptoms appear and medical therapeutics are ordered, clear and precise explanations are important. Particularly at these times, consultants must be alert to the possibility of reemergence of psychotic ideation. For example, it is not uncommon for schizophrenic patients on dialysis to incorporate their machines into their "physical" boundaries so that routine adjusting of the machine may be experienced as painful or as a molestation.

The first signs of relapse are loss of sleep, confusion, and changes of affect. Care must be taken to distinguish these signs from delirium. Physicians must also be careful not to rely solely on patients' histories or old charts for psychiatric diagnoses. Many patients whose illness was first diagnosed as schizophrenia have developed clear-cut bipolar affective disorders. Conversely, many people earlier diagnosed as manic have developed paranoid schizophrenia. A careful history from family, friends, and previous hospital charts should be compiled and checked against current symptomatology. When uncertain of the type of functional psychosis, the best treatment is a neuroleptic, given in divided doses in sufficient amounts to render patients slightly drowsy during the day and to enable them to sleep through the night. The best all-around neuroleptic for the acutely psychotic patient is haloperidol, 5 to 10 mg IM each hour or until the patient becomes drowsy, with a maximum daily dose of 30 mg. Initial doses of 10 to 30 mg have been used, but blood pressure must be carefully monitored at these doses. Patients can usually be changed to oral medication after the first 24 hours (see Chapter 5, on rapid neuroleptization).

The Onset of a New Functional Psychosis

The most likely cause of a functional psychosis in a patient on a medical/surgical ward is exacerbation of a dormant, but well-documented, mental illness or a delirium. But if the family and staff know of no past history of mental illness (and if delirium has been ruled out), the consultant can consider the onset of a new psychiatric illness of a functional nature.

The three most common disorders are brief reactive psychosis, schizophreniform psychosis, and dissociative reaction. The following case describes a brief reactive psychosis in a man with an underlying paranoid personality disorder.

> Mr. O., a 29-year-old single Latin-American unemployed dock loader, was admitted for workup of bloody diarrhea and fever of two weeks'

duration. On admission he appeared cheerful but quite tense. He was quite cooperative but volunteered little information about his personal life. He asked no questions when given the opportunity to do so by the admitting physician and showed no emotion when told he would have a sigmoidoscopy the following morning.

During the night, be became increasingly agitated, and by 7:00 A.M. he began yelling loudly that he was being attacked by some of the female nurses and aides. He became convinced that he was being singled out and spied on because of his sexual prowess. He was belligerent and tried to assault a dietary aide who entered his room. In the ensuing melee, he was subdued and sedated with two 5-mg doses of parenteral haloperidol given 15 minutes apart.

After two hours, he became calm and no longer heard voices taunting him. Maintained on oral haloperidol for the next three days, he confessed to one of his physicians that he was very fearful of the approaching colonic examination. Six days after admission, he was back to his usual self. The procedure was explained to him in detail. He was able to express his concern and, since he had formed a better alliance with his medical team, was able to tolerate the sigmoidoscopic examination without undue anxiety.

Psychiatrists must be careful to distinguish functional psychosis from delirium. Although insomnia, anxiety, agitation, and affective lability are common to both, other findings are more peculiar to one or to the other. Delirium is usually typified by disorientation; functional psychosis is not. Auditory hallucinations are more typical of functional psychosis, visual hallucinations are frequent in delirium. Fluctuating levels of consciousness, disturbance of attention, and impaired recent memory are also more typical of delirium. The history is another critical item. Although delirium begins abruptly, careful questioning of psychotic patients, their friends, and relatives often reveals the existence of prodromal symptoms over several weeks prior to the actual onset of delirium.

Once the diagnosis of functional psychosis is established, antipsychotic medication can be started. The goal of initial treatment is to eliminate the symptoms of psychosis without producing unnecessary side effects or interfering with the ongoing medical/surgical treatment. In this setting it is more important to use sufficient chemotherapy to ensure the continuity of medical/surgical treatment than it is to distinguish between schizophrenia and manic-depressive illness.

In addition to chemotherapy, every effort must be made to simplify patient's environment and to reduce environmental demands. Psychotic patients must be treated in safe and protected settings to ensure privacy and dignity as well as to hold disruptions to the usual ward routine to a minimum. Consulting psychiatrists must also adequately diffuse the fear and anxiety of the house officers and nursing staff treating these patients. Just as psychiatrists may not be familiar with the procedures for a cardiac arrest, medical ward nurses and staff are usually unprepared to deal effectively with acutely psychotic patients. Clear and unambiguous explanations of diagnosis and treatment can go a long way toward avoiding demands for immediate transfer of patients to psychiatric units. For the sake of future working relationships, it is also important to facilitate transfer when patients no longer need medical/surgical care. In some cases, the functional psychosis will subside as the medical illness subsides and will require only a brief period of maintenance medication. In other cases, psychiatric hospitalization and long-term drug treatment may be indicated.

In sum, acute psychosis and delirium are medical emergencies that require rapid, careful diagnosis by psychiatric consultants. Once the diagnosis is made, effective treatment can be instituted to alleviate the acute condition and the underlying conditions can then be evaluated. Consultants should also help relieve the house officers' and nursing staff's tension in this frequently frightening situation.

Suggested Readings

Anderson, W.H., and Kuehnle, J.D. (1981). Diagnosis and early management of acute psychosis. *New England Journal of Medicine* 305:1128–1130.

DeVaul, Richard A. (1981). Delirium: a neglected medical emergency. *American Family Physician* 24:152–157.

Folstein, M.F., Folstein, S.E., and McHugh, P.R. (1975). "Mini-mental state," a practical method for grading the cognitive state of patients for the clinicians. *Journal of Psychiatric Research* 12:189–198.

Lipowski, Z.J. (1983). Transient cognitive disorders (delirium, acute confusional states) in the elderly. *American Journal of Psychiatry* 140:1426–1436.

May, D.C., Morris, S.W., Stewart, R.M., Fenton, B.J., and Gaffney, F.A. (1983). Neuroleptic malignant syndrome: response to dantrolene sodium. *Annals of Internal Medicine* 98:183–184.

Murray, G.C. (1978). Confusion, delirium, and dementia. In *Massachusetts General Hospital Handbook of General Hospital Psychiatry*, ed. T.P. Hackett and N.H. Cassem, pp. 93–116. St. Louis, Mo.: C.V. Mosby.

Weiner, M.F. (1979). Haloperidol, hyperthyroidism, and sudden death. *American Journal of Psychiatry* 136:717–718.

CHAPTER 21

Alcohol Withdrawal

THOMAS P. BERESFORD, M.D.
DENNIS LOW, M.D.
RICHARD C.W. HALL, M.D.

Alcoholism must be suspected before alcohol withdrawal can be diagnosed and treated. A middle-aged derelict with terminal cirrhosis of the liver is atypical of the 5 to 10 million Americans who suffer from alcoholism. Most people suffering from alcoholism have families and jobs. They constitute the greatest untreated population suffering from a treatable illness in our time.

Alcoholism is an addictive illness whose signs are tolerance to alcohol *or* withdrawal symptoms on cessation of drinking *and* either the loss of control phenomenon when a drinking bout starts *or* a history of social decline associated with alcohol abuse. These four symptoms—tolerance, withdrawal, loss of control, and social decline—constitute the principal signs of addiction to alcohol. An episode of alcohol withdrawal is therefore a major diagnostic finding of the underlying illness of alcoholism.

Estimates of prevalence of alcoholism in general-hospital patients range from 14 to 50 percent. Patients in whom this condition is not recognized and who are therefore not treated are at considerably greater risk for developing the more serious complications of alcohol withdrawal such as seizures and delirium tremens.

Patients in the general hospital who suffer from alcohol withdrawal are likely to be troublesome individuals. Many discharges against medical advice are sought by patients suffering from alcohol abuse, especially when their alcohol withdrawal has been inadequately treated, leaving them no option but to seek relief from their discomfort by leaving the hospital to obtain alcohol.

Of those patients remaining in the hospital wth alcohol withdrawal symptoms, 7 percent are likely to develop withdrawal seizures and as many as 5 percent may experience delirium tremens. Death from withdrawal seizures is rare, but death occurs in 5 to 10 percent of untreated delirium tremens cases.

Diagnosis

Until recently, alcohol withdrawal was equated with delirium tremens. More careful observation of alcohol withdrawal has resulted in the delineation of the acute alcohol withdrawal syndrome as contrasted with other withdrawal phenomena such as seizures, hallucinations, and delirium tremens.

The acute alcohol withdrawal syndrome generally occurs within 6 to 12 hours of a precipitous drop in patients' blood alcohol level. To assess this situation, physicians must ask when patients had their last drink. The presence of alcohol in patients' blood does not rule out the possibility of withdrawal. A history of patients' recent drinking behavior obtained from families, friends, or from patients themselves may assist physicians, but the diagnosis of acute alcohol withdrawal syndrome rests on the physical examination.

The symptoms of acute alcohol withdrawal syndrome are those of sympathetic nervous system discharge: a pulse greater than 110 beats per minute, a mild increase in blood pressure, a degree or two increase in temperature (Fahrenheit), an increase in the rate of respiration, diaphoresis, fine tremor of the upper limbs, nausea and/or vomiting, and profound anxiety. More striking symptoms can include disturbances in tactile, auditory, or visual perceptions, visual hallucinations, and clouding of the sensorium. Clouding of the sensorium is an especially ominous sign.

Standardized assessment protocols for withdrawal symptoms have been designed by Gross and associates and by Shaw and associates. We recommend them for routine use because they offer a quantitative measure of the severity of the acute alcohol withdrawal syndrome that is helpful in clinical management. However, we caution that further research must be done with these instruments before clinicians will be able to place a prognostic value on quantitative symptom observations.

Uncomplicated acute alcohol withdrawal has a five- to seven-day course. During that time, patients may experience any or all of the above symptoms without developing withdrawal seizures or delirium tremens. Up to 40 percent of patients require pharmacotherapy. When in doubt, clinicians should use pharmacotherapy. Uncomplicated alcohol withdrawal, however, may be greatly ameliorated by supportive psychosocial contact.

Alcohol withdrawal seizures are generally of the grand mal type and occur most frequently about 24 hours after the last drink. They may, however, occur at any time during the alcohol withdrawal period. A history of previous alcohol withdrawal seizures is useful in establishing the likelihood of further convulsions. A negative history of seizures is of little importance.

The physical examination is especially helpful in assessing the imminence of withdrawal seizures. The presence of two or more beats of ankle clonus (produced by acute dorsiflexion of the foot) in the context of recent alcohol use suggests that a seizure will occur within the next few hours and demands aggressive treatment of the withdrawal syndrome. Patients who present with a history of withdrawal seizures must also be treated aggressively. Withdrawal seizures often occur in threes. Patients may undergo one or two seizures without complication only to die from asphyxiation or status epilepticus during the third seizure. Clinicians must, therefore, prevent seizures.

Delirium tremens, diagnosed by the observation of clouded sensorium, auditory or visual hallucinations, and a profound sympathetic discharge, most frequently occurs on the third day after patients' last use of alcohol. "DTs" may occur at any time during the alcohol withdrawal process, however, and have even been observed two weeks after cessation of heavy alcohol use. Because of the high associated death rate, delirium tremens is a medical emergency. Proper pharmacotherapy and supportive medical care must be initiated following admission to the hospital. Because these patients are often belligerent and provocative, physicians must pay careful attention to these patients' physical safety. Soft restraints and rapid sedation are often needed. Careful medical and nursing care for these patients must be continued, since this condition may take as long as two weeks to resolve.

Treatment

The treatment of alcohol withdrawal is symptomatic. The target symptoms are anxiety, tremor, and other symptoms of sympathetic hyperactivity. In withdrawal seizures, the target symptom is the seizure itself. In delirium tremens, the target symptoms include clouded sensorium, profound sympathetic hyperactivity, and hallucinations.

Prompt and early treatment of the acute withdrawal syndrome will obviate withdrawal seizures and delirium tremens. At present, we have no reliable clinical method of predicting which patients suffering from the acute alcohol withdrawal syndrome will develop withdrawal seizures or delirium tremens. Pharmacological intervention is therefore indicated when an acute alcohol withdrawal syndrome exists.

Standard treatment of the alcohol withdrawal syndrome entails use of long-acting benzodiazepines. Most patients can be treated with oral doses of diazepam or chlordiazepoxide. The aim of treatment is to aggressively administer sufficient amounts of benzodiazepine to give symptomatic relief. In our experience, the tachycardia, tremor, and anxiety associated with acute alcohol withdrawal syndrome offer the best index of treatment response. Patients should be given a large dose of a benzodiazepine within the first few hours—as much as 20 mg of diazepam *or* 100 mg of chlordiazepoxide. Patients should be monitored hourly and given as much of the benzodiazepine as needed to alleviate withdrawal symptoms without inducing somnolence. A maximum of 300 mg of chlordiazepoxide or 80 mg of diazepam may be given during the first 24 hours after a patient's last drink. Patients whose symptoms are not relieved at this dosage should be reassessed for intercurrent conditions before giving more of the drug. That dosage is rapidly tapered to a maximum of 200 mg chlordiazepoxide or 20 to 40 mg of diazepam on the second day, and a maximum of 100 mg chlordiazepoxide or 20 mg of diazepam on the third day. The benzodiazepine can be discontinued on the fourth day. Benzodiazepines have very long half-lives and will continue to exert an effect during days four and five of withdrawal. Their half-lives are significantly lengthened in elderly patients, who should be given smaller loading doses and smaller daily doses during the first three days of withdrawal. In elderly patients, the drugs may remain active as long as ten days to two weeks.

Symptoms of severe withdrawal such as tachycardia, fever, hypertension, gross tremulousness, hyperreflexia, clonus, clouded sensorium, and hallucinations are indications for initial treatment with intravenous diazepam—an initial injection of 10 mg IV followed by 5 mg IV every 5 minutes until the patient is calm or the signs of central nervous system hyperexcitability have abated. Oral diazepam in doses of 5 to 10 mg every 1 to 4 hours may then be administered.

For patients in acute alcohol withdrawal who also suffer from liver failure or emphysema, oxazepam, carefully titrated to reduce the target symptoms, may be the drug of choice. It is conjugated and removed by the kidneys, and its short duration of action facilitates the management of respiratory depression.

Avoid undertreatment. Patients must be carefully titrated during the first day of their withdrawal syndrome; they should not simply be placed on a routine of chlordiazepoxide, 25 mg q.i.d. General-hospital patients are often undertreated for their acute alcohol withdrawal and may therefore seek inappropriately to leave the hospital. Any patient with a history of excessive alcohol intake and symptoms of withdrawal who seeks to leave the hospital deserves a more careful treatment assessment before being allowed to leave.

Intramuscular injections of diazepam or chlordiazepoxide are contraindicated. Both of these agents are lipid-soluble, and they tend to remain crystallized in muscle tissue at the site of injection and are absorbed erratically.

Experimental evidence suggests that acute alcohol withdrawal syndrome may also be treated effectively with an intravenous loading dose of a benzodiazepine, such as diazepam, given on the first day of acute withdrawal, with no further benzodiazepine administration. Further data must establish the effectiveness of this technique before it can be recommended as standard pratice, however.

Patients who develop auditory or visual hallucinations deserve a careful trial of benzodiazepine with the addition of an antipsychotic agent if adequate benzodiazepine doses do not lessen or eliminate the hallucinations in 24 to 72 hours. Antipsychotics alone are not indicated for the treatment of withdrawal. They are used to control symptoms of hallucinations in a clear sensorium (i.e., alcoholic hallucinosis), which can occur during, or on cessation of, a prolonged drinking period. In the latter case, thioridazine is the drug of choice because it does not lower the seizure threshold. It is given in doses of 50 to 150 mg PO. Most of the other available antipsychotics lower the seizure threshold significantly, a great risk in patients with alcohol withdrawal. If thioridazine or mesoridazine is contraindicated for any reason, haloperidol appears to lower the seizure threshold less than other antipsychotic agents. Generally, the presence of an alcohol withdrawal syndrome is a relative contraindication to other antipsychotic agents. As the benzodiazepines are specific treatment for the syndrome of delirium tremens, antipsychotics are specific for the symptoms of alcohol hallucinosis. They should be gradually discontinued when the hallucinations and the alcohol withdrawal syndrome have ceased.

Finally, clinicians should presume that all patients in alcohol withdrawal are vitamin-deficient. Patients should be given 100 mg of parenteral thiamine prior to beginning parenteral glucose therapy and an additional 50 to 100 mg of thiamine daily by mouth. Otherwise, there is risk of brain-cell death because of impaired cellular glucose metabolism. In addition, it is wise to routinely administer a daily multivitamin tablet.

Overly aggressive replacement of the electrolytes, especially sodium, may result in permanent damage to the pons. Gradual replacement of electrolytes is best in patients suffering from alcohol withdrawal.

The following cases present common problems and principles. Fever and altered mental status require a lumbar puncture to rule out meningitis, even when the symptoms are mild or when meningismus is absent. Fever and altered mental status can be entirely due to delirium tremens, but a lumbar puncture must still be performed. Patients with chronic alcoholism must also be considered immunocompromised and susceptible to infections, as the following case demonstrates.

> Mr. P., age 47, was admitted with alcohol withdrawal tremors, mild disorientation, and a temperature of 101 degrees, with the presumptive diagnosis of impending delirium tremens. The neurological examination was within normal limits, and there was no nuchal rigidity. A lumbar puncture was not done on admission because of the lack of meningismus. On the second day of hospitalization a lumbar puncture revealed

pleocytosis. Antibiotic coverage was begun immediately, and *Escherichia coli* grew out of the spinal fluid culture.

On a rare occasion, the tremors that begin within 48 hours of the last alcohol intake will persist. Tremors may also be due to thyrotoxicosis, familial tremors, tardive dyskinesia, or Parkinsonism. Alcohol tremors may respond to a beta blocker, such as propranolol, as the following case illustrates.

> Mr. Q., age 56, was admitted to an alcohol rehabilitation program. His blood alcohol level was zero, but he had mild withdrawal tremors. He had a previous history of alcohol withdrawal tremors. There was no known history of familial tremors. After 30 days in the program, the mild tremors persisted. Thyroid studies were normal. The tremors responded to low-dose propranolol.

The next two cases illustrate that alcoholic individuals' seizures are not always due to alcoholism.

> Ms. R., age 42, was admitted after a grand mal seizure. She had a history of chronic alcoholism, and her current drinking could have accounted for a withdrawal seizure. Since this was her first seizure, the evaluation included an EEG and a lumbar puncture. The lumbar puncture was negative, but the EEG revealed a focus of epileptoid spikes. A thorough history revealed an earlier head trauma suffered in an auto accident that occurred when she was intoxicated.

Patients with alcohol dependence often experience seizures related to head trauma. Diphenylhydantoin (phenytoin) may be started immediately and withdrawn if the subsequent EEG is normal. An EEG should be done about two weeks after the seizure, as it may still be temporarily abnormal as a consequence of the seizure itself. Chronic phenytoin therapy is not recommended in the case of simple alcohol withdrawal seizure if the follow-up EEG is normal. The woman in this case did require chronic phenytoin therapy.

> Mr. S., age 60, was admitted after an observed grand mal seizure. His previous medical records revealed a long history of acute and chronic alcoholism, including withdrawal seizures. This seizure was presumed to be the same, and the patient was admitted in a state of postictal confusion. Upon improving, the patient vehemently denied any alcohol intake and claimed to have taken disulfiram for the preceding few months, both statements being substantiated by his daughter. The patient's blood alcohol level was zero on admission. The possibility of disulfiram encephalopathy was considered. An EEG revealed a pattern consistent with disulfiram encephalopathy.

Patients with affective or anxiety disorders sometimes drink in an effort to relieve symptoms. Similarly, patients with underlying thought disorders occasionally develop secondary alcoholism in an attempt to relieve their hallucinations. A detailed history of the course of the symptoms as well as the alcohol intake assist in separating primary alcoholism from alcoholism secondary to an underlying thought disorder, as seen in the next case.

> Mr. T., age 32, was admitted to an alcohol rehabilitation program. He gave a history of auditory and visual hallucinations related to his alcohol intake. This was initially judged to be alcohol withdrawal hallucinosis. During his stay in the program, the patient displayed a blunted affect and admitted to auditory hallucinations of threatening voices. A detailed history revealed that his auditory hallucinations began in his teenage years, prior to heavy alcohol intake. In fact, part of his heavy alcohol intake was to relieve the hallucinations, as the voices did not frighten him when he was inebriated. Treatment was then directed to his thought disorders.

Prompt diagnosis and recommendations for aggressive pharmacological intervention allow for a marked reduction in the morbidity as well as the mortality of the alcohol withdrawal syndrome. Once patients have been seen safely through the crisis of alcohol withdrawal, psychiatrists should begin or assist others in beginning the longer-term diagnosis and treatment of the underlying alcoholism and any other associated chronic illnesses.

Suggested Readings

Beresford, T.P. (1979). Alcoholism consultation and general hospital psychiatry. *General Hospital Psychiatry* 1:293–300.

Beresford, T.P., Low, D., Adduci, R., and Goggans, F. (1982). Alcoholism assessment on an orthopaedic surgery service. *Journal of Bone and Joint Surgery* 64A:730–733.

Beresford, T.P., Low, D., Hall, R.C.W., Adduci, R., and Goggans, F. (1982). A computerized diagnostic biochemical profile for the detection of alcoholism. *Psychosomatics* 23:713–720.

Frecker, R.C., Shas, J.M., Zilm, D.H., Jacob, M.S., Sellers, E.M., and Degani, N. (1982). Nonpharmacological supportive care compared to chlormethiazole infusion in the management of severe acute alcohol withdrawal. *Journal of Clinical Psychopharmacology* 2:277–280.

Greenblatt, D.J., Shader, R.I., Koch-Weser, J. (1974). Slow absorption of intramuscular chlordiazepoxide. *New England Journal of Medicine* 291:1116–1118.

Gross, M.M., Lewis, E., and Hastey, J. (1974). Acute alcohol withdrawal syndrome. In *The Biology of Alcoholism*, vol. 3, ed. B. Kissin and H. Begleiter, pp. 191–264. New York: Plenum.

Kaim, S.C., Klett, C.J., and Rothfield, B. (1969). Treatment of the alcoholic withdrawal state: a comparison of four drugs. *American Journal of Psychiatry* 125:1640–1646.

Sellers, E.M., and Kalant, H. (1976). Alcohol intoxication and withdrawal. *New England Journal of Medicine* 294:757–762.

Shaw, J.M., Kolesor, G.S., Sellers, E.M., Kaplan, H.L., and Sandor, P. (1981). Development of optimal treatment tactics for alcohol withdrawal: I. Assessment and effectiveness of supportive care. *Journal of Clinical Psychopharmacology* 1:382–390.

Whitfield, C.L., Thompson, G., Lamb, A., Spencer, V., Pfeifer, M., and Browning-Ferrando, M. (1978). Detoxification of 1,024 alcoholic patients without psychoactive drugs. *Journal of the American Medical Association* 239:1409–1410.

CHAPTER 22

The Diagnosis and Treatment of Depression in the Medically Ill

STEPHANIE CAVANAUGH, M.D.

A quarter to a third of all hospitalized medically ill patients experience feelings of depression. Behaviors and cognitions associated with depressed mood interfere at times with patients' ability to participate in medical care. Further, depression may result in increased medical morbidity and mortality.

Depression in medically ill patients appears to be distributed equally across sex, race, and socioeconomic groups. It is most common in patients who are severely ill, bedridden, in pain, not fully alert mentally, or confined to bed in the hospital for a prolonged stay.

Medically ill depressed people are as likely as physically healthy depressed people to report anhedonia, irritability, guilt, and the somatic symptoms of depression such as diurnal mood variation, work inhibition, fatigue, anorexia, vague somatic symptoms, and insomnia. Depressed medical patients, however, also differ from depressed psychiatric patients. Psychiatric depressives are more likely to report suicidal feelings and a previous history of depression. Medical depressives are more likely to experience anxiety, distinct depressed quality of mood, hopelessness, helplessness, self-pity, agitation, and psychomotor retardation.

Not all depression in depressed medical patients is caused by their physical illness. In 75 percent of these patients, the depression seems to be a consequence of the medical illness, but in 25 percent, the depression appears to antedate the physical illness.

Problems of Diagnosis

The diagnosis of depression in the medically ill is difficult. The stress of physical illness and hospitalization itself may cause a reactive depression, demoralization, or a grieflike reaction. Often, the most appropriate DSM-III diagnosis in the medically ill depressed is adjustment disorder with depressed mood. Typical depressive symptoms in medically ill patients include irritability, sadness, crying, mild dissatisfaction, mild discouragement about the future, and mild indecisiveness.

The somatic/vegetative symptoms of depression may also result from physical illness. Between 50 and 80 percent of medical inpatients experience psychomotor retardation, fatigue, anorexia, weight loss, insomnia, and somatic preoccupation at some time during their medical hospitalization. As depression worsens in the medically ill, the number of somatic symptoms experienced increases little. However, the intensity of somatic symptoms does increase as their depression becomes more severe.

Affective/cognitive symptoms are very useful in diagnosing depression in medically ill patients. The number and intensity of affective/cognitive symptoms in the medically ill increase linearly as the depression becomes more severe. Seven affective/cognitive symptoms are particularly discriminative for depression in the medically ill: sense of failure, loss of social interest, sense of punishment, suicidal ideation, severe dissatisfaction, severe indecisiveness, and frequent crying. Note, however, that mild dissatisfaction, mild indecisiveness, and occasional crying are common nonspecific findings in medical populations even without some type of diagnosable depression.

Specific Types of Depression in the Medically Ill

Depressed medically ill patients usually fall into two diagnostic groups: patients whose depressive symptoms are an adjustment disorder resulting from illness, and patients whose depressive symptoms are part of a major affective disorder. When depressed mood is a part of an adjustment disorder with depressed mood, the depressive symptoms usually diminish as the medical disorder improves. These patients also respond favorably to the passage of time, supportive interaction from staff, and/or psychotherapy. The severity of an adjustment reaction with depressed mood depends on patients' premorbid personalities, previous patterns of coping with stresses and loss, prior psychiatric history, adequacy of support systems, the physical discomfort caused by the illness, alteration in body image, and changes in societal roles. By contrast, medically ill patients with major depressive episodes usually do not lose their depressive symptoms as the medical symptoms abate, nor do they experience relief from support and/or psychotherapy. Instead, these patients also need antidepressant medication or electroconvulsive therapy.

Major Depressive Disorder

The DSM-III criteria for major depressive disorder are a useful framework for diagnosing depression in the medically ill, when modified for the contribution of physical illness.

Affective/Cognitive Symptoms

Predominant and persistent dysphoria and anhedonia are core symptoms of a major depressive disorder in the medically ill. In contradistinction to the experience of patients who have an adjustment disorder with depressed mood, in a major depression the sadness, depression, or anxiety does not lift as the medical illness improves or as support is given by family, friends, or medical staff. The nonpsychiatric physician notes that the dysphoria of depressed patients is more intense or persistent than that of other patients in the same situation. Patients may report that the quality of this mood is different from that experienced in previous hospitalizations or during periods of loss. Moreover, with the major depressive episode, patients may state that they no longer care what happens and may express hopelessness and helplessness. Patients' reports of predominant and persistent dysphoria are usually confirmed by histories obtained from families and medical staff. Often, however, it may take two or three diagnostic interviews to distinguish the predominant, persistent dysphoria of a major depressive episode from the variable dysphoria of an adjustment disorder with depressed mood.

Although many medically ill patients experience decreased interest in usual activities when ill or hospitalized, this anhedonia is not usually pervasive or severe. Further, most patients report pleasure from visits with family, friends, and medical staff. Pervasive loss of pleasure, on the other hand, particularly loss of interest in people, is symptomatic of a major depressive episode. Decreased interest in sex also reflects anhedonia in the medically ill. Often, the behavioral manifestation of anhedonia is withdrawal. Patients stay in their rooms and appear uninterested in their usual activities and medical care. Although many medically ill patients report that they feel worse in the morning, patients with a major depressive episode are observed by the nursing staff to be more dysphoric and anhedonic in the morning.

Often, the dysphoric, anhedonic patient with a major depression experiences *cognitive symptoms* of depression: loss of self-esteem, self-reproach, suicidal ideation, and severe indecisiveness. Patients with major depression feel bad about themselves as people, while patients with an adjustment reaction with depressed mood feel bad about their situation. In a major depression, patients may experience feelings of worthlessness, self-reproach, excessive or inappropriate guilt, a sense of failure, and a sense of being punished. Suicidal ideation or suicide attempts are infrequent in the medically ill and point strongly to major depression. Although mild indecisiveness is common in the medically ill, severe indecisiveness is a useful indicator of major depression in the medically ill. Difficulty in concentrating is not a useful symptom in discriminating major depression in the medically ill.

Somatic/Vegetative Symptoms

Mild somatic symptoms explainable by physical illness are not emblematic of a depressive disorder. Of nondepressed medically ill patients, 84 percent show somatic preoccupation; 81 percent, mild psychomotor retardation; 72 percent, work inhibition; 71 percent, fatique; 67 percent, insomnia; 61 percent, difficulty falling asleep; 59 percent, early awakening; 42 percent, weight loss; and 40 percent, anorexia.

When somatic symptoms are severe, persistent, out of proportion to the physical illness, and temporally related to the affective/cognitive symptoms of depression, such symptoms support the diagnosis of a depressive disorder. A careful history from families, nurses, medical staff, and the patient is required to distinguish the component of the somatic symptoms related to the physical illness and hospitalization from that related to depression.

Severe *psychomotor retardation and agitation* are excellent signs of depressive disease; nevertheless, they must be distinguished from the retardation or agitation of delirium and certain other conditions. Because lability of affect and dysphoric mood often accompany delirium, depression may be diagnosed inappropriately. A careful history and mental status examination, however, help establish the diagnosis of delirium. Mild psychomotor retardation is present in more than 75 percent of medically ill patients; severe retardation occurs most commonly in Parkinson's disease, renal failure, liver failure, and in critically ill patients with severe dysfunction in other systems. If such patients also complain of dysphoria and anhedonia, clinicians may have difficulty being certain about the diagnosis of major depression. The diagnosis is usually clarified when the medical condition improves, or when depressive symptomatology other than psychomotor retardation persists with psychomotor agitation. Agitation can also occur with anoxia, hyperthyroidism, corticosteroids, and levodopa.

Two other symptoms that challenge the psychiatric diagnostician are *anorexia and weight loss secondary to anorexia.* Nondepressed medically ill patients usually have an obvious reason for their anorexia: physical illness, hospital food, or medication. Nondepressed medical patients can usually imagine being interested in eating if they had their favorite food and were not ill, and they usually make an effort to eat to maintain their strength. On the other hand, depressed patients are rarely interested in food, find it tasteless, and cannot imagine enjoying their favorite food even if they were not ill. Finally, they may make no effort to eat even though they know it is important.

Mild insomnia is common in nondepressed medically ill patients. Patients with a major depression usually have insomnia out of proportion to the illness or the demands of hospital care. Frequently, such patients state, "I only sleep two hours," or "I don't sleep at all." A sleep record is helpful to document insomnia.

In summary, the diagnosis of a major depressive episode in the medically ill is best made using DSM-III criteria. Predominant and persistent dysphoria and/or anhedonia must be present for two weeks. In addition, at least four of the following cognitive symptoms must also be present nearly every day for two weeks.

1. Loss of interest or pleasure in usual activities (particularly loss of interest in people) or decreased sex drive.
2. Feelings of worthlessness, self-reproach, excessive or inappropriate guilt, and, most important, feeling like a failure or feeling punished.
3. Recurrent thoughts of death, suicidal ideation, wishes to be dead, or suicide attempt.
4. Severe indecisiveness.

Diminished ability to think, concentrate, or remember may be caused by an organic brain disorder and is not a useful symptom in making a diagnosis of a major depressive episode in the medically ill.

The preceding affective/cognitive symptoms are the best discriminators of a major depressive episode in the medically ill. The following vegetative or somatic symptoms, however, support the diagnosis of a major depression when they are severe, out of proportion to the medical illness, and temporally related to the affective/cognitive symptoms of depression.

5. Psychomotor agitation or retardation.
6. Anorexia and weight loss.
7. Insomnia.

Because fatigue and loss of energy are so commonly caused by physical illness, these vegetative symptoms cannot be used to make a diagnosis of major depression in the medically ill.

Special Problems

Patients who cannot communicate effectively because of organic brain syndrome or aphasia present special problems to physicians in diagnosing a major depression. Depression in these patients may present with withdrawal, frequent crying episodes, irritability, aggressive outbursts, refusal to eat or cooperate with medical care, psychomotor agitation or retardation, and change in sleeping patterns. After organic causes for the behavior have been ruled out, a diagnosis of depression should be considered. Although the dexamethasone suppression test may be helpful in establishing a diagnosis of depression in physically healthy psychiatric patients, physical illness and dementia may produce false-positive test results. Often, such patients must be treated empirically with a suitable antidepressant agent (see Chapter 6).

Organic Affective Disorders

Finally, organic causes of depression must be ruled out. Although numerous medical conditions and drugs have been associated with major depression, consultants should be particularly alert to these possible causes: hypothyroidism, vitamin deficiencies (particularly B vitamins), carcinoma of the prostate, carcinoma of the bowel, frontal lobe tumors, multiple sclerosis, lupus erythematosus, nondominant hemisphere strokes (first six weeks), and viral infections. These can present as, or be associated with, depressive disorder. Pharmacological agents that can contribute to or result in depression include: reserpine, alpha-methyldopa, beta-adrenergic blocking agents, and corticosteroids.

The following case histories contrast a major depressive episode (Mr. U.) with an adjustment disorder with depressed mood (Mrs. V.).

> Mr. U., a 55-year-old married businessman with insulin-dependent diabetes mellitus, was admitted to the hospital with pneumonia, congestive heart failure, diabetic foot ulcers, and renal insufficiency. The patient had had a myocardial infarction two years previously and had had multiple admissions for complications of his diabetes. He had no personal or family history of depression.
>
> During two months of hospitalization, the patient became increasingly despondent in spite of his improving medical condition. He recognized that he had coped well with his previous hospitalizations, but on this admission he felt unable to "bounce back." He described a "black cloud" that had settled around him. He showed decreased interest in his environment. He became withdrawn, neglected his personal hygiene, and participated passively in his medical care. The patient, whose wife and

children were very supportive, became gradually less cheered by their visits. He became concerned that he no longer felt anything for them. His concerns about his job, impotence, progressive renal failure, and being a burden to his family were realistic. But he began to dwell on feelings of worthlessness and had recurrent thoughts of wishing to die. He said his food tasted like cardboard. He slept but one hour per night and was too tired to participate in his medical care. The patient appeared markedly depressed and showed severe psychomotor retardation.

Mrs. V., a 48-year-old married woman with stage IV ovarian carcinoma, was readmitted to the hospital for her second treatment of chemotherapy. One month earlier she had undergone a colostomy to relieve a bowel obstruction secondary to peritoneal metastases. The patient stated she felt discouraged and angry about her illness, and she cried more than usual. She also expressed sadness about dying and leaving her husband and two teenage sons. The nurses reported that at times she was despondent and depressed. Still, at other times she was cheerful and smiled. She felt her colostomy bag made her dirty and was concerned that her husband found her unattractive. She felt increasingly tired as a result of her illness and the chemotherapy, and experienced a great sense of loss when she was forced to quit her job because of her deteriorating physical condition. On occasion she felt useless when she was too tired to do simple household tasks. She was glad to see family, friends, and hospital staff, and her mood improved from their visits. She enjoyed reading. She had little appetite, saying, "I think my taste buds have been killed by the chemotherapy and hospital food." She did attempt, though, to force herself to eat. She had some difficulty falling asleep and woke early, when nauseated. She had no psychomotor retardation or agitation, nor did she experience persistent self-reproach, feelings of worthlessness, excessive or inappropriate guilt, or a sense of being punished.

Treatment

Somatic Therapies

Antidepressants are essential in treating a major depressive disorder in the medically ill, but they must be used carefully because their absorption, rate of distribution, metabolism, and excretion are altered by age, weight, physical illness, and drug–drug interactions. Useful guidelines in prescribing antidepressants for the medically ill are:

1. Begin with half the usual dose.
2. Increase the dose half as rapidly.

3. Plateau at half to three-quarters of the usual dose for five days, and observe for side effects.
4. After five days at a constant dose, obtain an antidepressant plasma level.
5. Adjust the final therapeutic daily dose on the basis of the plasma level and side effects; use the lowest therapeutic plasma level with tolerable side effects.

Older patients, cachectic patients, and patients with cardiovascular, liver, or kidney disease require smaller loading and steady-state doses.

The anticholinergic side effects of antidepressants may adversely affect patients with organic brain disorder, narrow-angle glaucoma, respiratory disease that is worsened by thickened secretions, constipation, impending functional or mechanical ileus, urinary retention, or benign prostatic hypertrophy, and patients taking other anticholinergic drugs. On the other hand, the anticholinergic side effects of antidepressants may be helpful for patients with Parkinson's disease, peptic ulcer, and diarrhea. In approximate decreasing order, the anticholinergic potency of antidepressants is amitriptyline, imipramine, doxepin, nortriptyline, desipramine, maprotiline, and trazodone. Maprotiline lowers the seizure threshold and may cause seizures in vulnerable patients.

The cardiovascular side effects of antidepressants are an important consideration in treating a major depressive disorder in the medically ill. Orthostatic hypotension is the most common cardiovascular side effect. Amitriptyline and imipramine cause the most orthostatic hypotension; desipramine, nortriptyline, doxepin, maprotiline, and trazodone cause much less orthostatic hypotension. An increase in heart rate of 5 to 10 beats per minute is common early in treatment with amitriptyline, imipramine, desipramine, and nortriptyline; doxepin and maprotiline cause a smaller increase in heart rate, and trazodone causes almost no increase.

Most antidepressants are quinidine-like; they increase cardiac conduction time, depress cardiac contractility, and are antiarrhythmic. Amitriptyline, imipramine, nortriptyline, and desipramine are the most quinidine-like; maprotiline and doxepin have less quinidine-like effects on the heart, and trazodone has no such effects. The quinidine-like antidepressants are potentially hazardous for patients with conduction defects and should be used carefully in patients with congestive heart failure and patients who are using beta-adrenergic blocking agents (e.g., propranolol, quinidine, and procainamide) as these have a negative ionotropic effect on the myocardium.

Occasionally, during the loading phase of antidepressant therapy, desipramine (and, more rarely, imipramine and nortriptyline) may cause a transient blood pressure increase or premature ventricular contractions (PVCs) in the patient with a history of hypertension or ventricular arrhythmias. If, however, the drug can be continued safely to therapeutic levels, the blood pressure and PVCs usually fall below pretreatment levels. Trazodone at steady state has also been associated with increased PVCs.

Antidepressants may therefore be given to many patients with cardiovascular disease if the proper drug is chosen. Amitriptyline and imipramine should be avoided in this population; desipramine, nortriptyline, maprotiline, doxepin, and trazodone are the most useful in patients with cardiovascular disease. Cardiovascularly impaired patients treated with antidepressants should be carefully monitored, with frequent observation of vital signs and repeated electrocardiograms until steady state is reached. Patients with unstable cardiovascular disease may require a cardiac monitor early in treatment. Guanethidine and clonidine should not be used with antidepressants, as the latter block the ability of the former to lower blood pressure.

Sedation can help or harm medically ill patients. The more noradrenergic drugs—desipramine, maprotiline, and nortriptyline—usually cause little sedation. Imipramine is somewhat sedating. And the serotonergic drugs amitriptyline, doxepin, and trazodone are highly sedating. Although treating a major depressive disorder requires therapeutic levels of antidepressants, serotonergic drugs in low doses are often helpful in patients with mild depression accompanied by anxiety, pain, and severe vegetative signs. Amitriptyline *or* doxepin, 50–75 mg at bedtime, *or* trazodone, 50–150 mg at bedtime, is helpful to promote sleep, increase appetite, decrease anxiety, and decrease pain.

Monoamine oxidase (MAO) inhibitors are rarely used in the hospitalized medically ill because of the need for a tyramine-free diet and the hazardous interaction with meperidine and sympathomimetic drugs, including alphamethyldopa, levodopa, and dopamine. However, MAO inhibitors are useful when other antidepressants have failed, particularly with atypical depressions. Although these drugs have little effect on the cardiac conduction system or the myocardium, they have anticholinergic side effects and may also cause significant orthostatic hypotension. MAO inhibitors are contraindicated in patients with congestive heart failure and liver disease.

Electroconvulsive therapy, although rarely necessary, can be used when the depression is life-threatening or is refractory to antidepressants, or when the medical condition or its treatment precludes the use of antidepressants (see Chapter 23 for a fuller discussion of electroconvulsive therapy).

Psychotherapy

Patients with a major depressive disorder are often not amenable to psychotherapy until the depressive symptomatology has been reduced by antidepressants. Nevertheless, such patients require a milieu on the medical ward conducive to improvement of the depression. The medical staff and the patients' families must be empathic and supportive while encouraging self-care, grooming, socialization, and eating. Physical therapy and occupational therapy are helpful. Depressive cognitions, particularly hopelessness, helplessness, and worthlessness, need to be challenged gently, and patients need to be assured that their depression will lift. When the depression begins to lift, psychotherapy can help patients deal with their illnesses or with other stressors in their lives.

In developing relationships with depressed medically ill patients, therapists should be warm, empathic, noncritical, and nonjudgmental, and should demonstrate concern for patients' plights. Patients who are ill and hospitalized often have a number of difficult psychological tasks. They must cope with separation from family, friends, job, and all that is familiar. Also, change in bodily function, painful diagnostic procedures, and anxieties about the outcome of the illness must be endured. Further, patients' illnesses often cause them to function differently from the way they had functioned previously in their family, job, and social environment. Assessment of patients' previous success in coping with stress and loss often provides useful insights into methods of coping with current stresses and losses.

After therapists assess patients and the difficulties they must face, therapists and patients define the problems that can be practically addressed in psychotherapy. The focus of the therapy is the "here and now." The past is not utilized except as it relates to the present. Transference is not interpreted except as it pertains to current issues. Therapists can help patients express painful affects and mourn the losses of function, role, and in the case of dying patients, loss of life and separation from loved ones. Therapists support patients' healthy defenses and coping mechanisms. Finally, therapists help patients find practical solutions and focus on what they can do rather than on what they cannot do. Family involvement in such psychotherapy to promote open communication and problem solving is essential. After such brief psychotherapy, psychologically healthy patients and family can usually carry on without further need for intervention. The case examples presented earlier in this chapter are illustrative.

> Treatment of Mr. U.'s depression required therapeutic levels of antidepressant medication and psychotherapy. The patient's medical condition was carefully assessed at the time antidepressants were considered. Desipramine was chosen because it is alerting, has quinidine-like effects, causes little orthostatic hypotension, has few anticholinergic side effects, and does not lower the seizure threshold. Because the patient had a history of congestive heart failure, his vital signs and weight were carefully monitored during antidepressant treatment to be certain that the desipramine did not depress cardiac muscle contractility.
>
> Desipramine was started at 25 mg at bedtime and increased by 25 mg every other day until a daily dose of 75 mg was reached. The patient's

pulse increased from 75 to 85 beats per minute, and the patient experienced no orthostatic hypotension. Daily EKGs were normal, and chest x-ray and physical exam showed no increase in heart size. The patient complained of no anticholinergic side effects. Because the patient had mild renal failure, his desipramine dose was kept at 75 mg per day for five days, reaching a plasma level of 165 mg/ml. The dose was not increased because his plasma level was within therapeutic range and his depression was showing signs of response.

After Mr. U.'s first week at therapeutic plasma levels, his mood and appetite improved somewhat, he had more energy, and he became more outgoing. During the initial ten days of his drug treatment, family and staff encouraged him to eat, improve his personal hygiene, participate in his medical care, and socialize. His feelings of worthlessness and suicidal thoughts were gently challenged. He was reassured that his mood would continue to improve.

During the next two weeks of hospitalization, as the signs and symptoms of the patient's depression improved further, the psychiatrist addressed the patient's concerns about his work, progressive renal failure, impotence, and sense of being a burden on his family. Two conjoint sessions were held with Mr. U. and his wife to deal with these issues. At the time of discharge, 3½ weeks after treatment was started, the patient's depression had remitted. He required no psychotherapy after discharge. Three months following his discharge, his desipramine was gradually decreased by 25 mg every three weeks. He had no recurrence of symptoms after desipramine was discontinued.

Mrs. V.'s depression was treated psychotherapeutically. She identified her colostomy bag, fatigue, feelings of uselessness, and probable death within the next year or two as the issues she wished to discuss. The patient had met previous stresses by developing a concrete, practical plan and doing something positive about the situation, but had often contended with painful affects by burying herself in her work.

In her individual psychotherapy, she discovered her feelings that the colostomy bag made her feel imperfect and conflicted with her need for cleanliness. As she worked through this issue, she began to realize that she, not her husband, found herself unattractive. That insight, plus highly ritualized care of her colostomy bag, helped her deal with the narcissistic injury of her change in bodily function. Of greater importance were her loss of the satisfaction she obtained from her job and the uselessness she felt when unable to complete tasks at home. Constructive ways to deal with her fatigue were suggested, such as not expecting too much of herself, obtaining extra help at home, organizing her day creatively, and prioritizing her activities. Thus, she would have more energy to deal with what was important to her and her family. A redefinition of her role in the family was also positive.

The mourning issues related to Mrs. V.'s terminal illness were dealt with in the context of family sessions. She outlined what she wanted to teach her sons before she died. She identified those parts of her role to be taken over by her husband after her death. She made audiotapes on various subjects, to be used by her family after her death.

Mrs. V. ate better when the family brought food from home; her sleeping difficulties responded well to a benzodiazepine hypnotic and an antiemetic. At the time of discharge, she felt at peace and "on the track again," and reported that her sadness had abated considerably. Her anorexia and fatigue improved only slightly.

Suggested Readings

Ayd, F., and Frank, J. (1981). New antidepressant drugs. *Psychiatric Annals* 11(11):11–17.

Cassem, N. (1982). Cardiovascular effects of antidepressants. *Journal of Clinical Psychiatry* 43:22–28.

Cavanaugh, S. (1983). The prevalence of cognitive and emotional dysfunction in a general medical population using the MMSE, GHQ, and BDI. *General Hospital Psychiatry* 5:15–24.

Cavanaugh, S., Clark, D.C., and Gibbons, R.D. (1983). Diagnosing depression in the hospitalized medically ill. *Psychosomatics* 24:809–815.

Marshall, J.B., and Forker, A.D. (1982). Cardiovascular effects of tricyclic antidepressant drugs: therapeutic usage, overdosage, and management of complications. *American Heart Journal* 103:401–414.

Moffic, H.S., and Paykel, E.S. (1975). Depression in medical inpatients. *British Journal of Psychiatry* 126:346–353.

Preskorn, S.H., and Irwin, H.A. (1982). Toxicity of tricyclic antidepressants—kinetics, mechanism, intervention: a review. *Journal of Clinical Psychiatry* 43:151–156.

Schwab, J.J., Bialow, M.R., Brown, J., and Holzer, C.E. (1967). Diagnosing depression in medical inpatients. *Annals of Internal Medicine* 67:695–707.

Stewart, M., Drake, F., and Winokur, G. (1965). Depression among medically ill patients. *Diseases of the Nervous System* 26(8):479–485.

Wahl, C. (1972). The technique of brief psychotherapy with hospitalized psychosomatic patients. *International Journal of Psychoanalytic Psychotherapy* 1:69–82.

CHAPTER 23

Electroconvulsive Therapy in Consultation Psychiatry

CHARLES A. WELCH, M.D.

Electroconvulsive therapy (ECT) continues to be an indispensible psychiatric treatment. In spite of the recent advances in antidepressant medication, there is still a population of patients for whom ECT is the only effective therapy. After several decades during which ECT was inappropriately prescribed for a variety of disorders, its use has become more restricted and specific. In response to critics inside and outside the medical profession, there has been a decrease in the cavalier use of ECT and a decrease in its availability, even under appropriate circumstances.

Indications

The most common indication for ECT is a major depressive disorder in patients who either cannot tolerate or are unresponsive to an adequate trial of antidepressants. The symptoms that predict a positive response to ECT are the vegetative signs of major depression. These include anorexia, weight loss, agitation, psychomotor retardation, early-morning awakening, anergia, anhedonia, social withdrawal, guilt, impaired concentration, and diurnal mood variation, with worsening in the morning and improvement in the evening. In addition, symptoms do not change in response to external circumstances. The prognosis is better when these symptoms occur as part of an acute illness in patients with a good premorbid adjustment. The prognosis tends to be poorer when these symptoms are lifelong or occur in the presence of chronic hypochondriasis, chronic pain, or evidence of a serious personality disorder.

The criteria for an adequate drug trial depend on the individual patient. For young, physically healthy individuals a serial trial of two or three agents at therapeutic doses at adequate blood levels is reasonable. On the other hand, elderly, chronically ill people should not have more than one drug trial because this type of patient's medical status deteriorates rapidly during a depressive illness. The elderly are particularly prone to postural hypotension and other autonomic side effects of antidepressants, and drug trials are sometimes quite risky.

ECT is indicated as a primary treatment in three conditions: depression leading to a medical emergency, delusional depression, and catatonia. Some patients present after a protracted depressive illness with over 50 percent weight loss, malnutrition, and exhaustion from lack of sleep. It is unethical to subject these patients to a three-week trial of medication when a more prompt treatment response can be obtained. Delusional depression responds poorly to tricyclics. Although preliminary data suggest that the concurrent use of a tricyclic and a neuroleptic may improve response rates, ECT remains the most effective treatment for the delusionally depressed, with a response rate equal to that of the depressive population in general. Catatonia is also exquisitely sensitive to ECT, particularly when it accompanies an affective disorder. Although treatment with a neuroleptic is reasonable for patients who are known to be schizophrenic, ECT is the most effective primary treatment when an affective disorder is present. Because of the serious potential complications of catatonia, including pulmonary embolism, fluid and electrolyte imbalance, pneumonia, and muscular contractures, prompt resolution of catatonia is imperative.

The use of ECT in schizophrenia has been well studied. ECT is often dramatically effective for neuroleptic-refractory younger patients experiencing a first or second episode of psychosis. Many of these patients are suffering from a schizophreniform psychosis and may be more appropriately classified as affectively disordered than schizophrenic. For chronic schizophrenic patients with an established history of unremitting psychosis, ECT is only transiently effective and does not affect the basic course of the illness.

Efficacy trials have demonstrated that ECT is more effective for severe depression than placebo or sham ECT and more effective than either tricyclics or MAO inhibitors. Most drug trials find a response rate of about 75 percent and 65 percent with tricyclics and MAO inhibitors, respectively, whereas ECT has a response rate of 85 to 90 percent in similar patients. Recent advances in drug therapy, particularly the use of higher doses and the development of more readily tolerated psychotropic agents, have led to drug response rates closer to that of ECT. On the other hand, many patients are refractory to high drug doses for extended periods of time. These patients respond readily to ECT. Failure to respond to drugs does not portend a poor response to ECT in the melancholically depressed patient.

Mode of Action

Although the mechanism of action of ECT is unknown, it has been clearly established that a generalized grand mal seizure is the effective component of the treatment. Efficacy is unrelated to degree of memory loss, the intensity of the stimulus, or the psychodynamic meanings of the treatment to the patient. Length of seizure and generalization of seizure are the only factors that have been conclusively related to efficacy.

The functions affected by ECT are mediated primarily by the thalamus and hypothalamus: sleep, appetite, activity, and the experience of pleasure. It is likely that the grand mal seizure alters receptor sensitivity in the diencephalon. Although alpha-adrenergic, cholinergic, and serotonergic receptors are probably involved, it is also likely that changes occur in the receptor sites for large-molecular-weight polypeptides.

Risks and Side Effects

ECT is probably the safest treatment for major depression, with procedural mortality of less than 1 per 100,000 treatments. On the other hand, certain cardiopulmonary stresses do occur. Ventricular ectopy is common, with irregular beats occurring in up to 40 percent of patients. These are benign, last only a few minutes, and disappear promptly after the treatment. They occasionally require management with a lidocaine drip. Most patients sustain a two- to three-minute increase in blood pressure immediately following the seizure, presumably caused by increased circulating catecholamines. Blood pressure may rise to as high as 240/140. When the rise in blood pressure is higher or more sustained, it should be moderated with a prophylactic dose of an intravenous antihypertensive agent. The best drug for this purpose is nitroglycerine at a dose of 30 mg in 250 ml of 5 percent dextrose in distilled water. It should be administered as a constant infusion beginning before seizure induction. While allowing effective, reversible control of blood pressure, nitroglycerine also increases cardiac perfusion, a particularly desirable effect in the elderly.

The principal side effects of ECT are anterograde and retrograde memory impairment: both may be permanent for the events immediately before and after the course of ECT. Events that occurred most recently tend to be forgotten, whereas events occurring in the more distant past are less affected. Anterograde deficit presents as difficulty remembering names, phone numbers, appointments, and daily events in the days following ECT. The impairment tends to be cumulative, increasing with the number of treatments. Bilateral ECT produces much more retrograde and anterograde impairment than unilateral ECT. Patients treated with unilateral ECT often experience no subjective or observable memory disturbance. Some patients treated with bilateral ECT complain of permanent memory impairment. Attempts to demonstrate this impairment objectively with neuropsychological testing have found no cognitive deficit six to nine months following the last treatment. This discrepancy is probably due to the limitations of the testing, and it is likely that patients given large numbers of bilateral, high-energy treatments do suffer long-term or even permanent cognitive deficits.

Contraindications

The only absolute contraindication to ECT is a myocardial infarction within the preceding six weeks. The anesthetic risk in such a circumstance is prohibitive. In treating a major depressive disorder, the benefits of ECT outweigh the risks in almost every other medical condition. For some years, ECT was thought to be contraindicated in the presence of a brain tumor. The assertion was based on a limited number of case reports of patients who did not have depressive illness, but were suffering from an undiagnosed tumor and deteriorated with ECT. More recently, ECT has been shown to be effective and safe for patients suffering from major depression in the presence of an intracranial tumor.

Consent

Perhaps the most difficult issue in contemporary ECT is patient consent. Many depressed patients are unable to give informed consent because of delusional negativism and paranoid thinking, or because of incapacitation due to catatonia, psychomotor retardation, or severe medical debilitation. Formerly the signature of the next of kin was adequate in these situations, but now most states require a court hearing and prohibit treatment without patient consent, except by a judge's order. Although these legal restrictions are intended to protect patients, they often result in unnecessary delay and expense to patients and their families. A good working relationship with patients' families and the court can simplify and speed this process immeasurably.

Technique

The technique of ECT has evolved significantly over the past ten years. A typical anesthetic dose is 50 to 100 mg of methohexital sodium and the same dose of muscle-paralyzing succinylcholine chloride injected intravenously in rapid succession. The patient is ventilated with 40 percent oxygen. Because of the large metabolic demands of the seizure, care is taken to vigorously oxygenate the patient before and after the seizure. Because of the small, but definite, risk of cardiopulmonary emergencies, complete resuscitation equipment should be available. A well-equipped treatment room is adequate for young, healthy people, but elderly or debilitated people should be treated in an operating room or in a recovery room in a general hospital.

The first major variable in technique is electrode placement: The treatment electrodes may be placed bilaterally or unilaterally. Unilateral placement (see Figure 3) results in a dramatic decrease in the amount of cognitive impairment, but 80 percent of the ECT done in this country is still administered bilaterally because it is believed to be more effective. Of the more than 35 comparisons of unilateral and bilateral ECT, the more rigorously designed studies tend to show equal efficacy. On the other hand, some investigators continue to find greater efficacy with bilateral ECT. It is more difficult to trigger generalized seizures with a unilateral stimulus, and this may account for the lower efficacy with the unilateral technique reported

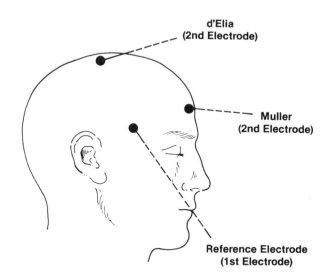

FIGURE 3.
The two most commonly used unilateral electrode placements are the d'Elia and the Muller placements. The d'Elia placement is more efficient in the induction of seizure activity, requiring about a third as much energy as the Muller placement, with no loss of efficacy. As would be expected, significantly less posttreatment confusion occurs with the lower-energy stimulus.

by some investigators and clinicians. However, the routine use of bilateral placement is probably unjustified, and because of its side effects the technique should be reserved for patients who fail to respond to unilateral stimulation.

The second major variable in technique is the stimulus wave form (see Figure 4). Traditionally, a 60-cycle-per-second sine-wave impulse has been used, but recently the use of low-energy, brief-pulse stimulus has been increasing. The brief-pulse wave form is much more efficient in triggering seizure activity. Generalized seizures may be induced with a third to a quarter of the current required with sine-wave stimulus. This results in a marked reduction in the cognitive side effects of the treatment. The extensive literature comparing the efficacy of these two wave forms shows that they are equally effective.

During the treatment, it is imperative that the seizure be monitored to assure a generalized grand mal seizure of at least 15 to 20 seconds. Shorter seizures appear to be less effective. The newer ECT apparatuses include a two-lead EEG, which gives an accurate measure of the duration of seizure activity. The seizure appears as 3-cycle-per-second spike-and-wave tracing, which usually ends abruptly at the end of the seizure. However, the EEG can be misleading, in that ineffective partial or unilateral seizures are indistinguishable on the tracing from generalized seizures. Consequently, it is advisable to use a second monitoring technique. This can be accomplished

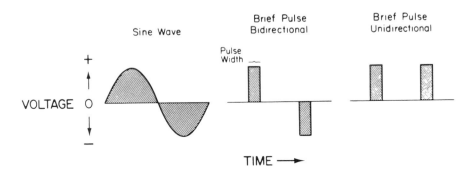

FIGURE 4.
Brief-pulse waves consist of a sudden deflection from O voltage to one pole and, after a short interval, an equally sudden return to O voltage. The pulse width, frequency of pulses, and total duration of the stimulus may be adjusted at the discretion of the clinician. Although the average energy requirement for sine-wave ECT is in the range of 70 watt seconds per treatment, brief-pulse ECT usually requires only 10 to 15 watt seconds to induce a generalized seizure. There is a commensurate decrease in posttreatment confusion and memory impairment, both retrograde and anterograde, with brief-pulse ECT.

by placing a blood pressure cuff on the arm ipsilateral to the stimulus and, immediately prior to the injection of succinylcholine, inflating it above systolic pressure. This leaves the ipsilateral arm unparalyzed during the treatment itself. If the seizure is generalized, it crosses the diencephalon to the motor cortex of that arm and convulsive activity will be observed in that hand. This does not, however, give an accurate measure of seizure duration. Electrical seizure activity usually persists for 5 to 10 seconds after physical convulsive activity ceases, but it may persist as much as 30 seconds longer. Although the technique outlined is cumbersome, there is no way to ascertain that generalized seizures of adequate length are being induced without the concurrent use of these two monitoring techniques.

The highest medical risk period immediately follows the treatment. When the patient has not yet fully regained consciousness and respiratory drive is compromised, close observation of blood pressure, pulse, and respiratory function is necessary. Younger patients treated with the brief-pulse unilateral technique may be fully alert and conversive five minutes after their treatment, but older patients or those treated with more cognitively devastating techniques may require several hours before they can be safely left unobserved.

The dose-response curve of ECT has not been accurately established, but a total of 6 to 8 treatments given 2 to 3 times a week suffices for most patients. Some patients with major depression require as many as 15 treatments, but this is quite unusual. At the other extreme, patients occasionally require as few as 2 or 3 treatments, particularly young patients with bipolar illness who occasionally switch suddenly from depression to mania after a small number of treatments. The use of more than 15 treatments in one series is unlikely to be of benefit, and suggests the possibility of a misdiagnosis.

The total seizure time required for a series has not been accurately determined and probably varies from patient to patient. Several investigators have effectively given more than one seizure per treatment session, in the hope of inducing a more prompt remission. Typically, three or four seizures are given sequentially to an anesthetized patient during the course of the session, which may last up to an hour. This technique of multiple-monitored ECT appears to effect a more prompt remission, but the total number of seizures is larger and the cognitive deficit is greater and may last longer. The indication for routine multiple-monitored ECT has not yet been established.

Following a course of ECT, the one-year relapse rate without maintenance medication is greater than 50 percent. The limited studies of maintenance medication indicate that maintenance therapy with amitriptyline, imipramine, phenelzine, or lithium reduces the one-year relapse rate to 15 to 20 percent. There is no clear preference among these drugs in terms of efficacy, and the choice should be made in relation to the diagnosis and the medical condition of the patient. The monoamine oxidase inhibitors are extremely well tolerated, even by elderly patients. For those who can responsibly follow the dietary precautions (see Chapter 6), these are probably the best post-ECT maintenance medications.

This chapter concludes with a case history illustrating the efficacy of ECT followed by maintenance medication.

> Mrs. W., a 68-year-old housewife, was brought to the emergency room by her family because of a change in mental status. She had been active, had shopped for herself and her husband, had cleaned house, and had taken an active interest in cooking, knitting, and socializing with her friends and family. She had been an avid gardener and enjoyed reading. About two months prior to her presentation at the emergency room, she suddenly began to lose interest in her usual activities. She sat alone for extended periods during the day, and avoided social contact. Three weeks later, she developed early-morning awakening and anorexia, which eventually resulted in a 40-pound weight loss. One week prior to her arrival at the hospital, she became confused, did not recognize her neighbors, and became unable to keep track of the most elementary details of household function.

> Her admission physical examination revealed a gaunt, fatigued-looking woman. Her blood pressure was 100/60 supine, with a drop to 80/40 standing. Aside from poor skin turgor and emaciation, physical and neurological examinations were entirely normal. On mental status examination, she was unable to give the year, the date, the name of the hospital, or her reason for being there. She repeated, "It's hopeless. There's no use doing anything." Her affect was markedly constricted, with neither laughter nor crying. There was no evidence of hallucinations, and there was no loosening of associations. Her speech was retarded, and there was some agitation, with hand wringing and pacing.

> She was admitted to the medical service for a full workup. Her CT scan and EEG were normal, and aside from hypovolemia and malnutrition, there was no evidence of any other metabolic abnormality. Her dexamethasone suppression test was positive, demonstrating nonsuppression at 8 A.M. and 4 P.M., with cortisol values greater than 5 mg/ml (see Chapter 6 for further discussion). She was transferred to the psychiatry service, where she received a three-week trial of imipramine, at 250 mg/day, monitored with blood levels. During that time, she required periodic intravenous hydration but, with vigorous staff encouragement, was able to maintain adequate nutrition. After three weeks with no response to medication, a course of ECT was recommended by the staff.

> After tapering off her tricyclic medication, the patient received a series of seven unilateral, nondominant, brief-pulse stimuli, with adequate seizure monitoring. By the fourth treatment she started to show improvement in her vegetative symptoms, and by the end of the series her symptoms were in full remission. Before she had sat mutely in her room; now she bustled about the ward, helping to prepare meals, taking care of

other patients, and offering motherly advice to the younger patients. Three days following her last treatment, her dexamethasone suppression test had returned to normal. The following day she was started on tranylcypramine, 10 mg t.i.d.; a week later she was discharged home to the care of her family. She was offered the option of ongoing psychotherapy, but she declined. She reported that she was enjoying life again and saw no need for psychotherapy. She returned for follow-up visits at bimonthly intervals, and the tranylcypramine was successfully discontinued at the end of one year.

Suggested Readings

d'Elia, G., and Raotma, H. (1975). Is unilateral ECT less effective than bilateral ECT? *British Journal of Psychiatry* 126:83–89.

Fink, M. (1982). Prediction of outcome in convulsive therapy. *Psychopharmacology Bulletin* 18:50–56.

Glassman, A.H., Perel, J.M., Shostak, M., and Fleiss, J.L. (1977). Clinical implications of imipramine plasma levels for depressive illness. *Archives of General Psychiatry* 34:197–204.

Ottosson, J.O. (1960). Experimental studies of the mode of action of electroconvulsive therapy. *Acta Psychiatrica Scandinavia* (suppl.), 145.

Price, T. R. P. (1982). Short- and long-term cognitive effects of ECT. *Psychopharmacology Bulletin* 18:81–100.

Report of the Task Force on Electroconvulsive Therapy of the American Psychiatric Association (1978). No. 14. Washington, D.C.

Welch, C.A., Weiner, R.D., Weir, D., Cahill, J.F., Rogers, H.J., Davidson, J., Miller, R.D., and Mandel, M.R. (1982). Efficacy of ECT in the treatment of depression: wave form and electrode placement considerations. *Psychopharmacology Bulletin* 18:31–35.

Woodruff, R.A., Goodwin, D.W., and Guze, S.B. (1974). *Psychiatric Diagnosis*, pp. 25–44. New York: Oxford Press.

CHAPTER 24

The Chronic Pain Patient

NELSON HENDLER, M.D.

Chronic pain is a most vexing problem for patients and their physicians. Because there are frequently no objective organic accompaniments of many pain complaints, psychiatrists' chief diagnostic tool is the clinical interview. In order to adequately assess chronic pain patients, special care must be given to establishing rapport. Adequate time must be allowed for taking a detailed history and asking specific questions about the nature, duration, and time of onset of the pain complaints, in addition to open-ended interviewing that elicits personality dynamics.

Development of rapport is important because these patients have often had unproductive or negative experiences with physicians. Many of these patients, because of their pain or as part of their personality structure, demand, complain, or behave in a passively aggressive or dependent manner. Many have become addicted to narcotics. It is easy for physicians to be judgmental and dismiss their complaints as part of a personality disorder or an addictive process.

From the patients' perspective, there is a different set of problems. First and foremost, pain suggests that something is physically wrong. Because of this, there is much fear and anxiety associated with persistent pain. After seeing multiple physicians, there is also a great deal of hostility and anger toward physicians, because of failure to diagnose, repeated referral, and occasional declarations of "I can't find anything wrong with you; it's all in your head." This produces resentment, and referral to a psychiatrist is final confirmation that their treating physicians have not believed them or that their treating physicians think they are "crazy." In effect, referral to a psychiatrist is the ultimate insult. It signals the end of traditional medical interventions; the real doctors are giving up.

Acute Pain versus Chronic Pain

The treatment of acute pain differs importantly from the treatment of chronic pain. Acute pain is strongly influenced by people's psychological state at the time the painful stimulus occurs. The perception of acute pain has less to do with the personality traits of individuals than their psychological preparedness for the experience of pain, or the psychological significance of the event that produces the pain. Therefore, it is conceivable that well-adjusted people, poorly prepared for surgery, would have as much anxiety prior to surgery as histrionic people who were well prepared for the surgery. The perception of pain, especially from surgical procedures, can be greatly reduced by educating patients about the extent and type of surgery they will undergo, preparing individuals for the amount of pain to be experienced after surgery, and judiciously using psychoactive agents. Narcotic and nonnarcotic analgesics, and transcutaneous electrical stimulation, are perfectly acceptable for the treatment of acute postsurgical pain. Hypnotics, on the other hand, do not relieve pain and may instead produce an agitated delirium. At times, prochlorperazine, used for postoperative nausea, produces akathisia and other untoward reactions. The use of any pharmacological agent for the continued treatment of postsurgical pain is probably uncalled for on the basis of our understanding of wound healing and repair. On rare occasions, the psychological changes associated with the pain-producing event do result in posttraumatic neuroses, producing the rare patient who has a pure psychogenic pain.

Diagnosis of Chronic Pain

Chronic pain patients can be divided into two broad categories— patients with objective pain and patients who exaggerate their pain.

Objective Pain Patients

The objective pain patient has clear organic pathology documented by x-ray, electromyogram, nerve conduction velocity studies, thermography, computerized tomography scan, myelogram, or physical examination. Objective pain patients experience four stages of chronic pain. The first, or acute, stage lasts up to two months. During this stage, no apparent psychological changes occur because patients expect to get well. The second, or subacute, stage lasts two to six months. During that time, patients become concerned and frightened. In previously well-adjusted individuals, this produces a reaction that resembles hypochondriacal concerns. In fact, if well-adjusted individuals with chronic, persistent pain complete a Minnesota Multiphasic Personality Inventory (MMPI) during the subacute stage, scales 1 and 3 (hypochondriasis and hysteria) may be elevated (see Chapter 34, on psychological testing).

If pain persists for more than six months, patients enter the third, or chronic, stage of chronic pain. This period may last from six months to eight years. During this stage, previously well adjusted individuals may become depressed and may experience sexual difficulties, sleep disturbance, increased drug use, and increased anxiety. MMPIs completed during this stage of the chronic pain process often have elevated scales 1, 2, and 3, with scale 2 (depression) more elevated than scales 1 and 3. In fact, clinicians should be suspicious of patients who are not depressed after they have had pain longer than six months.

After patients have had pain for three years or more, they enter the fourth, or subchronic, stage. By the time that they have entered this stage, depression has resolved, but the somatic concerns still persist. Patients usually say that they have grown accustomed to the pain, although it still bothers them. Typical MMPI profiles during this stage are elevated scales 1 and 3, with the return of scale 2 to normal as depression resolves.

It is important to remember that a patient may drift between one or another of these four stages at certain times in their experience with chronic pain; these stages are guidelines, not a rigid diagnostic framework. The following case presents a typical picture of objective pain.

> Mr. X., a 38-year-old disabled police officer, had been married for 15 years and had four children. When he was referred for psychiatric consultation, he complained of pain in his neck and back that had followed an on-the-job injury that had occurred when he had tried to make an arrest without using a night stick 2½ years earlier. The CT-metrizamide-myelogram showed a definable lesion. The patient had been scheduled for anterior cervical fusion and diskectomy, but was so tearful and depressed that the orthopedic surgeon and the neurosurgeon requested a psychiatric consultation before surgery.
>
> The patient's history revealed no drug use, alcohol abuse, sexual difficulties, marital difficulties, or emotional disorder. Prior to the injury, he had had no difficulty with erection or ejaculation and had had sexual relations two to three times a week. He coached little league baseball, had no financial difficulties, and spent most of his free time with his family. His hobbies were cabinetmaking and woodworking.
>
> The patient had gone through stages of (1) expectation that the pain would get better, (2) anxiousness because no one could diagnose the source of the pain, (3) anger when told by physicians, "It's all in your

head," because of earlier negative x-rays, and (4) depression about "being half a man," because of financial difficulties, irritability, and reduction of sexual activity to once a month. He had difficulty with erection because of the pain, and lack of interest in sex because of depression. He did not use narcotic medication because he "had seen what drugs could do to you" in his work as a police officer. He had tried diazepam and oxycodone for a week but discontinued them because they were not helping.

On psychological testing, he had elevated scales 1, 2, and 3 on the MMPI (hypochondriasis, depression, and hysteria). On the Hendler Screening Test for Chronic Back Pain Patients, the patient scored 11 points, placing him well within the objective pain patient category.

On the basis of the patient's history and test results, doxepin, 150 mg at bedtime, and perphenazine, 2 mg q.i.d., were recommended to improve sleep, reduce depression, and alleviate anxiety. Group psychotherapy with other chronic pain patients and family counseling were recommended for a two- to three-month period before surgery. During this course of therapy, the patient's depression lifted, and he tolerated the surgical procedure of fusion and diskectomy well. After surgery, he required an additional three months of follow-up psychotherapy and marital counseling. His pain diminished, and two years postoperatively he was back at work on light duty.

Exaggerating Pain Patients

Exaggerating pain patients are quite different from objective pain patients. Usually, their premorbid adjustment is poor. They often have a history of multiple marriages, drug or alcohol abuse, sexual difficulties, and other indications of social adjustment problems prior to the onset of pain. They frequently do not have clear-cut, objective indications of organic pathology. This does not mean that they are imagining the pain. Rather, their disability from the pain is out of proportion to what one would expect in the absence of severe physical damage.

Exaggerating pain patients deal with pain according to their personality type (personality types and associated behaviors in a medical setting are discussed in Chapter 13). People with histrionic personalities may use pain in order to get attention or avoid unpleasant tasks. Tense, perfectionistic individuals may worsen their own pain by increased muscle tension. They are usually quite upset because they are no longer perfect or because they cannot function as they did prior to developing pain. Patients with organic brain syndromes may use pain to explain a loss of intellectual functioning, which may be a far more socially and personally acceptable way to explain their deficits than memory loss. Passive-dependent individuals may find pain a convenient excuse for not functioning in situations they find difficult to manage. Only rarely (in less than 0.1 percent of the cases) does a clinician see a depressive equivalent, a conversion disorder, or Briquet's syndrome. The following case illustrates an exaggerating pain patient.

Mrs. Y., a 35-year-old white woman, was three years into her third marriage. She had a son by her first marriage who lived with his father because "the kid wanted to."

She complained of pain in her back following a fall while skiing three years earlier. EMG and nerve conduction and velocity studies were unremarkable. Orthopedic and neurosurgical consultants found no physical disorder. In order to rule out the possibility of a central disc, she underwent a CT-metrizamide-myelogram, which was helpful. She was then referred for psychiatric evaluation with the diagnosis of "hysterical pain" to see whether there was a psychogenic component to the pain.

During the psychiatric consultation, the patient revealed that she had suffered her skiing injury two months after her marriage to her third husband, who had been very understanding of her disability from persistent back pain. Because of her back pain, they had sex infrequently, but he fully appreciated her problem because he was 15 years older than she and "less interested in sex than he used to be." She had always had difficulty with orgasm. Their sexual contact had been approximately twice a week prior to the injury, and afterward it was reduced to once a month. She described her back pain as an aching pain in the lower back radiating into the right buttock. Past history revealed that she had made a suicide attempt prior to her second divorce. She denied any other physical complications or operations. Her hobbies were shopping and watching television.

The patient was taking diazepam, 5 mg q.i.d., and oxycodone, "only four pills a day, when the pain is unbearable." She denied suicidal ideation, depression, or irritability. She was very complimentary to the physician who was examining her but made derogatory comments about previous physicians.

The patient scored 22 points on the Hendler Screening Test for Chronic Back Pain Patients, placing her within the exaggerating pain patient category. Her MMPI scores revealed elevated scales 1 and 3 (hypochondriasis and hysteria) and a normal scale 2 (depression). The secondary gain from her symptoms appeared to be reduction of sexual activity and an excuse for her inactivity. Withdrawal from diazepam and oxycodone was recommended, along with the suggestion that oral doxepin, 50 mg at bedtime, and oral perphenazine, 2 mg t.i.d., be used to help the patient sleep and to reduce some mild anxiety. Because of the diagnosis of myofascial pain, a trial with naproxen, 250 mg t.i.d., and carisoprodol (Soma), 350 mg q.i.d., and repetitive trigger-point injections were recommended. Couples counseling was suggested but refused by the patient, as was group psychotherapy.

At 18-month follow-up, the patient had not received much benefit from trigger-point injections. She had received only four injections and had not taken the psychotropic medication recommended. However, she did use the naproxen and carisoprodol on occasion. The pain in the low back and the right buttock persisted, as did the relationship she had with her husband. It was felt that confrontation would be counterproductive, and that the patient had achieved a steady state in her marital relationship.

This case study illustrates the features generally seen in an exaggerating pain patient. However, psychiatrists should recognize that patients with a poor premorbid psychological adjustment can become physically ill, and physicians are obliged to rule out all possible etiologies for pain complaints before considering an emotional etiology.

Psychological Tests

The Hendler Screening Test for Chronic Back Pain Patients* is specifically designed to assess the validity of patients' complaints of pain, regardless of preexisting personality traits, and appears more accurate than the MMPI for this group of patients. In a recent study, 79 percent of the patients whose scores did not exceed 17 points on the Hendler Screening Test had definite physical abnormalities as measured by six objective tests; 100 percent of the patients with scores of 21 or more were found not to have any severe physical abnormalities, again as measured by the six objective tests. This does not indicate that patients scoring 21 points or more on this screening test do not have pain. Instead, it indicates that patients scoring 21 points or more on this test probably do not have a surgically correctable lesion, but may have minimal physical discomfort as a result of muscle strains, myofascial syndrome, or the like.

Management

In-hospital treatment of chronic pain involves getting patients out of bed and rewarding them for activity and self-care. A rehabilitation program begins with a level of activity that patients can tolerate; activity is gradually increased in length and degree and consists of occupational therapy, physical therapy, and recreational therapy. Patients are praised for each positive step they make.

---

*Permission to use this test may be obtained by writing Nelson Hendler, M.D., Mensana Clinic, 1718 Greenspring Valley Road, Stevenson, Maryland 21153, or by writing Medicomp, Inc., 845 Margaret Place, Shreveport, Louisiana 71101; both have this test available as part of a computer-scored and -interpreted, integrated psychological testing package.

Psychiatrists have several specific treatment techniques at their disposal. Group psychotherapy probably makes the most effective use of psychiatrists' time. With a homogeneous population, a great deal of mutual support can be derived from members of the group. In a short-term setting (i.e., less than a month), group therapy sessions should be held for an hour, two, three, or more times a week, with the group serving educational and exploratory functions. In an outpatient setting, groups should meet for an hour and a half weekly and should serve supportive and interactive functions. In both settings, groups are open-ended, taking in new members and experiencing "graduations" regularly. Artificial time limits for the number of sessions are not set. In my experience with such groups, patients can derive benefit from as few as 12 sessions. Some patients, however, find it necessary to have group support for three to four years. Optimal benefit is usually achieved after one or one and a half years of group participation.

Couples therapy and family therapy are highly recommended in conjunction with group psychotherapy. At present, only anecdotal reports support the contention that hypnosis is an effective management technique for chronic pain patients (see Chapter 35 for a fuller discussion of hypnosis on the medical and surgical wards). However, if one accepts the premise that a therapeutic intervention should not be directed toward removing the pain entirely, but rather toward helping patients in pain function better, then training patients in the use of relaxation techniques or biofeedback techniques, which can provide some degree of improved pain tolerance, can be beneficial (see Chapter 36 for a discussion of these techniques). In some instances, biofeedback techniques, such as electromyographic biofeedback for muscle tension headaches, can be a direct benefit and a definitive treatment technique. The use of acupuncture for chronic pain patients is fraught with difficulties, since the technique seems to provide reduction in acute pain, but not chronic, persistent pain. Along the same lines, transcutaneous electrical stimulation can help chronic pain patients, but its usefulness depends on patient compliance and acceptance. In addition, only neuritic pain seems to respond well to this type of intervention.

Psychiatrists can be of further benefit by advocating the appropriate use of pharmacological agents. The chronic administration of narcotics, benzodiazepines, and hypnotics often creates more problems for patients than its cures. Narcotics are indicated in chronic pain of nonmalignant origin if (1) the amount of medication taken does not escalate, (2) patients are able to function with the medication and unable to function without it, (3) there is no indication of intellectual impairment from the medication, and (4) one physician, and one physician only, is the source of the narcotic medication. The use of narcotics in patients with cancer pain usually does not escalate unless there is a clear-cut worsening of the malignancy, such as metastasis to bone. However, chronic pain patients often state that narcotic medications don't help the pain, but instead produce a euphoria that helps them ignore the pain. Indeed, memory loss and reduced intellectual functioning have been found in approximately a third of patients on chronic narcotic medications. Finally, physicians should be aware of the accepted medical practices within their own communities: In some states the long-term prescription of narcotic medications for patients without malignancies may be construed as excessive prescribing of narcotic drugs.

Psychiatrists should also be familiar with the mechanism of action of benzodiazepines. Drugs such as oxazepam, chlordiazepoxide, diazepam, prazepam, clorazepate, and lorazepam seem to have addictive potential, as well as a tendency for abuse. Although they are effective antianxiety agents, they are not intended for long-term (more than four months) use, and intellectual impairment, memory loss, and electroencephalogram changes compatible with sedative drug effects have been noted in many patients taking these medications. Moreover, they may interfere with the neurochemical processes of natural sleep and, from a theoretical point of view, may enhance the perception of pain. Benzodiazepine hypnotics such as temazepam and flurazepam also exhibit these effects. Other hypnotics have even more deleterious side effects and a greater potential for abuse.

To prescribe medication rationally, psychiatrists should understand normal sleep, pain perception, and anxiety and depression. One common denominator is that serotonin promotes normal sleep, reduces the perception of pain, and has antianxiety and antidepressant qualities. Therefore, drugs that enhance serotonin activity within the central nervous system are recommended. These medications include some tricyclic antidepressants and the newer bicyclic and tetracyclic antidepressants. Benzodiazepines seem to inhibit serotonin action. Thus a tricyclic antidepressant, given at bedtime, may assist patients in sleeping, reduce the perception of pain, and reduce anxiety and depression. Dosage will depend on patients' age, tolerance of certain side effects, and idiosyncratic reactions. By the same token, phenothiazine tranquilizers, especially in conjunction with the antidepressants just mentioned, provide some additional benefit for patients with chronic pain. Thorough discussions of the psychopharmacological rationale for these recommendations can be found in the suggested readings at the end of this chapter.

Conclusion

Chronic pain is a complex disorder, and psychiatrists must consider myriad factors influencing patients' behavior, from the sociological to the pharmacological, from the psychological to the medical. Work with chronic pain patients is time-consuming and demands a constantly investigative approach, but it can be both challenging and rewarding.

Suggested Readings

Blumer, D. (1975). Psychiatric considerations in pain. In *The Spine*, ed. R. Rothman and R. Simeone, pp. 871–906. Philadelphia: W.B. Saunders.

Hendler, N. (1981). *Diagnosis and Nonsurgical Management of Chronic Pain.* New York: Raven Press.

Hendler, N. (1982). The anatomy and psychopharmacology of chronic pain. *Journal of Clinical Psychiatry* 43:15–20.

Hendler, N., Derogatis, L., Avella, J., and Long, D. (1977). EMG biofeedback in patients with chronic pain. *Diseases of the Nervous System* 38:505–509.

Hendler, N., Viernstein, M., Gucer, P., and Long, D. (1979). A preoperative screening test for chronic back pain patients. *Psychosomatics* 20:801–808.

Hendler, N., Viernstein, M., Shallenberger, C., and Long, D. (1981). Group therapy with chronic pain patients. *Psychosomatics* 22:335–340.

Melzack, R., and Chapman, C.R. (1973). Psychological aspects of pain. *Postgraduate Medicine* 53:69–75.

Pilling, L., Brannick, T.L., and Swenson, W.M. (1967). Psychological characteristics of psychiatric patients having pain as a presenting problem. *Canadian Medical Association Journal* 97:387–394.

Sternbach, R.A. (1974). *Pain Patients: Traits and Treatment.* New York: Academic Press.

Sternbach, R.A., Murphy, R.W., Akeson, W.H., and Wolf, S.R. (1973). Chronic low back pain: "the low back loser" *Postgraduate Medicine* 53:135–138.

The Patient's Milieu:
A Systems Approach

Illness impinges on more than the mind and body of the patient, and the course and treatment are influenced by factors in the patient's family, hospital, and religious and cultural environment.

The patient's family is a part of the illness. The family reacts to those aspects of illness that threaten family integrity and alter family roles, and therefore the needs of the family must often be addressed as part of the patient's treatment. In a sense, the patient's family extends in the hospital to include those with professional concerns, the physicians and nurses. They, too, have needs that must be addressed in the course of psychiatric consultation, and the effectiveness of the psychiatric consultant depends in large measure on how well the psychiatrist understands the needs of the staff, their philosophy of patient care, and the points at which the needs of the patient and staff are congruent or in conflict.

Other aspects of the milieu that the patient brings to the hospital are religious and cultural concerns, which make up a large part of an individual's set of values. Although not a routine part of psychiatric or medical examinations, awareness of a patient's religious and cultural values facilitates the patient's integration into the hospital environment and enables adjustment of staff attitudes and procedures so as to enhance cooperation and mutual respect.

M.W.

CHAPTER 25

Upset and Upsetting Families

DON R. LIPSITT, M.D.
MERNA P. LIPSITT, M.S.W.

The presence or absence of a family plays a role in every patient's illness. Family support, or its undermining influence, often changes the clinical course of illness. Failure to attend to families may prolong or complicate treatment, create turbulence, and frustrate physicians' treatment efforts. Appreciating families and their values or dilemmas can enhance therapeutic effectiveness and provide unexpected professional gratification.

This chapter calls attention to some of the ways families respond to illness in their members and the influence of these responses on both patients and staff. The process is not one-sided. The psychiatric consultant must keep in mind that although competent staff are usually sensitive to the needs and anxieties of patients and families, staff behavior does precipitate some disruptions. We therefore speak of systems in which problems may arise in *any part* of them and, by complex communications and feedback loops, evolve into major disturbances.

Family uniqueness has so far deterred successful classification of family responses to illness. While family researchers continue their attempts to categorize levels of family pathology and responses in the face of crisis, the psychiatric consultant does well to approach patients and their families on a case-by-case basis, for cultural, ethnic, religious, and socioeconomic differences modify individual responses. Careful family histories of every patient will reveal that there is no such thing as a "noncontributory family history." The following vignette demonstrates the utility of this case-by-case approach.

Mrs. Z., a 57-year-old housewife with emphysema that had been stable, surprised her pulmonologist when she urgently requested hospitalization for increasing dyspnea of 2 to 3 days' duration. Her pulmonary function did not appear to have changed, yet she was unresponsive to her usual medications. Knowing that Mrs. Z. was not one to seek hospitalization, her physician urged the doubting medical resident to grant her admission for further evaluation and treatment.

Once in the hospital, the patient improved, seemingly confirming the admitting resident's hunch that she could have been managed as an outpatient. He was mildly annoyed. Intermittently, the patient complained of tightness in the chest, dyspnea, and tremulousness. Having elicited a past history of alcohol abuse and heavy smoking, the medical resident suspected the patient of renewed activity in these areas, in spite of the patient's proud insistence that she had "kicked" the habits by sheer will power over ten years ago. Staff described and noted in the chart that she complained, was demanding, and was difficult to get to know. When she began joking in ways they described as crude, sexual, or obscene, they tagged her as eccentric. House officers, more and more offended by her behavior, found excuses to avoid her on rounds and failed to explore possible roots of her behavior or further aspects of her personal history.

The patient's complaints escalated. Yet there was little change in her respiratory condition, and hospital discharge was suggested. She developed new complaints of weakness and fatigue and insisted that she could not possibly go home. Her husband, reached by phone, said she was too sick to come home. Then, the staff's mild annoyance, curiosity, and occasional amusement turned to anger. The patient was presented on medical-psychology rounds as a management problem, with a request for assistance in planning her discharge. The presenting medical resident commented that most of her family history was noncontributory, although her husband had a history of smoking and drinking.

The patient agreed to be interviewed by the attending psychiatrist. She proved to be a formidable interviewee—joking, digressing, and questioning the importance of inquiries about her family and home life. Though tempted at times to terminate the interview, the psychiatrist persisted until she became more participatory. She revealed an intense pride in her children, all but one of whom had married and achieved respectable positions. The son who remained at home was a 16-year-old high school student who worked part-time in a fertilizer factory, a job she held in great disdain and spoke of with great reluctance and an awkward attempt at humor. With considerable embarrassment, she described the strident, at times violent, disagreements between herself and her husband over this son, who attempted to mediate between them. She condemned her husband for drinking and smoking, then came to his rescue by describing him as a really good man.

The suggestion from the interviewing psychiatrist that these mixed feelings about her husband and son might have aggravated her respiratory condition brought self-recriminatory remarks about how she needed "a good kick in the ass" from time to time. She broke into tears as she told how she always felt she could handle her family, how she was always good for a laugh and could take care of herself, but "Now they've had enough of me. I'm no good to them and no good to myself; they're fed up with me at home."

When asked if she had anyone she could talk to about the way things were at home, she revealed that she was closest to a sister-in-law suffering from cancer who had gone rapidly downhill the week before the patient was admitted, and now was hospitalized in a terminal state. The patient looked sad and appeared to be fighting tears but denied that this was a big loss for her. As the interview ended, she said that her breathing was easier, that she felt better, and that she wouldn't mind if someone came back to talk with her again. A social worker returned to help her mourn the loss of her sister-in-law and find new ways to deal with her resentment toward her son and her husband.

Family Dysfunction and Illness

As the vignette demonstrates, family adaptation to chronic illness may achieve a delicate equilibrium over time. Attending the balancing of pressures are regressions, anxieties, and coping defenses such as those experienced by the identified patient in the family. Some families have difficulty tolerating illness just as patients do, and often, through covert and overt interactions, the members begin reacting to each other through frustration, resentment, bitterness, anger, and, ultimately, outright rejection. Our emphysematous patient was upset about her husband's smoking. She had rid herself of the habit because of its deleterious effect on her health, but how could she deny this "good man" his pleasure? She contained her resentment, directing it at her young son, with whom she was disappointed, and, in turn, responded with a worsening of her breathing as well as further disruption of the family.

Anxiety and Distress

Failure of understanding leads to anxiety in physicians and other staff as it does in patients and their families. Without a thorough history of life events preceding patients' episodes of illness and admission to the hospital, it is sometimes impossible to comprehend patients' distress. In the vignette, the patient was anxious because she tended to deny the seriousness of her illness and therefore could not adequately explain her current exacerbation to herself or her physicians. Before the consultant shared with the staff information about the patient's familial conflicts, they saw no reason for the patient's behavior. The consultant's clarification helped the staff to tolerate her behavior, respond to her eccentricities appropriately, and thereby decrease her outbursts. Aside from trying to cope with the imminent loss of her only confidant (her sister-in-law), she herself did not recognize the importance of this woman's role in maintaining homeostasis in her family and her illness. The patient experienced respiratory relief following empathic interest, questioning, and listening.

Staff Reactions

Failure to comprehend how the family setting exacerbates illness often promotes premature labeling in place of thorough evaluation and accurate diagnosis. From the moment Mrs. Z. entered the emergency room, the medical resident questioned her need for admission. His resentment at being overridden by the attending's recommendation sowed the seeds for a negative attitude toward the patient.

The patient's "need" to be punished by her family can also provoke "punishment" from staff. As complaints escalated, a series of dysfunctional relations developed between patient, nurses, and house staff. When she was presented as a management problem on psychiatry attending rounds, the patient's own anger was obvious, and it seemed clear that a mutual standoff had been created by cumulative negative attitudes, resentments, and hostilities, and that hospital discharge seemed the only option to staff. The resident's presentation made it clear that there had been no further effort to elicit more personal or family history beyond the admitting workup. Upset patients not only upset their families but also upset the caretaking staff to the point that good care is compromised.

Sometimes in the furor or commotion caused by an upsetting family, even consulting psychiatrists can lose track of the fact that reactions in staff often mirror patient-family interactions. The patient's distress in this case led to repercussions in staff similar to those in her family. The patient's efforts to establish closeness by joking, arguing, or provoking punishment caused further distancing, withdrawal, and rejection by both family and staff. The helplessness and frustration experienced by both in attempting to maintain their own essential functions and self-esteem commonly lead to despair, readily transmitted to the patient and transmuted into clinical depression. Repetitive experiences of seemingly inexplicable frustration and turmoil among staff may give rise to feelings described by some as occupational burnout.

Interviewing Family Members

It is often important for the consultant to interview members of a patient's family, and it is certainly essential if the family is an upset or upsetting one. Consultants should bear in mind that patients vary in their ability as historians and that the nuances and colorations of medical histories change according to the perception of the storyteller. A consultant should not be fooled into thinking that a family's absence at visiting hours is always indicative of familial discord and friction. It may also indicate illness in the spouse or other family members. Commonly, family members indicate that they are too angry, guilty, ashamed, relieved, or frightened to participate in the patient's hospital experience. Family members who are otherwise very caring and supportive are sometimes too upset by the increased regression, dependency, pain, and anxiety to spend much time at the patient's bedside. On other occasions, family members may overdo their visiting and caring, as though to erase any negative feelings they may have. Interviewing family members can help eliminate the guesswork about family behavior, attitudes, perceptions, and emotional reactions. Such clarification can be of great help to the on-line medical and nursing staff.

A family that has had earlier bad experiences with doctors or hospitalizations may appear testy and uncooperative, with an edge of suspiciousness and distance. The members challenge physicians or nurses to prove their interest and caring by bearing with the patient in spite of blatant hostility. The consultant needs to empathize with the battered staff and then remind them that a response in kind is certain to preclude any effective working relationship. The staff's giving up too soon or avoiding the patient cuts off opportunities to expand on the patient's history, form a clearer picture of the problems, and develop a better alliance. The staff's being upset with the patient, who is already upset, deprives the patient of health-promoting interventions and deprives the staff of the gratifying experience of seeing the patient respond favorably to their ministrations—although this is not always the outcome with a truly dysfunctional family, whose members may need to scapegoat the staff to diffuse or deflect their own distress.

Guidelines

The vignette illustrates a number of system repercussions originating in patients, families, physicians, and nursing staff. Harmonious balance between all elements of the system usually results in patients being considered "good," while unharmonious relationships promote the designation "bad." It is the consultant's task to discover techniques to convert upsetting situations into health-promoting experiences. The consultant can offer the medical and nursing staff the following guidelines:

1. Recognize that a family history is never "noncontributory." Each family has its characteristic strengths, weaknesses, cohesiveness (or divisiveness), rigidity or flexibility in coping with family problems, availability (or unavailability) to members in trouble, capacity to support and encourage, and level of tolerance for sickness. Although each member of a family may vary from the mode, the family as a system can be assessed in global terms as supportive or nonsupportive, denying or accepting, cooperative or resistant, available or distant, and so on. Seeing a family collude with a patient to deny the presence of serious illness helps the physician know that considerable education and support of both family and patient will be needed to assure compliance with medical recommendations.

2. Utilize contacts with patients on rounds and diagnostic tests to expand on personal and family history. An approach that demonstrates the physician's and staff's awareness of the patient's reality as much more than the current illness helps to preserve the patient's sense of self, dignity, and identity. Acknowledging the importance of the patient's life—and learning about the patient's life—before the illness curtails the regressive impact of dehumanization often experienced with illness and hospitalization. It also provides clues to family roles in the onset and course of the illness, useful to the physician in promoting a rehabilitative family setting for the patient's return home.

3. Remember that families, as well as patients, become anxious when a family member is sick and hospitalized. Reactions of individual family members may be colored by closeness to, identification with, anger toward, or guilt concerning the patient. Where individual members and whole families stand in the life cycle (e.g., childhood, adolescence, midlife, senescence) will strongly affect the quality and pattern of response to illness. Furthermore, the role of each member changes as the family constellation shifts or encounters adversity. The degree of family disruption often depends on the hospitalized member's role in the family.

   The seeming nuisance of repeated phone calls from family members may be an expression of appropriate anxiety. Limit setting based on empathic understanding, explanation, education, and support is preferable to resentment, abruptness, and punitiveness.

   It is surprising how little knowledge patients and their families have about particular illnesses, even after they have presumably been informed about them. At times, anxiety blocks understanding of medical explanations, especially if the explanation is given in a matter-of-fact, rather than an empathic, manner, as the following case illustrates.

Mr. A., a 68-year-old architect from a proud, genteel family, had an illness accompanied by delirium. In this state, he shouted expletives and remarks about the medical staff that shamed and humiliated his wife. Besides expressing fear that he would remain abusive, Mrs. A. spent considerable time apologizing to the staff, explaining that her husband really didn't mean what he said and that he had never talked like that to anyone before.

The wife's distress and embarrassment were not initially decreased by a cursory explanation from a staff member that delirious people often say odd things, but they were decreased by the consultant's calm, empathic attention and her explanations of the transient nature of the delirium and of the lack of intent, awareness, or personal significance of the patient's remarks. The consultant also was able to point out that the staff did not take such outbursts personally, and she hoped that Mrs. A wouldn't either.

Explanations about the behavioral repercussions of illness enhance the supportiveness of family members by allaying their fears, guilt, distortions, and anxieties.

4. Learn to use a family's strengths in patient care. Enlist the family members who seem most able to feed, walk, or talk with the patient. In large families, where each member wants equal time with the physician, it may be useful to hold a family conference in which one member whom the family accepts as an authority is assigned to be the spokesperson and communicator for the entire family. In this way, time is saved, family cohesiveness is promoted, and physicians can more efficiently attend to treating patients. In some situations, it may be necessary to encourage visiting by members who seem repelled or rightened by illness. On the other hand, family members may visit excessively, sometimes motivated by guilt. In such instances, the staff may need to give permission to visitors to take time off, and to reassure family members that they will be more helpful to the patient if they rest and relax.

5. Develop flexibility that allows for effective interventions with individuals of various personality types, as illustrated by the following vignette.

Mrs. B., a 76-year-old widow with Parkinson's disease, had had several hospital admissions. On one of them her son called the hospital and angrily told the nurse that if his mother's medication wasn't straightened out, he would take further steps of his own. She attempted to reassure him about his mother's treatment, but his menacing tone and attitude upset her. He demanded that the physician call him after seeing his mother that day.

A psychiatric consultation had been requested because of the patient's complicating depression, and the nurse reported her encounter to the psychiatrist. The woman was moderately depressed, but had shown considerable strength and adaptability as her illness worsened and she became more disabled. She lived alone and tried to manage everything herself, including the complex medical regimen of eight different pills and different times.

The consultant's discussion with the patient revealed her distress over her son's recent divorce, her own increased dependence on him, and her regret that she now needed him to visit her twice a week (instead of once) to help her with transportation to town and household tasks. Arrangements were made for her to be seen in psychiatric follow-up and a phone call was made to her son. He was angry, contentious, and challenging. The psychiatrist gave a nondefensive explanatory response about his mother's treatment. The son's concern about the number of drugs his mother took became more understandable after his allusion to a friend's addiction to diazepam. He was also upset about his mother's increasing dependency, a clear threat to his own wish to deny his own dependency needs. A review of the nature of her illness and the nonaddictive nature of the individual medications seemed to mollify him; reassurance that his mother was a very strong and courageous person elicited the more congenial retort, "She sure is; she's put up with me for forty-five years."

Later that week, the floor nurse reported that the son was friendlier and more cooperative when he next appeared at his mother's bedside. Acknowledging the needs of the patient's son and facilitating his expression of distress helped avert a disruption of the patient's treatment.

6. Know that help is available. Trying to fulfill all the functions alluded to here might soon overwhelm most house officers. Most general hospitals (especially those with teaching affiliations) have social workers and psychiatric nurses to assist the psychiatric consultant. Caring for some upset and upsetting families requires the moral support and reinforcement of a team capable of bearing the emotional burden. The availability and skills of consultants of various disciplines often depend on the institutional structure and individual programs.

A Final Word

Family members who upset, or become upset by, the patient and the staff must be considered as much a part of the system as the patient's symptoms and illness. The consultant needs to remind the staff that the patient is not the only one with problems. The consultant can demonstrate that a thorough family history contributes to understanding the context in which illness has occurred. A staff that can accommodate to, rather than avoid, upset and upsetting families will cultivate better relations with patients and their families, a more collaborative staff effort, and a health-promoting approach to all illness.

Suggested Readings

Anthony, E.J. (1970). The impact of mental and physical illness on family life. *American Journal of Psychiatry* 127:138–146.

Costell, R.M., and Reiss, D. (1982). The family meets the hospital: clinical presentation of a laboratory-based family typology. *Archives of General Psychiatry* 39:433–438.

Lazarus, R. (1977). Psychological stress and coping. In *Psychosomatic Medicine*, ed. Z.J. Lipowski, D.R. Lipsitt, and P. Whybrow, pp. 14–26. New York: Oxford University Press.

Lewis, J.M. (1980). The family matrix in health and disease. In *The Family: Evaluation and Treatment*, ed. C.K. Hofling and J.M. Lewis, pp. 5–44. New York: Brunner/Mazel.

Lipsitt, D.R., and Lipsitt, M.P. (1981). The family in consultation-liaison psychiatry. *General Hospital Psychiatry* 3:231–236.

Mailick, M. (1979). The impact of severe illness on the individual and family: an overview. *Social Work in Health Care* 5:117–128.

Parkes, C.M. (1972). *Bereavement: Studies in Grief in Adult Life*. New York: International Universities Press.

Richardson, H.B. (1945). *Patients Have Families*. New York: Commonwealth Fund.

Steidl, J.W., Finkelstein, F.O., Wexler, J.P., Feigenbaum, H., Kitsen, D., Kliger, A.S., and Quinlan, D.M. (1980). Medical condition, adherence to treatment regimens, and family functioning. *Archives of General Psychiatry* 37:1025–1027.

Steinglass, P., Gonzalez, S., Dosovitz, I., and Reiss, D. (1982). Discussion groups for chronic hemodialysis patients and their families. *General Hospital Psychiatry* 4:7–14.

Weakland, J. (1977). "Family somatics"—a neglected edge. *Family Process* 16:263–272.

CHAPTER 26

Working with the Nursing Staff

PAUL C. MOHL, M.D.

Patients' emotional problems occur within a complex social system. Each hospital unit is a relatively self-contained unit with its own norms, roles, values, expectations, and standards of behavior. Requests for psychiatric consultation may indicate that the group organization has been disturbed in some fashion. The consulting psychiatrist may be expected to restore homeostasis. Thus, to be effective, the psychiatrist must evaluate and sometimes deal with the system in order to treat the patient.

The nursing staff is more than a single element in a complex hierarchy. Nurses are the only permanent members of the system. Patients are admitted and discharged; physicians make rounds and disappear; the nurses remain. Thus they become the culture bearers. They socialize physicians, patients, administrators, and psychiatric consultants into appropriate roles and behavior. Anyone who has been gently but firmly told by a nurse, "We don't keep depressed patients here. We transfer them," appreciates the power of that process.

Working with Nurses during Evaluation

Talking with the nurse(s) is part of the evaluation of patients. Nurses frequently possess more information than do primary physicians; and they make different kinds of observations. Nurses have more direct contact, talk more with patients, interact more with family members, and see patients at more varied times of the day. Nurses are often more aware of dysphoric states, behavior problems, and the need for psychiatric consultation than patients' physicians, as the following case illustrates.

> A psychiatric consultant was asked to see Mr. C., a 72-year-old widower, for "depression and insomnia." The primary physician could report only that the patient seemed withdrawn and demanded nursing attention at night. On evaluation, the patient was not depressed and had a normal mental status examination. The day nurse, however, reported that the night nurse had noted that the patient seemed "a little off, confused." That led the consultant to return in the evening, at which time the patient displayed decreased cognition and clouded sensorium. An organic mental disorder was diagnosed and appropriate management and workup were recommended.

Nurses also have more opportunities to know patients personally and thus can save the consulting psychiatrist's time in identifying the central issues, as shown in the next case.

> A psychiatric consultant was requested for Mr. D., a 45-year-old lawyer who had recently suffered a myocardial infarction and who had become particularly anxious. The cardiologist focused his discussion on the symptoms, cardiac risks of uncontrolled anxiety, and need for adequate medications. The nurse described the patient's anxious need for comforting and then recalled that the patient had twice mentioned that his father had died of a myocardial infarction. The psychiatric consultant was able to focus rapidly on the issue of the patient's father and began brief insight/supportive therapy for the patient's unresolved grief during the initial evaluation.

Physicians' requests for consultation are usually organized within a medical framework: signs, symptoms, diagnoses. However, what provokes a particular consultation at a particular time is often the patient's disruption of the social system or its key members. As the culture bearers, nurses are more likely to address those issues than are physicians. They are much more likely to comment that "these patients make us uncomfortable." The wise psychiatric consultant attends to all comments, especially the nurses', for information about the unit social system. It may take careful listening to determine that the unit social system is being challenged by a particular patient. For example:

> A consultant was asked to see Mr. E., a 23-year-old single store clerk dying of a malignant thymoma. The oncologist felt the patient was depressed and needed psychiatric support. The nurse reported that the patient was tearful at times and added that on morning rounds the patient had responded to the social greeting, "What are you up to?" by saying he was struggling to accept death. The nurse described this in a manner as if to say, "See! That proves there's something wrong!" At that

point, the psychiatrist began to suspect that the problem lay more with the unit norms than with the patient. Indeed, the patient was actively but appropriately grieving. He had more than enough family support available and did not require further intervention.

Although psychiatric consultants must be careful about suggesting interventions that conflict with social system mythology, a patient care conference with the nurses helped in Mr. E.'s case to modulate norms against overt grieving, men crying, and nurses feeling sad. An equally effective intervention might have involved regular psychotherapeutic visits to the patient, thus shielding the unit staff from the challenge to its established way of dealing with feelings. The important issue in such a case is recognizing that the central issue is a destabilized social system. The psychiatrist can select an intervention directed toward reestablishing the former homeostasis or establishing a new one.

Another issue that can lead to a request for a psychiatric consultation is unresolved disagreement within the medical team. This hidden conflict will rarely be expressed in the written consultation request, but it may be expressed in face-to-face discussion. It becomes apparent most often in the conflicting observations and reports of different team members, as we see in the next vignette.

> A liaison psychiatrist working with an oncology unit noticed that she often received requests to help treat depression, withdrawal, or decreased motivation when part of the team was not prepared for the death of a terminal patient but when other team members had accepted that the patient would soon die.
>
> After considerable frustration, spending much time evaluating patients and finding those evaluations unhelpful, she began identifying these cases early in the consultation process by asking the referring physicians and nurses for their estimates of prognosis. When there was a large discrepancy in their estimates, she met with the physician and nurses together before seeing the patient. Frequently, this meeting resolved the need for consultation. Eventually, she suggested a regular meeting between the oncologist and the nursing care coordinator to review and discuss the level and vigor of care for all patients. This effectively resolved the conflict within the system.

Finally, sometimes nurses fully understand what is going on with a patient, but primary physicians are unwilling to accept their ideas and opinions. The psychiatric consultant helps by translating the nurses' information into medical/psychiatric terms, thus authenticating and validating the nurses' communications.

To summarize, nurses have much information about the patient and about the social system's reaction to the patient. In order to approach the consultation maximally informed, the psychiatric consultant should discuss the request with the nurses and should evaluate information about the patient at a content level and should evaluate information about the medical team's response to the patient at a process level.

Working with Nurses to Implement Treatment

Nurses rarely have the time to talk with patients at length, but when they do, their already-established rapport makes them valuable adjunct therapists. The psychiatric consultant may use these adjunct therapists in formulating or implementing a treatment plan. This has been accomplished on physical medicine units, coronary care units, oncology units, and obstetrical units. Nurses may offer support groups for stroke patients, or do individual supportive work with depressed, anergic patients. Coronary care nurses usually have an educational role. Nurses may give information to and counsel spinal cord injury patients concerning sexual difficulties (see Chapter 33, on spinal cord injuries). For nurses comfortable with the role, it is just a short step to supportive counseling for anxious or depressed patients. Here, the consultant can back up nursing staff by providing informal supervision. Moreover, the consultant sometimes encourages nurses to carry out their educational functions in a group setting. In such circumstances, group support may become a valued offshoot of their efforts. Oncology nurses are effective death and dying counselors and family support group counselors. Obstetrical nurses can promote griefwork following poor-outcome deliveries. In all these situations, proper supervision and support from a liaison psychiatrist are essential. (For further discussion of specialty support wards for patients, see Chapters 29 to 32.)

Developing nurses as a resource for implementing therapy often requires the coordinated effort of an established liaison program, as seen in this example.

> A psychiatric resident participated in the weekly team staffing on a rehabilitation unit and initiated a support group for stroke patients. When she left the consultation service, the nurses took over under the supervision of a staff liaison psychiatrist. A spinal cord support group was formed, and later a sexual counseling program was initiated. Thus, with an effort of one or two hours per week, far more patients were treated than could be dealt with in routine consultation. Without the initial liaison effort, the nurses might never have become involved.

Nurses are also important to the treatment process as key members of the patient's immediate support system. In many instances, the nurses' reactions to the patient and their response to the patient's needs determine the level of the patient's adaptation to the illness and hospitalization. Nurses' ability to deal with an antisocial patient's provocative acting out will often prevent its escalation. Their provision of nonrejecting but firm limits to a borderline patient can prevent psychotic fragmentation. Their empathizing with a narcissistic, entitled perfectionist may lead to compliance instead of rageful noncompliance. And their willingness to meet the needs of a regressed patient may prevent prolonged withdrawal and depression. (For further discussion of personality types and their behaviors in medical settings, see Chapter 13.)

Thus in many consultations the nurses become the primary objects of recommendations concerning the patient's basic needs, motives, and feelings. It is important that the consultant's comments and suggestions evoke an empathic response in the nurses. A set of specific, concrete recommendations can then be spelled out and implemented effectively. In the first of the following two examples, the evocation of an empathic response was central. In the second, detailed behavioral suggestions were required.

> Ms. F., a 25-year-old taxi driver with a borderline personality disorder was being treated for seizures on a neurology unit. She was splitting the nursing staff, provoking hostile rejection, alternately clinging to and raging at them. In his note, the psychiatric consultant detailed her chaotic developmental history, which included abuse as a child, sexual molestations, and repeated abandonment. He then wrote:
>
> 1. Her reactions have nothing to do with our current behavior. We are all stand-ins for everyone who abused and abandoned her.
> 2. She is a 15-month-old masquerading as a 25-year-old. Respond to her as you would to any ambivalent, empty, fearful, angry 15-month-old.
> 3. See how this works. I'll check back and set up a conference if further help is necessary.
>
> The conference was never necessary. The nurses intuitively assumed a firm but empathic stance and became more tolerant of the patient's affective swings, and their concern helped modulate her behavior.

> Mr. G., a 50-year-old married truck driver with a Guillain-Barré syndrome, became quadriplegic. After a month in the ICU, the patient's family decreased their visits. A month later a consultation was requested to deal with the patient's depression and withdrawal. The patient had regressed, relating apathetically to the nurses, rejecting their offers to turn on the radio, bring in a television, or to read a newspaper. He had no vegetative signs of depression but seemed not to care about anything. The psychiatrist made the following recommendations on the basis of his presumption that the patient was experiencing a conservation-withdrawal response.
>
> 1. Accept and tolerate this patient's need to regress. Touch him as often as possible, more than is required by your regular nursing care. Talk with him whether he responds or not. Tell him what's

happening on the unit (his home now) and in the world. Try to be soothing, as with a sick child.

2. Reestablish a good diurnal variation. Keep lights off from 11 P.M. to 7 A.M.; absolutely minimal nursing activities during that time. Lights should be on all other times and something should be happening—radio, TV, visitor. Do this despite his requests to be left alone.

3. Assume responsibility for keeping him "in contact." Keep a calendar and a clock highly visible, and keep familiar objects from home at the bedside, including fishing magazines (his hobby). Read to him from them twice a day for 5 to 10 minutes. Show him the pictures. Have a radio or TV on or someone talking to him virtually all day.

4. Suggest to his family that they set up a rotational schedule (it is a large family) so that someone can be here almost every day for 30 to 60 minutes.

The nurses were able to implement this plan. The patient's regression stabilized and then reversed as he awaited the abatement of his illness. Despite very slow physiological change, the patient returned to his prior level of interaction within two weeks.

The Specific Needs of Nurses

Much emphasis has been placed on the vulnerability of nurses to "burnout," but it is not always entirely clear what is meant by this term. Nor is it clear that nurses are more susceptible than are other professional or nonprofessional workers. It is clear to all who work in hospitals that many nurses seem unhappy, angry, disillusioned, and unfulfilled.

There are two major hypotheses about nurses' vulnerability to burnout. One involves job stresses. Nurses are far more intimately and personally involved with patients than other health care workers. Thus the impact of debilitated, ill, dying patients, and of stressed, emotionally demanding families is profound. Furthermore, nurses are on the front line, recognizing and responding to crises. Yet often they lack authority for initiating or maintaining standards of caregiving despite their personal feelings of responsibility to the patient. Finally, they work irregular shifts as part of a hospital bureaucracy, and lack the autonomy and power of physicians.

The other hypothesis involves nurses' roles within the health care system. Unlike physicians, nurses have very little control over their work situations. Much of what they do is spelled out in physicians' orders or in bureaucratic procedures. A complicating feature is the sex-role issue of nurses (mostly women) who take orders from physicians (mostly men) in a climate in which women are struggling to achieve equality. And, of course, nurses' remuneration levels are vastly different from physicians'.

A veritable industry providing support for nurses has arisen. Supporting nurses is justified partly by the inherent need, partly as consulting psychiatrists' role in serving the patients by serving the system, and partly to improve care to the patients through increased nursing knowledge and efficiency. Attention was first paid to the problems of nurses in intensive care settings. Although general medical units are probably as stressful as intensive care units, the continuing focus of consultation psychiatrists has been on specialized units such as coronary care, oncology, and renal dialysis. An area of high-stress nursing that has received even less attention than general medical and surgical units is chronic care. This includes nursing homes and long-term rehabilitation units. In these settings, nurses' involvement with patients and families is very intense and demanding. Emotional factors are an important determinant of treatment outcome, but nurses have little training in that area.

A major intervention offered by psychiatrists is support groups. In these meetings a substantial proportion of the nursing staff (or the entire nursing staff) of a given unit meets weekly with a consulting psychiatrist. Support groups usually begin as discussions of direct, clinical problems. The leader of the group has much latitude from that point forward, however. Some groups remain at that level, perhaps extending the group task to dealing with countertransference problems with specific patients. Other groups attend to more general support issues, not always related to specific patients. This may include teaching specific stress-management techniques, allowing ventilation, or building group cohesion.

Some consulting psychiatrists have sought to use support groups to change the system. This may involve trying to alter the unit culture in the direction of more therapeutic norms, or it may involve work on communications problems and intrastaff conflict. Regardless of the stance and direction taken by the leaders, most have reported success with most or all of their groups.

Despite the extensive literature on and experience with support groups, they may not be the most effective nor efficient method for dealing with the needs of the nursing staff. Direct consultation may be just as useful.

If a problem involves only nurses' difficulties in dealing with a particular patient, consultation by a psychiatric nurse may be very effective. Many hospitals make this possible by using nurses from their psychiatric inpatient units for consultation with medical-surgical nurses. Other hospitals include psychiatric nurse clinicians as members of the psychiatric consultation service or as part of the nursing service itself. Such direct nurse-to-nurse consultation is very effective and more efficient than a psychiatric consultation as long as the problem is limited to a nurse's countertransference or other problem managing a patient. It is no substitute for careful psychiatric diagnosis and treatment. The medical-surgical nurse, the psychiatric nurse, or the nurse clinician may not be in a position to recognize the boundary between a nursing problem and a psychiatric problem. Thus, if this model is used, a consulting psychiatrist should actively supervise the psychiatric nurse.

Another model involves direct consultation between the psychiatrist and head nurses. The potential value of this model is suggested by the finding that stress levels among nurses on a given unit correlate (inversely) with staff support, not with the type of unit, work load, or group cohesion. Staff support is the degree to which each nurse feels supported by the head nurse. The best intervention may therefore be to assist the head nurse in supporting the unit nursing staff, as shown in the next vignette.

> A consulting psychiatrist was approached by the medical intensive care unit head nurse to assist the nursing staff in dealing with burnout. Informal conversation with nursing staff revealed conflicts with physicians, administrative problems, competitiveness, hypervigilance, and stress symptoms. Two group meetings revealed, in addition, a deep alienation between the head nurse and her staff. They respected her, but yearned for a more personal, listening relationship with her. She believed that supervisors should maintain distance from their supervisees. Subsequently, in a 1½-hour individual session with the consultant, she explored ways of being a good supervisor while offering a genuine, personally involved relationship to her staff. Informal follow-up at 6 and 12 months with the head nurse and staff nurses revealed significant improvement in their relationship, and a significant decrease in the staff's other problems.

The consulting psychiatrist can offer education to nurses. Nurses receive little schooling in behavioral science. Thus it is not realistic to expect them to easily recognize or distinguish the major psychiatric disorders or to appreciate different personality patterns. Nor is it realistic to always expect medical-surgical nurses to know effective ways of relating to problem patients or the transference/countertransference issues that are involved. Education in basic psychological mechanisms and processes is commonly needed and well received. Active participation by consulting psychiatrists in nursing in-service programs is also important.

Conclusion

Nurses are crucial to psychiatric consultation. Their roles within the unit social system put them in a position to facilitate or undermine the consultant's efforts. Their observations often clarify clinical problems. Their frequent contact with the patient and family members make them invaluable in implementing a treatment plan. Meeting their needs can become an important part of the consulting psychiatrist's efforts. Educational support, direct consultation, and support groups can all be used to achieve this.

Suggested Readings

Caldwell, T., and Weiner, M.F. (1981). Stresses and coping in ICU nursing I. A review. *General Hospital Psychiatry* 3:119–127.

Dubovsky, S.L., Getto, C.J., Gross, S.A., and Paley, J.A. (1977). Impact on nursing care and mortality: psychiatrists on the coronary care unit. *Psychosomatics* 18:18–27.

Gunther, M.S. (1977). The threatened staff: a psychoanalytic contribution to medical psychology. *Comprehensive Psychiatry* 18:385–399.

Karasu, T.B., and Hertzman, M. (1974). Notes on a contextual approach to medical ward consultation: the importance of social system mythology. *International Journal of Psychiatry in Medicine* 5:41–49.

Mohl, P.C. (1980). Group process interpretations in liaison psychiatry nurse groups. *General Hospital Psychiatry* 2:104–111.

Mohl, P.C. (1981). A review of systems approaches to consultation-liaison psychiatry: the need for synthesis. *General Hospital Psychiatry* 3:103–110.

Mohl, P.C., Denny, N.R., Mote, T.A., and Coldwater, C. (1982). Hospital unit stressors that affect nurses: primary task vs social factors. *Psychosomatics* 23:366–374.

Rosini, L.A., Howell, M.C., Todres, I.D., and Dorman, J. (1974). Group meetings in a pediatric intensive care unit. *Pediatrics* 53:371–374.

Schulman, B.M. (1975). Group process: an adjunct in liaison consultation psychiatry. *International Journal of Psychiatry in Medicine* 6:489–499.

Torem, M., Saravay, S.M., and Steinberg, H. (1979). Psychiatric liaison: benefits of "active" approach. *Psychosomatics* 20:598–611.

Weiner, M.F., and Caldwell, T. (1981). Stresses and coping in ICU nursing II. Nurse support groups on intensive care units. *General Hospital Psychiatry* 3:129–134.

CHAPTER 27

Religious Concerns

THE REVEREND ROBERT L. DAVIS

The religious beliefs of patients and their families strongly influence their adaptation to illness, hospitalization, and medical personnel. Adaptive religious beliefs that support self-esteem and provide personal direction in a context of health can become maladaptive during periods of ill health and hospitalization.

American culture has assumed many of the values and norms of its religious communities. Whether or not people have grown up in deeply religious homes, the influence of religious symbols is usually apparent. Many of the 300 separate religious groups in America have lost their clarity and their sense of their own history. The result has been a blending of religious symbols and ideals, more obvious in the less confessional religious bodies and in geographical regions where religious belief has been overwhelmed by survival needs or political influence. In these instances, cultures and subcultures become more influential in people's lives than religious beliefs. Thus, if life is suddenly threatened, people may be inclined to depend on the belief system of their subculture as if it were the belief system of their religious group. For example, hospital chaplains are regularly called on to baptize infants of Southern Baptist couples when the children's lives are in danger. This occurs despite the fact that the Southern Baptist Church does not believe in infant baptism; it believes only in adult or "believers" baptism. In a community with a specific ethnic heritage such as an Italian-American community, the basic beliefs of most community members may be most similar to those of the Roman Catholic Church. Roman Catholic beliefs become integrated into the subculture in a way that produces people who are

"Baptist-Catholic," "Lutheran-Catholic," "Presbyterian-Catholic," and so forth. In communities that grew out of a distinct pioneering spirit, such as those found in the panhandle of Texas, where people have survived dust-bowl storms and dry-land farms, the religious and political tone tends to be a "work righteousness" or "proof-is-in-the-product" mind set. Thus people of varying religious beliefs incorporate into their belief systems values of their region and subculture. In fact, many cannot distinguish between their religious beliefs and commonly held community beliefs.

Added to this phenomenon is the fact that many religious denominations, such as United Methodist and Presbyterian, hold openness to new ideas as a significant value. Although that openness is appealing to many, it brings about a poor pluralism that results from people not knowing their own religious history well enough to make informed comparisons. When this is the case, it is almost impossible to differentiate between religious and cultural attitudes. The belief system that often emerges is a combination of belief based on religious scripture and tradition, on folk tales that have become a part of an oral tradition in the subculture, on regional survival needs or heroes, and at times on responses to having been oppressed.

Psychiatrists evaluating patients must take seriously their patients' religious preferences, but they must avoid making too many generalizations about them. Especially in a time of personal crisis, it may be difficult to distinguish between the influences of religion and of culture. Thus the significant point is to ascertain the meaning and power patients grant their religion as they attempt to "order" life, even if this meaning or power is couched in cultural terms.

Generally speaking, people aligned with a liberal Protestant denomination or with reformed Judaism are most open to scientific information, to change, and to experimentation. They are typically more comfortable with pluralism than with dogmatism. The responsibility for making decisions in reference to medical treatment clearly belongs to each individual. These people are inclined to operate from an internal locus of control. Their religions provide certain guidelines for making decisions, but individuals decide ultimately. In contrast, but in varying degrees, people belonging to more fundamentalist or orthodox religious groups are more inclined toward an external locus of control. Conflicts between religious belief and medical practice are more common in these people because the faith group has usually developed stronger, and often rigid, doctrines. People's motivation for belonging to these groups often lies in their need to move against or to be set apart from more dominant cultural patterns. These religions thus claim timeless truths and their own unique way of making sense of life. In times of crisis, members of liberal faiths tend to become diffuse and confused; followers of dogmatic religions tend to become even more dependent on external value systems and are therefore more resistant to new ideas or practices, quick decisions, and change.

Given the basic tendencies just outlined, the most important factor may be the commitment people feel to their beliefs, and the way they use them in crisis, instead of the actual beliefs of their source. The clinician may therefore find it helpful to identify significant religious themes that cross denominational and cultural classifications.

Important Religious Themes

Advent or "End-of-the-World" Teachings and Practices

The word *advent* is commonly used in Christian tradition to mean the season of the Christian year when people anticipate and celebrate the coming or birth of Jesus. Adventists, however, believe a second coming of the Messiah will happen in their lifetime. When that occurs, Adventist believers expect that they and other like believers will become the empowered, whether on Earth or in Heaven. Two religious groups strongly identified with Adventist theology are Seventh Day Adventists and Jehovah's Witnesses.

The Seventh Day Adventists' origin may be traced to Baptist minister William Miller, who calculated the date for the Second Coming of the Lord to be October 22, 1844. Many prepared for the occasion that was afterward labeled "The Great Disappointment"; it was the last definite date set by the movement's leadership. These Adventists became "Seventh Day Adventists" following the leadership of Ellen Harmon White, who believed the Ten Commandments to represent the character of God and emphasized worship on Saturday instead of Sunday, the first day of the week.

For health care professionals, the most significant teachings of the Seventh Day Adventists concern diet, health, and medical care. They are vegetarians and have been creative in developing meat substitutes. They abstain from drinks containing caffeine or alcohol. Obesity is not acceptable to them. They have established a number of programs of preventive health care, own hospitals throughout the nation, and operate the Loma Linda Medical School.

The Jehovah's Witnesses were founded by Charles Taze Russell around 1870. Russell taught that the end of the world would come during the year 1914. Their doctrine changed when that did not happen. They believe that millions of people now living will never die. They reject the idea of priesthood and have developed a group relationship with God in which all members are considered ministers. Jehovah's Witnesses tend to resist any external encroachment on their lives, whether from government agencies, health care teams, or other organized religions. This resistance is often seen in relation to public education of children, payment of taxes, military service, and treatment of the sick. Jehovah's Witnesses are not likely to accept the authority of doctors. Legal measures used in committing patients for psychiatric care are usually challenged on religious grounds. Sterilization is forbidden and contraception is discouraged. Hypnosis is considered an evil practice. Jehovah's Witnesses are best known for their interpretation of Leviticus 17:10 in their New World Translation: "God told Noah that every living creature should be meat unto him, but that he must not eat the blood, because the life is in the blood." From their publication *Jehovah's Witnesses and the Question of Blood* comes this quote from the Bible: "a human does not sustain his life with the blood from another creature" (Gen. 9:3–4). When the life of an animal is taken, the blood representing that life is to be "poured out," given back to the life giver (Lev. 17:13–14). And as described by the Apostolic Council, Christians are to "abstain from blood," which applies to human blood as well as animal blood (Acts 15:28–29). There are no exceptions to the rule of blood and blood transfusions. Since 1944, when their prohibition of blood transfusion went into effect, there have been court cases in which the power of the State was invoked against their religious tradition when physicians deemed a life to be at stake.

A further problem for psychiatrists attempting to work with Jehovah's Witnesses is their adherence to a belief system that encourages believers to invite persecution and prompts them to take a condescending position in relation to others' beliefs. Resistance to medical care may also be a way to express their belief that they are immune to death.

In summary, these two Adventist groups have responded very differently to a similar belief system. Jehovah's Witnesses use their belief in the Second Coming to reject authority and to deny death. Seventh Day Adventists, following "The Great Disappointment," have begun to affirm the reality of death and to look for ways of extending and enhancing life. They see themselves as moving toward conservation of life rather than martyrdom.

Sacramental-Liturgical Teachings and Practices

During the first century, the Christian Church was formed to "embody" Christ's teachings. It developed a structure for caring for children, widows (often left without care in those days), the needy, and the oppressed. Such teachings were so greatly misinterpreted in the first and second centuries that Christians were persecuted severely. The persecutions continued until Constantine took the Roman throne in A.D. 313. He had his troops baptized and so laid the groundwork for Rome's becoming the established seat of the Church. A hierarchy of deacons and priests, utilizing creeds, doctrines, and sacraments, became custodians of the Church, which was deemed "God's kingdom on earth." The Roman Catholic Church, the Greek Orthodox Church, the Russian Orthodox Church, and the Anglican Church each developed a system of discipline that takes into account the major events and common crises of the human life cycle. This system is called the sacramental system. The seven sacraments common to these groups parallel the stages in human social development from birth to death:

1. Baptism (at birth).
2. Confirmation (at 12 or 13).
3. Eucharist, or the Mass (weekly and at high holy days).
4. Penance (confession to a priest as needed, but at least once a year).
5. Orders (initiation to priesthood, deaconate, or into an order of sisters).
6. Marriage (only by a priest).
7. Sacrament of the Sick (administered by a priest when a person is ill or when death is imminent).

Psychiatrists should be aware that all these sacraments can have medical implications. These sacraments focus all the concerns of these churches having to do with sex or procreation, contraception, abortion, divorce and remarriage, euthanasia, and so forth. Since the "rules are clear," many people struggling with current societal norms, individual thought, and value setting feel guilty, unclean, or sinful. Many members of the clergy are helpful; many are not. When left with unresolved feelings of guilt, many believers become depressed, and some become indifferent not only to the "rules" of the church but also to those of society at large.

Although the sacraments may be fewer than seven (more often two: Baptism and the Eucharist, or Holy Communion) or no sacraments at all, the basic assumptions and beliefs of many Protestant church members will be quite similar to members of the sacramental-liturgical churches. Some Protestant churches never intended to be separated out. United Methodism, for example, began with the Anglican Church as a movement toward social reforms, spiritual piety, and evangelistic concerns. Although it became a church denomination in America during the Revolutionary War, it bears much in common with its Anglican parent.

The basic belief systems—cultural and religious—concerning marriage, sexuality, divorce, child rearing, and death do not differ greatly among most Protestants and Catholics. Most Protestants, in accepting these ideologies (at whatever level), have done so without developing a system of enforcement and instruction. Therefore, these individuals are bound with a heavy burden of certainty that their place in heaven or hell is assured by the way they behave in these matters. Thus many Protestants are laden with conflicting demands and guilts without, for example, the social or liturgical resolution offered by the Catholic Church. It is curious that some of the more fundamental believers who find Catholicism objectionable have themselves built denominational structures upon their own interpretation of "sacraments" and practice. They emphasize being "born again" through conversion from sin to a profession of faith as a resolution to the inner conflicts.

The psychiatrist should be alert to the possibility that obsessive-compulsive rumination and depressive self-rejection may collect around symptoms having their roots in religious teaching, whatever the denomination.

Deliverance and Ethnic Teachings and Practices

The religious experience of people who have lived their lives in oppression is marked by a longing for deliverance. The Jews are one of the oldest and most powerful ethnic groups whose religion has focused on a theme of deliverance—from bondage in Egypt, from Babylonian captivity, and from the Holocaust under Hitler. Family ties are usually close and often present unique family dynamics. Much of the energy of celebration, sadness, or anger that might become generalized in its expression in other subcultures is focused within the "safety" of the Jewish family.

Reformed Judaism leaves most decisions that would affect medical treatment to individual discretion. Conservative and Orthodox Judaism prefer to keep strict dietary laws. At death, they prefer that a family member close the eyes of the deceased, that the clothes the person is wearing at the time be left intact or, at least, buried with the person (especially if the clothes contain any of the person's blood). An autopsy may be performed when legally necessary, but the deceased person must be buried within 24 hours after death.

A newer religious group formulated around the deliverance theme is the American Black Muslims. Their religion makes an effort to meet problems of pride, identity, and deliverance from associations with slavery and discrimination. Much of their believers' religious expressions will appear hostile and threatening, with distinct bitterness toward white authority.

Spiritual Gifts and Spirit Possession Teachings and Practices

Pentecost Sunday falls on the fifth Sunday after Easter in the Christian year. This was a time when, according to the second chapter of Acts, the Holy Spirit descended upon the Apostles, granting them various gifts related to God's attributes. The Pentecostal Church focuses much attention on the "gifts" of the Holy Spirit: gifts of healing, glossolalia (speaking in unknown tongues), and power over demons. Most emotional illnesses and some physical illnesses—especially physical illnesses that affect movements—are interpreted as the result of demonic possession. Thus Pentecostals have healing sessions and often seek to exorcise these demons. Although these activities could conceivably be successful with certain hysterical conditions, such methods may be very harmful to people who are becoming psychotic. Generally speaking, Pentecostals in our society understand people's problems as evidence of the war between good and evil: God and the devil. More often than not, these people approach life from a "one down" position. Pentecostal churches attract many of their numbers from socially and economically depressed areas. The strong emphasis on "otherworldly" rewards and judgment on those who do not believe the same way may be a way of saying: "Although we do not have the 'goods' in this life, we have the power where it really counts." These people are often rigid and hostile to health care professionals.

Of course, not all Pentecostals have rigid personalities; nonetheless, many Pentecostals and other "fundamentalists" are perceived as unbending. They tend to see things only in terms of right or wrong, good or bad, black or white. There is little appreciation for the "gray areas" of life. There is a very low tolerance for ambiguity. Children of such rigid, fundamentalist parents are often excellent candidates for developing psychopathy. In adolescence, when faced with life's ambiguities, they begin to feel they cannot "win." They have not been taught the difference between thought and action, feelings and behavior, and they begin to feel it is as wrong to have feelings as to act on them. There are many problems with human sexuality, as an example. Such scriptural quotes as "As a man thinketh in his heart, so is he" or "If a man so much as look upon a woman in lust, he has as much as committed adultery" are examples. Thus a young man who has normal feelings of sexual arousal and who does not act on those feelings may feel as guilty as if he had acted on them. The adolescent, after a number of similar instances, may begin to feel "damned if he does, and damned if he doesn't." He may unconsciously decide, then, to establish his own rules for behavior: rules that may be very egocentric.

And, of course, the very struggle with "evil spirits" in the world raises the possibility of a paranoid disorder.

Positive Thinking and Health Teachings and Practices

There is a joke about a Roman Catholic priest, a rabbi, and a Christian Science practitioner having died and gone to Hell. The priest and the rabbi, in trying to understand why they were in Hell rather than Heaven, remembered times when they had broken dietary laws; the former ate steak on a Friday during Lent, and the latter ate ham during Passover. After discussing their dilemma for a time, they turned to the Christian Science practitioner and asked: "Why do you think you are here?" He responded, "Oh, I'm not really here." Christian Scientists believe evil, pain, sickness, and even death exist only in the mind.

The Church of Christ Scientist was founded by Mary Baker Eddy in 1879. Christian Scientists consider people who seek medical attention as unenlightened or without faith. Christian Science's key teachings are that God is totally supreme, that matter is nothing, and that the only reality of sin, sickness, and death are their *seeming* reality to the mind. For them, the best treatment is, with the assistance of a Christian Science practitioner, to deny the reality of pain, sickness, or death. Actually, practitioners have much success in treating psychogenic illnesses. However, Christian Scientists may not discriminate between functional and organic disorders, and they often feel guilty for taking any medication, for seeing a physician, and certainly for being admitted to a hospital, even when the illness is clearly life-threatening. Drugs or other medical modalities are seen as poor substitutes for becoming a part of the Divine Mind, which is eternal and transcends pain and death.

The mental health professional does well to remember what was stated earlier about the confusion that is often generated when people in crisis begin to draw from any available resource as they attempt to deal with their anxiety. Any or all of the tenets of the religious groupings outlined here may be available for a person for healthy or unhealthy use. Knowing the religious background of the patient can help the psychiatrist, but only as an indicator or a beginning point of reference.

The Hospital Chaplain

Where trained hospital chaplains are available, it is often a good idea to call on them for assistance in evaluating patients' use of religion or religiosity in coping with crisis.

Clinical pastoral education is an interfaith, interdenominational graduate education program that integrates studies in behavioral sciences and theology into a pastoral care/pastoral counseling ministry.

Trained hospital chaplains usually have completed at least a Bachelor of Arts or equivalent degree (four years), a Master of Divinity or equivalent degree (three or four years), and at least one full year of internship/residency in clinical pastoral education. Chaplains are also members in good standing of a denominational or religious body and have completed at least three years in the ministry before becoming certified as hospital chaplains. If chaplains are certified chaplain supervisors (or teaching chaplains), they have completed at least two more years' residency and have met the requirements of regional and national certification committees. Trained chaplains can be important members of the health care team.

Because the training required for ordination of clergy varies from denomination to denomination, the psychiatrist may, in attempting to work with some patients' pastors, experience some limitations in the pastors' ability to deal with psychiatric issues. It is even possible that the clergy may be antagonistic toward the psychiatrist. For this reason, the psychiatrist may want to use the trained chaplain as a liaison person with patients' pastors, priests, or rabbis.

Chaplains attempt to approach patients holistically. They make every effort to see patients as persons of worth and dignity, rather than as diagnosed illnesses. Chaplains will often be involved with patients' families and thus may gain a different perspective of the patients than psychiatrists who interview only the patients. Chaplains can serve as liaisons between patients' pastors and physicians and between patients' families and physicians. Chaplains can also ascertain whether the patients' use of religious language is part of their upbringing or results from illness.

Because some people trust science and not religion and others trust religion and not science, psychiatrists and chaplains who have already developed a working relationship will often be able to discern which of them will be trusted by which patient. Very often, pastors (chaplains) will be seen as "homefolk" and therefore will be trusted by patients who might not trust psychiatrists. There is great symbolic power in the role of the clergy. Sometimes that power is used judgmentally and undermines self-worth; sometimes the power embodies grace and forgiveness, as shown in the following case example.

Mrs. H., age 25, was brought to the emergency room by her husband, who reported that she had been withdrawn and had refused to eat or drink since she had been dismissed from the hospital following a hysterectomy. She not only refused proper nourishment but stayed in bed (although she had been told that inactivity could delay her recovery) and was noncommunicative.

The primary emergency room physician began treating the patient's dehydration and called for a psychiatric consultation. The psychiatrist was able to elicit conversation from the woman who, during the course of the interview, had mentioned several times that "God is punishing me." The patient did not want to accept medical treatment because she felt she deserved to be punished.

The psychiatrist called for the hospital chaplain who, in talking with the patient, learned that she was a Roman Catholic who felt her hysterectomy had not been essential to her physical survival and, therefore, that she had gone against "God's commandment" by having the surgery. After visiting with the patient, who continued to talk more freely, the chaplain, a Protestant, obtained the patient's permission to contact a Roman Catholic priest. The chaplain discussed the situation with the priest and then introduced the priest to the patient. The priest heard the patient's confession and offered her forgiveness through absolution, after which the patient agreed to accept medical treatment.

Every situation is different. The better the working relationship that psychiatrists develop with chaplains, the more helpful can be their team effort in working with patients and their families.

Suggested Readings

Cavenar, J.O., and Spaulding, J.G. (1977). Brief communication: depressive disorders and religious conversion. *Journal of Nervous and Mental Disease* 165:209–212.

Cohen, R.J., and Smith, F.J. (1976). Socially reinforced obsession: etiology of a disorder in a Christian Scientist. *Journal of Consulting and Clinical Psychology* 44:142–144.

Frank, J. (1961). *Persuasion and Healing*. Baltimore: Johns Hopkins University Press.

Hulme, W.E. (1981). *Pastoral Care and Counseling*. Minneapolis: Augsburg.

Oates, W. (1978). *The Religious Care of the Psychiatric Patient*. Philadelphia: Westminster Press.

Pruyser, P.W. (1976). *The Minister as Diagnostician*. Philadelphia: Westminster Press.

Watchtower Bible and Tract Society (1977). *Jehovah's Witnesses and the Question of Blood*. Brooklyn, N.Y.: Watchtower Bible and Tract Society.

Weintraub, W., and Aronson, H. (1974). Patients in psychoanalysis: some findings related to sex and religion. *American Journal of Orthopsychiatry* 44:102–108.

CHAPTER 28

Cultural Concerns in Consultation Psychiatry

THOMAS M. JOHNSON, PhD.
ARTHUR KLEINMAN, M.D., M.A.

People are taught by their culture how to interpret and communicate about symptoms, from whom to seek care, how to explain illness etiology and pathophysiology, how serious and long-lasting the problem is, and what to expect from treatment.

An appreciation of the differences in styles of communication and codes of etiquette for physician-patient interaction is important in working with culturally diverse patients.

This chapter provides guidelines for working with patients whose medical practices and attitudes toward health care differ from those of their caregivers. The reduction of barriers to communication and understanding is essential to increasing the quality and effectiveness of care, as seen in the following examples.

> A 65-year-old black grandmother is seen in psychiatric consultation because of "depressed affect." She avoids eye contact by lowering her gaze and responds minimally to direct questions. Does her behavior result from her thyroid condition, a recurrence of "schizophrenia" for which she was hospitalized for ten years two decades previously, an affective disorder, or a culturally patterned response to authority figures?

> A 33-year-old Chinese clerk presents to the emergency room with complaints of tiredness, weakness, dizziness, anorexia, weight loss, and insomnia of six months' duration. His physical examination is within normal limits, but he refuses to accept a diagnosis of depression, instead ascribing his problems to "not enough blood." What is a useful approach to such a patient?

A 23-year-old single Hispanic mechanic has pneumonia and manic symptomatology. He has a history of bipolar affective disorder and is taking lithium. He reports that his mood is "too hot" and that the lithium makes him "too cool" so that he takes it with garlic each day. What is the best way to ensure that he will follow a prescribed lithium regimen after discharge?

Assessing Patients from a Cultural Perspective

There is as much cultural heterogeneity within ethnic groups as there is between them; physical appearance must not be confused with ethnic identity. Members of any ethnic group vary in the extent to which the distinctive characteristics of their ethnic heritage influence their behavior. Ethnic identity is defined as *behavioral* when the distinctive values, norms, beliefs, and language of the ethnic group powerfully shape interaction with others in and out of the ethnic group. Ethnic identity may be considered *ideological* when there is only nominal identification with one's cultural heritage and the distinctive customs and beliefs of the ethnic group are unimportant in daily life. Ideological ethnicity tends to be found in upwardly mobile ethnics of higher social class. Behavioral ethnicity is frequently associated with the lower social classes.

In general, the less an ethnic group member is acculturated to American culture, the more ethnicity will influence that person's health care practices and interaction with health care practitioners. The major predictors of less acculturation include (1) low level of formal education, (2) recent immigration at an older age, (3) segregation (from the larger population) within an ethnic social network, (4) lack of experience with American medical services, (5) rural origins, and (6) frequent returns to the country of origin.

Cultural Factors in Clinical Interaction

Communication and Language

When using a translator, the psychiatrist arranges the clinical setting to make this person as unobtrusive but involved as possible. It is useful to instruct the translator that all questions and eye contact will be directed at the patient but that pauses will be frequent to allow for translation. The translator can then be positioned to the side of the psychiatrist or the patient but still feel part of the team.

Translators are often members of the same ethnic group as patients. Cultural codes of etiquette may make it difficult to discuss certain topics or for translators to be in the same room with patients and their physicians. For example, many Hispanics are reluctant to talk about genital or excretory functions, or to be in view of people who are partially dressed.

When working with patients who speak no English, nonverbal forms of communication, such as a reassuring touch on the arm, are very important. Although the patient does not understand what the physician says, tone of voice and facial expression can be highly reassuring. Clinicians who know only a few words of the patient's language can use them, even if ungrammatically, to communicate acceptance of ethnic background.

In working with ethnic patients who speak some English but are not truly bilingual, it is important to remember that stress and anxiety diminish fluency in a second language. Also, in the clinician's eagerness to communicate, it is common to speak more loudly rather than more slowly, which may suggest hostility instead of concern to the patient. It is also important to be tolerant of ethnic patients' hesitant English; many ethnic group members work hard to learn English, take pride in their abilities, and are offended by impatience. Finally, ethnic patients often understand more English than they read or speak, but thoughts of an emotional or psychological nature are particularly difficult to express in a second language.

American blacks and Appalachian whites often speak dialects of English, using words or phrases such as "risins" (boils), "the smothers" (dyspnea), "racks" (dentures), or "coming on" (menstruating). Psychiatrists working with patients who speak dialects of English should refrain from trying to emulate such speech patterns but should feel comfortable employing ethnic terminology if technical terms cause misunderstanding or discomfort.

Culture and Clinical Behavior

Although a firm handshake is a sign of good character in Anglo culture, it is a sign of aggression to most Native Americans, who usually "pass hands" with only a light touch. Similarly, eye contact among Anglos signifies interest, while for Native Americans and Appalachian whites it is a hostile invasion of privacy. Although some discomfort may occur between blacks and whites because a white listener tends to maintain eye contact while the black speaker allows his or her eyes to wander, the opposite tends to be true among blacks. Among Hispanics, eye contact is expected and considered a sign of real interest. Among some less acculturated Filipinos, eye contact reassures the patient that the practitioner is not a witch, because witches cannot tolerate direct eye contact. For black patients, a "cut eye" (abrupt termination of eye contact) can be an insult, and rolling eyes upward and to the side may be a way for black adolescents to indirectly signal anger. Older black patients may habitually avert the eyes and head in the presence of whites, a culturally derived practice that can be misinterpreted as a sign of depression or personality disorder.

People from middle-class white culture in this country tend to value "conversational efficiency," in which discussion quickly focuses on needed information. This approach may offend Hispanics, who often prefer a period of socializing prior to the elicitation of clinical information. Further, Hispanic patients tend to respond better to nondirective questioning and will talk more freely after an initial social interchange. With Asian groups, however, a concrete, directive approach to interviewing will be more productive, although open-ended questions can be employed to avoid yes or no answers. Patients of Asian origin characteristically do not talk freely, feeling that those who do are seeking attention, or that by not thinking things through carefully they might say something embarrassing and "lose face." Asian cultures value emotional restraint, leading to the stereotype of the stoic Oriental, while Middle Eastern cultures encourage emotional expression.

Explanatory Models and Clinical Reality

Because cultural beliefs dictate how people think, talk, understand, expect, and behave with their symptoms, steps must be taken to understand lay explanatory models of illness. Many cultural groups attribute sickness to characteristics of the blood (for example, too much, too little; too thick, too thin; dirty or stagnant; too high or too low). Among Chinese, Haitians, Mexicans, and Puerto Ricans, disease can be precipitated by an imbalance, causing the body to be "hot" or "cold" (this can be caused by eating too much of certain foods), and treatment must compensate for this imbalance. Drafts or air currents cause respiratory problems and joint pain in susceptible individuals (when perspiring, after childbirth, with a fever); and hospitalized patients with this explanation of illness may be preoccupied with the air around them.

Most ethnic groups include psychological and situational states (stress, grief, worry, loss, family disruption) as causal factors in disease. Full discussion between patient and psychiatric consultant of such etiological variables and their implications for treatment is often warranted, since inattention to this information often undercuts compliance. Other common elements of ethnic explanatory models include hexing and witchcraft among blacks, spirit possession and "attacks" among Puerto Ricans, herbal remedies and diet among Chinese, spiritual and natural harmony among Native Americans, polluted and pure parts of the body among Gypsies, semen loss and weakness among Southeast Asians, and the "evil eye" among Italian Americans. It is essential that the psychiatric consultant maintain an awareness of, and a sensitivity to, ethnic disease concepts, whatever they may be.

Patient-Practitioner Interaction

Middle- and upper-class urban white patients and their physicians often share a cultural orientation that values egalitarian relationships and recognizes a liberated role for women. But egalitarianism and informality are unacceptable to most rural ethnic patients. Among them, the elderly are accorded great respect, and social interaction between the sexes is more rigidly controlled. When working with such patients, standards of etiquette should be carefully observed. Among traditional Hispanic patients, for example, there are specific standards of modesty for women. Subjects such as sexuality, venereal disease, and birth control are particularly sensitive and are better discussed between patient and physician of the same sex. Any discussion of problems concerning genitals, particularly of a male Hispanic child, is better conducted with the father than with the mother.

An egalitarian relationship between patient and physician is unacceptable to most Asians, whose culture demands respect and deference toward those with special training or education. Age is also respected, so young physicians working with older Asian patients should make formal introductions before asking any questions or beginning any procedure. Other cultures share this code of etiquette toward the elderly, and patients from these groups may not relate well to casually attired or informal white psychiatrists. Young black patients may view white psychiatrists as representing an oppressive, racist majority and may be especially defensive about interaction styles that heighten status differentials or, conversely, that are seen as preferential or patronizing.

Ethnic patients also have distinctive beliefs about the propriety and efficacy of certain clinical practices. Gypsies consider that part of the body above the waist differently from that below: The former is "pure" and the latter is "polluted." Many ethnic and lower-class patients expect to receive injections when they seek medical help. If such treatment is denied them, they feel their problem is not being taken seriously. Yet another potential difficulty occurs when attempting to elicit personal information from some Native American patients, or from their family members. In Navajo culture, for example, there is extreme reluctance to reveal personal information. Not even a close family member has the right to discuss personal matters about someone else. This practice can be frustrating to the consultant who is attempting to elicit a patient's history from a family member, but in an emergency a spouse or other relative will usually try to give a history, especially if the psychiatrist gives full attention and listens unhurriedly.

Finally, it is important to remember that most illness episodes are dealt with in the context of the family, regardless of ethnic background. This may involve special diets, foods, herbs, massage, exercise, religious treatment, and prescribed or nonprescribed medications. Ethnic patients also may consult with folk practitioners such as *curanderos* among Hispanics, rootworkers and spiritualist ministers among blacks, herb doctors and acupuncturists among East Asians, voodoo specialists among Haitians, and medicine men among Native Americans. It is common for patients to engage in lay healing practices and to consult traditional health practitioners while simultaneously seeking health care from physicians. It is essential that the consulting psychiatrist be aware of patient use of traditional cures and curers. It is equally important not to convey disapproval or deny the importance of these traditional methods.

Ethnicity and Psychiatric Epidemiology

There are ethnic differences in the incidence of various diseases. Whites are more frequently diagnosed as depressed than blacks; and blacks account for more schizophrenic diagnoses, proportionally, in this country. Although alcohol use and associated problems are less common in Chinese Americans, there is a higher suicide rate in this group, particularly among women. Puerto Rican males are at the highest risk of suicide of any ethnic subgroup, with suicide rates twice that of whites or blacks. Among Puerto Rican ethnics, drug use is a more integral part of the culture, common in all strata, and should be considered more seriously in the differential diagnosis of such patients. Native American groups have a high prevalence of alcoholism and inhalant abuse, although there is much intertribal variability.

Mexican Americans have a relatively low prevalence of psychoses and a relatively higher prevalence of affective symptomatology. The causes of these differences are unclear, but they may be related to low utilization of psychiatric facilities by Hispanics or to a social buffering in which family members and alternative healers play an important role in care.

Several other unique features of ethnic-group membership also influence psychiatric diagnosis. Social class and life-style differences can be so striking that they appear pathological. For example, extreme apathy or indifference may be a response to chronic marginality and blocked mobility rather than character disorder. The flamboyant, grandiose, or eccentric language used by street people of some ethnic groups may sound psychotic to the clinician, but it may actually be culturally patterned and normative. Finally, among recent refugees, who are at increased risk for depression and other psychiatric disorders owing to the stresses of migration and acculturation, behavioral disorders may reflect underlying parasitic disease or tuberculosis, and culture shock can produce transient, florid paranoid states.

Treating Patients

Presentation of Symptoms

In many ethnic groups, somatic complaints are common presenting symptoms of psychiatric disorder or psychosocial problems. Somatization is particularly characteristic of Asian ethnic groups, and discussion of psychological issues can be difficult because mental illness is highly stigmatized. This fact is reflected in the paucity of psychological terms in the vocabularies of many such patients: Cambodians, for example, have no word for depression. Such patients may complain of pain, tiredness, or insomnia but deny a psychological basis for symptoms. Even if symptoms are attributed to psychosocial situations, there is often a reluctance to accept therapies that do not include medication.

Other cultural groups such as Italian Americans, Hispanics, or Middle Easterners may present symptoms with great emotionality, leading an unwary psychiatrist to assume greater emotional instability than is actually present. Many Italians feel that suppressing emotions can lead to illness and that emotionality is an essential part of disease prevention and treatment. Crying is common among such ethnic-group members in situations for which such behavior would be inappropriate by Anglo standards. Hispanic patients, especially recent arrivals from rural areas, may present with culturally authorized "attacks" that are a socially effective, often expected, response to family stress.

Some ethnic patients present with culture-specific disorders for which there are no recognized correlates in psychiatric nosology. Mexican Americans, for example, may complain of *empacho*, a digestive dysfunction attributed to consuming the wrong foods or eating when not hungry. *Empacho* is thought to cause constipation or death. "Gas in the stomach" and "fever in the stomach," the complaints associated with *empacho*, are indicated by extreme thirst and are treated by ingesting copious amounts of liquid. Another specific complaint, "*mal ojo*" (evil eye), is characterized by headache, insomnia, nervousness, weeping, feverishness, and is blamed on a strong person exerting power over a weaker person. "*Susto*" (fright), a disorder with gastrointestinal and vegetative signs, is caused by traumatic social events or life experiences. A similar syndrome affects Chinese Americans, who also recognize a disorder called "*koro*," a fear that the penis will withdraw into the body and cause death. Chinese-American and other South Asian adolescent males also suffer an acute anxiety state associated with semen loss, which leads to somatic complaints.

Attempts to divide such disorders into component parts for treatment, to interpret them in terms of psychodynamic concepts peculiar to Western psychiatry, or to translate them directly into DSM-III terms will often lead to incomplete or unacceptable treatment.

Help Seeking and Compliance

The major factor underlying delay and noncompliance is disagreement about the meaning of symptoms and about appropriate treatment. Because of different explanatory models, ethnic patients may have entirely different understandings about their illnesses and different expectations for treatment. The psychiatrist's insistence on the importance of a symptom that is not recognized as significant in the patient's explanatory model will not be welcomed by the patient, and prescribed treatment that does not fit the lay explanatory model of etiology and pathophysiology will not likely be followed.

To the psychiatrist, delay in seeking treatment for medical symptoms may suggest pathological denial, but many ethnic patients seek medical care only after prolonged consultation with family members and visits to alternative practitioners who are culturally prescribed.

Elicitation of Explanatory Models

A culturally sensitive psychiatric consultation begins with an exploration of the patient's explanatory model. The approach to the patient demands open-ended, empathic, but persistent questioning to determine what the patient believes to be the cause of the illness, its pathophysiology, expected clinical course, and prognosis, and the type of treatment that should be administered. Helpful questions are:

1. What do you call your problem?
2. What do you think has caused your problems?
3. Why do you think it started when it did?
4. What does this sickness do to you? How does it work?
5. How serious is this illness? How long will it last?
6. What kind of treatment is best for this illness?
7. What results do you expect from treatment?
8. What are the chief problems your illness has caused you?
9. What worries you most about being sick?

Explanatory models are particularly important for consulting psychiatrists because consultation work often involves mediation among patients, their families, physicians, and native practitioners. The consulting psychiatrist can use this explanatory-model framework to act as a go-between. The psychiatrist uncovers incongruities in models that impede understanding, and "translates" for patients and their physicians.

Negotiation

In the negotiation model, patients and their families are accorded ultimate responsibility for decisions, while the physician serves as an expert advisor. Although such an egalitarian or "patient-centered" approach is not acceptable to some ethnic patients because of culturally dictated deference to authority, clinicians who determine patient expectations through eliciting explanatory models will know when to use a negotiated approach.

The following are guidelines for negotiation:

1. Elicit the patient's explanatory model and delineate psychosocial problems associated with symptoms.
2. Present the medical or psychiatric explanatory model, guided by the patient's model and employing terms or concepts used by the patient in articulating his or her model.
3. Acknowledge incongruities between models and compromise both patient and clinician models to achieve congruence.
4. Decide on mutually desired or compromised treatment on the basis of the physician's expertise and the patient's explanatory model.
5. Provide ongoing monitoring. Be alert to the need to renegotiate clinical issues and aspects of the patient-caregiver relationship.

Clearly, not every clinical interaction with ethnic patients will afford consulting psychiatrists the opportunity to fully elicit explanatory models or negotiate treatment expectations. However, this should not be a major concern and should not dissuade clinicians from following the suggestions presented here. Moreover, this approach to culturally sensitive care is a skill that requires practice. Any demonstration of cultural sensitivity will increase rapport, in addition to increasing understanding of the culturally based assumptions and practices that are part of the ethnic patient's illness.

Suggested Readings

Freebairn, J., and Gwinup, K. (1979). *Cultural Diversity and Nursing Practice* (Instructor's Manual). Irvine, Calif.: Concept Media.

Harwood, A. (1981). *Ethnicity and Medical Care.* Cambridge, Mass.: Harvard University Press.

Johnson, T.M. (1981). Interpersonal skill in physical diagnosis. In *Physical Diagnosis: An Introduction to Clinical Medicine*, 16th ed., ed. J. Burnside, pp. 11–26. Baltimore: Williams & Wilkins.

Katon, W., and Kleinman, A. (1980). Doctor-patient negotiation and other social science strategies in patient care. In *The Relevance of Social Science for Medicine*, ed. L. Eisenberg and A. Kleinman, pp. 253–279. Boston: D. Reidel.

Kleinman, A. (1980). *Patients and Healers in the Context of Culture.* Berkeley: University of California Press.

Kleinman, A. (1982). Teaching of clinically applied medical anthropology on a psychiatric consultation-liaison service. In *Clinically Applied Anthropology*, ed. N.J. Chrisman and T.W. Maretzki, pp. 83–115. Boston: D. Reidel.

Kleinman, A., Eisenberg, L., and Good, B. (1978). Culture, illness and care: clinical lessons from anthropologic and cross-cultural research. *Annals of Internal Medicine* 88:251-258.

Press, I. (1982). Witch doctor's legacy: some anthropological implications for the practice of clinical medicine. In *Clinically Applied Anthropology*, ed. N.J. Chrisman and T. W. Maretzki, pp. 179-198. Boston: D. Reidel.

Weidman, H. (1982). Research strategies, structural alterations, and clinically applied anthropology. In *Clinically Applied Anthropology*, ed. N.J. Chrisman and T.W. Maretzki, pp. 201-241. Boston: D. Reidel.

Specialized Units

General hospitals often house specialized patient care units whose unique patient populations require special treatment procedures and whose staffs operate in concert to produce milieus different from other areas of the hospital. We have selected four such specialized areas for discussion: the medical intensive care unit, the burn unit, the renal dialysis/transplant unit, and the spinal cord unit. Each of these units has a different focus. Medical intensive care units usually deal with short-term patient care. Burn units deal with patients who have painfully disfiguring burns and who interact with staff over long periods of time. On renal dialysis/transplant units, patients are chronic and have brief episodes of hope that are dashed by the progression of their illnesses, by the failure of transplanted kidneys, or by complications of the technology that is required to keep them alive. On spinal cord units, patients must learn to make a transition from activity to passivity, and then to activity again as the rehabilitation process goes on.

Each of these units is a small community. Psychiatrists need to know the specialized ways in which these units work and the means by which to influence these environments. Because these units frequently deal with people who are severely ill and have poor prognoses, psychiatrists, in their work in these units, must also find ways to deal with their own feelings about the severely ill and to help reinforce the morale of the staff when they become overwhelmed by the severity of their patients' problems or when they begin to project some of their own feelings onto patients and their families.

F.G.

CHAPTER 29

The Intensive Care Unit

LINDA GAY PETERSON, M.D.

The general medical or surgical intensive care unit offers thorough, often exhaustive, patient monitoring and treatment in an environment that can be impersonal and confusing. Televisions, phones, and personalization of patient rooms with cards and other amenities are frequently absent. The ICU is commonly windowless; the pervasive noises are the beeps of monitors and the whirring of respirators. "Codes" performed for cardiac and respiratory arrest are ordinary experiences. Into this environment are thrown the frightened, ill patient, the patient's family, the specialized nurse, and the anxious physician.

These elements commingle to create special psychiatric needs, as illustrated in the following case.

Mrs. I., age 45, was admitted to the hospital because of behavior change, increased blood pressure, and laryngitis. On the third day of hospitalization, the patient stated she would jump out the window if her husband didn't remove her IV. He refused and she jumped. Following that, a psychiatrist was called.

On examination, her speech was difficult to understand because of her hoarseness. She denied suicidal or homicidal ideation. She thought that a voice might have told her to jump out of the window, but she denied hearing voices at the time of the examination. The patient was agitated and in constant purposeless motion. Although oriented in all spheres, she could recall none of three objects at three minutes. Her recent memory was impaired, but her remote memory was intact. She could not subtract serial threes or sevens; she could repeat four digits forward but none backward. Her judgment appeared fair and her insight into her medical condition was good.

The patient was at times cooperative, although her memory and higher-level intellectual functions were impaired, and at times bizarre, obviously hallucinating, and agitated.

A complete workup to identify the etiology of the patient's organic brain syndrome was performed. Her husband reported a personality change of at least a year's duration. A CT scan showed marked cerebellar and brain-stem atrophy, consistent with a diagnosis of olivopontocerebellar degeneration.

On daily doses of up to 30 mg of parenteral haloperidol, she showed some improvement in her delirium. However, close supervision and restraints were frequently necessary.

Mrs. I.'s psychotic episode is typical of the complex cases the consultant evaluates in the ICU. The patient's psychological makeup and brain dysfunction may significantly contribute to his or her psychological difficulties, but factors outside the patient and the illness must also be considered, including the patient's family and the ICU staff.

Evaluating the Patient

Mrs. I. had several biological causes for abnormal behavior. She may have had neuronal damage in her cerebral cortex as well as her cerebellum, olivary nuclei, and pons. She was also hypoxic and hypercapnic. And as with many ICU patients, she had received several medications with analgesic and anticholinergic properties. In her case, there was no acute change in electrolyte balance, no cardiac or renal dysfunction of recent origin, no evidence of delirium tremens, nutritional deficiencies, vitamin deficiencies, or trace metal deficiency—all of which are common among chronically ill patients whose critical status may necessitate transfer to an ICU.

Admission to the ICU often causes fear. Mrs. I. later recalled feeling quite frightened when told she was going to the intensive care unit. She thought it meant that she would be on a respirator for the rest of her life. Shortly before she jumped out the window, she had witnessed a cardiac arrest in the bed next to hers. In her confusion, she had thought the patient was being murdered by the staff.

The patient's interpretation of transfer to intensive care and the events that transpire there may induce anxiety, depression, or a brief reactive psychosis. The patient's perception of the environment also may influence the course of an existing delirium or dementia.

Sedative drugs, sleep deprivation, and the lack of normal orienting cues such as clocks and calendars may cause some patients with clear sensoria to misinterpret stimuli. Most patients report their ICU experience as positive and the monitors as reassuring, but when asked about specific events that occurred during their stay, they report gross misunderstandings. One patient described the intubation of another patient in this way:

> First, I thought Mr. J. was gargling. Then I saw them put something down his throat, a sword. Of course, it couldn't have been a sword, but he sure looked white. I'm sure it helped him, but I don't know why it was so sharp.

The Suicide Attempter

Assessment of suicidal patients is described in Chapter 3. The usual issues are whether the patient is an immediate suicide risk and needs an around-the-clock sitter while in the ICU, whether the patient requires psychotropic medication, and whether transfer to the psychiatric unit is indicated.

Suicide attempters often distress the nursing staff. The nurses are apprehensive about the patients' harming themselves or others, especially if they are intoxicated and emotionally labile following an overdose. Often, these concerns are alleviated by the psychiatrist's direct feedback to the primary nurse and the head nurse about potential risk and needed interventions. ICU physicians often have a limited understanding of psychiatric disorders and view suicide attempters as morally weak. They tend to be angry with them for occupying a bed that could be occupied by someone who is "really sick." Case-by-case didactic teaching can increase the medical staff's knowledge of suicidal behavior and of effective interventions for those psychiatric disorders most common in suicide attempters. This in turn increases their understanding of the psychiatrist's recommendations and allows them to view these patients as ill and deserving of compassion and careful medical attention.

The staff also have negative feelings about suicide attempters because they see them at a time of maximum distress and, therefore, do not develop a rapport with them as people. Suicidal patients may make physicians feel helpless, vulnerable, and hopeless, causing physicians to withdraw from them. This is a problem in a teaching hospital, whose house staff may find the act of a suicide attempt antithetical to their new role as healers. Frank discussion of this type of staff reaction and the psychological factors leading to a suicide attempt can improve the care of these patients.

Delirium

Organic mental disorders are the most common causes of disruptive behavior in the ICU. After determining that the patient has an organic brain syndrome, the next step is diagnostic evaluation. The following is a list of checkpoints to be assessed in screening causes of delirium.*

1. MEDICAL INFORMATION
   Prior psychiatric history
   Withdrawal: alcohol, barbiturates, benzodiazepines, meprobamate
   Drugs: steroids, levodopa, amphetamines, psychotropics, digitalis, lidocaine, anticholinergics, cimetidine
2. VITAL SIGNS
   Blood pressure
   Temperature
3. ROUTINE LAB STUDIES
   Hematocrit, mean corpuscular volume greater than 96 μ^3, vitamin B_{12}, folic acid
   Erythrocyte sedimentation rate, antinuclear antibody titer
   Electrolytes, magnesium, calcium, phosphates
   Blood urea nitrogen
   Blood glucose
   Thyroxine, triiodothyronine
   Oxygen pressure (arterial)
   Carbon dioxide pressure (arterial)
   Liver function tests, ammonia
   Venereal disease report
4. SPECIALIZED STUDIES
   Electrocardiogram
   Electroencephalogram
   Skull roentgenograms
   Brain scan
   Computerized tomography scan
   Cerebrospinal fluid protein, cells

The importance of routinely assessing *all* these parameters cannot be overstated. The next step is to improve environmental factors, thereby increasing the patient's reality contact. Nurses are instructed to orient the patient hourly, restrain the patient, check mental status once or twice each shift, and contact the medical staff if there is any deterioration. If there is any question of the patient's removing intravenous lines or tampering with other monitoring devices, restraints should be used. Having a family member stay

---

*After Cassem, N. (1978). The setting of intensive care. In *Massachusetts General Hospital Handbook of Consultation–Liaison Psychiatry*, ed. T.P. Hackett and N.H. Cassem, p. 325. St. Louis, Mo.: C.V. Mosby.

with the patient if possible or playing soft music on the radio may also help decrease agitation and confusion.

The final step in management is the use of a psychotropic agent (usually an antipsychotic) to decrease agitation. Depending on the patient's medical problems, there may be specific reasons to choose a particular antipsychotic. In general, haloperidol is a good choice. It has minimal anticholinergic activity. Given parenterally, it acts in 15 to 30 minutes and has a 14-hour half-life. An epinephrine-filled syringe should be kept at the bedside in case laryngospasm occurs as an idiosyncratic reaction. Used orally, the onset of action may be slightly slower and the half-life is about 24 hours. Haloperidol should be administered in a dose of 2 to 10 mg every 30 minutes until the initial target symptoms are under control. Once adequate sedation is achieved, half the total dose used to calm the patient should be given at night for the next day or two. If agitation reemerges, an additional 2 to 5 mg may be needed, but once a patient is past the acute episode, improvement should continue if the underlying medical problem has been resolved. The haloperidol dose can then be reduced over two to three days, with a maintenance dose of 1 or 2 mg nightly over the next week.

In rare instances, a patient may develop a paradoxical response to the haloperidol, particularly in doses over 40 mg, and become more agitated and distressed. In this case, the drug should be stopped and a piperazine phenothiazine or thiothixene should be used. Most patients will be well controlled on less than 40 mg of haloperidol per day. Doses greater than 60 mg per day do not improve patients' behavior significantly. If 40 to 60 mg of haloperidol is insufficient, the aforementioned drugs might be tried. Alternatives include more-sedating phenothiazines such as chlorpromazine 25–50 mg intramuscularly or short-acting barbiturates such as sodium amytal, 250 mg administered intravenously over 5 to 10 minutes (refer to Chapter 5 for more information on rapid neuroleptization).

Substance abusers cause a number of psychiatric problems in an ICU. Withdrawal from alcohol, prescribed medications, and street drugs is probably their greatest difficulty. Unsuspected alcoholic patients who have had emergency surgery may experience delirium tremens after three to seven days in the hospital, often while still in the ICU. This creates diagnostic difficulty, because there may be a concomitant organic brain syndrome secondary to electrolyte imbalance, hypoxia of pulmonary origin, infection, or narcotic or anticholinergic toxicity. Therefore, careful review of the patient's prehospital history and postoperative course are essential to an accurate diagnosis and to appropriate treatment. An added confounding factor is the practice of routinely treating ICU patients with cimetidine to prevent peptic ulceration. Cimetidine can cause psychotic symptoms and delirium, particularly in patients with severe debilitation, renal or hepatic insufficiency, or alcoholism. Furthermore, minor tranquilizers seem to increase the half-life of cimetidine.

Effective management of the hallucinating, agitated, delirious patient also includes preventing self-harm, as the vignette about Mrs. I. illustrated. The use of soft restraints and, if necessary, mittens to keep patients from removing intravenous tubing, endotracheal tubes, or other devices is important. Frequent orienting by nurses and family, and reassurances about the meaning of the unfamiliar noises and activity, can reduce confusion and keep patients more calm and comfortable. If patients are delirious from drug or alcohol withdrawal, treatment with a cross-tolerant agent should be used (for further discussion, refer to Chapter 21, on alcohol withdrawal).

The Anxious Patient

For patients who are agitated because of severe anxiety, a benzodiazepine such as diazepam, 5 to 10 mg PO or IV, is useful while monitoring carefully for respiratory depression. After patients become calmer, they should be encouraged to discuss their underlying fears. Often, patients are frightened mainly by their transfer into an ICU. When the staff tries to reassure them that everything will be all right, it increases their distress; patients often assume that they are being duped and that they are going to die. Some patients need to feel in control of their care. A sense of helplessness can be very anxiety-provoking to people who are accustomed to controlling their environment and who have low levels of interpersonal trust. Techniques for diminishing tension can be taught, including relaxation techniques, breathing techniques, visual imagery, and self-hypnosis. Because these same patients are often reluctant to accept psychological help and may minimize the importance of a psychological intervention, the need to use these techniques for their *physical* recovery must be stressed.

Dealing with Personality Disorder

Patients with personality disorders may have great difficulty dealing with severe medical illness (for further discussion, see Chapter 13, on coping styles and behaviors). Those with histrionic or antisocial personality styles are likely to have the most difficulty tolerating the structured environment and the limitations on their mobility caused by the ICU regime. They may be perceived by staff as demanding, overreacting to pain, or mentally ill because of their tendency to dramatize their needs. They may become extremely agitated or violent, or complain of hallucinations or illusions, to get attention. They may manipulate their caregivers in other ways. The consulting psychiatrist helps these patients to communicate in more acceptable ways.

Case conferences encouraging nurses to set consistent limits with these patients and supporting nursing staff's refusal to tolerate abuse help diminish patients' acting out.

Demoralization and Depression

Transfer to intensive care can cause a failure in coping, especially when there are differences among patient, family, and staff concerning the perception of the patient's illness. For example, patients may see themselves as terminally ill and not want to undergo further heroic treatment efforts, but the staff and family's impression may be different. Neither side may wish to acknowledge the difference of opinions, and as a result, communication breaks down. This part of the problem can be dealt with by patient, family, and staff having a meeting with the psychiatrist to discuss the situation. In addition, patients may need to confront their own grief over loss of health, approaching death, or other perceived losses. It can be useful to reconstruct the illness from its onset and carefully review the patient's thoughts, feelings, and behavior up to the present, and then rehearse with the patient how he or she might handle the potential outcome of the current situation. Often, the patient has learned bits and pieces about the problem from the medical staff but has not pieced all the information together or begun to deal with the likely outcome of treatment and its effects on quality of life and longevity. By systematically investigating the patient's thoughts, wishes, and feelings, an opportunity is provided to integrate conceptions and establish a framework that allows the patient to feel more at ease both alone and with others.

Antidepressants may be useful for patients who have vegetative symptoms of depression. Trazodone is useful because of its low anticholinergic side effects, but it causes sedation and hypotension. It is used in twice the dose of tricyclics such as amytriptyline. A tricyclic antidepressant can also be used, provided EKG, blood levels, and side effects are followed closely with each dosage change (for further discussion, see Chapters 6 and 22).

Dealing with the Family

The patient's family may be in conflict with the nursing staff or may be coping poorly with having a family member in intensive care. Placement in intensive care signals critical illness, and to many people, it is equated with a decreased likelihood of recovery. In addition, the ICU's operations are not always comprehensible. Reasons for limited visiting hours may not be understood. Contacting the patient, nurse, or doctor in this setting may be difficult, and the various monitoring devices and tests may appear more like torture devices than necessary medical adjuncts. Witnessing a cardiac arrest or other emergency may be very frightening for a family member.

Individual or family sessions with the psychiatric consultant or other members of the health care team help to provide a better grasp of the environment. Group sessions for families of ICU patients are especially helpful. They may be led by any health care team member with psychological expertise, and the psychiatrist may be needed only to supervise or consult or to conduct the sessions on adjustment to catastrophic illness. These family groups require careful structuring to prevent them from becoming merely an arena for the recital of frightening stories. Education by members of the ICU team can increase families' knowledge about the care of their loved ones. A respiratory therapist can explain pulmonary toilet procedures, a nurse can talk about special care issues, and the unit's senior physician can discuss problems common to most patients. Describing the patient's experience of reactions to, and needs in, intensive care often improve the family's ability to give support. For example, a family's efforts to shield a family member in intensive care from bad news often make the patient feel even more isolated and helpless. Families are therefore encouraged to include all their members in routine matters (for further discussion of patients' families, refer to Chapter 25).

Working with the Staff

ICU staffs cope efficiently with cardiac and respiratory emergencies, but they may feel less capable of managing behavioral emergencies. The consultant must therefore provide clear instructions for investigating biological etiologies for behavior change, instructions for management of symptoms, and careful guidelines for nursing staff for dealing with the patient and the family.

ICU staff morale is frequently high because of the team work, high visibility of team members, and high levels of competence on the job. Because of the more intense team work, most doctors have a high regard for ICU nurses' skills. Important stresses for ICU nurses are heavy work load, inadequate support, limited feedback from senior staff, crowding, and noise. In addition, they have feelings about being involved in life-and-death decisions, and they experience frustrations over dealings with severely ill patients, highly stressed families, and anxious house staff.

Nursing-staff support groups that allow for systematic exploration of patient-care issues, relationships with other staff members, and personal issues relevant to the group members' activities in the unit are an effective means to deal with nursing stress. Support groups allow nurses to explore their options for behavior in various situations and tend to increase their sense of control of their working environment. These groups can be led by a member of the consultation team or by the nurses on the unit with supervision by the psychiatric consultant (refer to Chapter 26 for further discussion).

When a psychiatric consultation has been generated by the ICU attending physician's personal reactions to a very ill patient or by a physician's ethical dilemma, tactful, thoughtful discussion with the referring physician about the psychiatrist's perception of the situation may be useful in facilitating the attending physician's own resolution of the problem.

Similarly, when a particularly troublesome death occurs (see Chapter 30) and the staff does not have a built-in review process, the psychiatric consultant can help members of the ICU team discuss the case constructively. This minimizes the risk that residual feelings will interfere with the care of other patients.

In sum, the constant pressure of life-and-death issues in the ICU knit patients, their families, and staff into an emotionally intense relationship. The consultant must be aware of the issues and interactions for each part of the system while attending to the biopsychosocial problems of the patient.

Suggested Readings

Hackett, T.P., and Weisman, A.D. (1960). Psychiatric management of operative syndromes: I. The therapeutic consultation and the effect of noninterpretive intervention. *Psychosomatic Medicine* 22:267–282.

Hackett, T.P., and Weisman, A.D. (1960). Psychiatric management of operative syndromes: II. Psychodynamic factors in formulation and management. *Psychosomatic Medicine* 22:356–372.

Jones, J., Hoggart, B., Withey, J., Donaghue, K., and Ellis, B.W. (1979). What the patients say: a study of reactions to an intensive care unit. *Intensive Care Medicine* 5:89–92.

Kimball, C.P. (1979). Psychotherapeutic intervention in acute medical situations. *General Hospital Psychiatry* 1:150–154.

Lindemann, E. (1944). Symptomatology and management of acute grief. *American Journal of Psychiatry* 101:141–148.

McKegney, F.P. (1966). The intensive care syndrome: the definition, treatment, and prevention of a new "disease in medical progress." *Connecticut Medicine* 30:633–636.

Nichols, K.A., Springford, V., and Searle, J. (1981). An investigation of distress and discontent in various types of nursing. *Journal of Advanced Nursing* 6:311–318.

Thompson, II, T.L., and Feinberg, L.E. (1980). Evaluation of postoperative changes in mental status. *Postgraduate Medicine* 67:277–287.

Tune, L.E., Holland, A., Folstein, F., et al. (1981). Association of postoperative delirium with raised serum levels of anticholinergic drugs. *Lancet* 2:651.

Weiner, M.F., and Caldwell, T. (1981). Stresses and coping in ICU nursing: II. Nurse support groups on intensive care units. *General Hospital Psychiatry* 3:129–134.

CHAPTER 30

The Burn Unit

NORMAN R. BERNSTEIN, M.D.

The immediate problems of burn care involve hospitalization and treatment of shock, followed by prevention or treatment of infection and management of pain and delirium. Many patients are not in acute pain immediately after a burn injury because nerve endings have been burned away. The discomfort is often soreness rather than acute pain. However, as treatment progresses, tubbings, debridement of wounds, and dressing changes all cause extreme pain and anguish.

Burns exude fluid and are sites for serious infection. Patients must be isolated. Staff must take sterile precautions. Masking, scrubbing, and gowning are required. Burn patients also have eating problems because they are lethargic and uncomfortable and can find very little to fight against aside from feedings. The psychiatric consultant is often asked to help patients establish a caloric and protein intake high enough to permit healing, frequently two or three times a person's normal intake.

There are many problems for the staff, including experimental approaches to treatment, new methods of isolation, and new antibiotics. Medications for local and general anesthesia are constantly changing. New types of immobilization, new kinds of pins and wires and improved respirators, and redesigns of burn units' airflow to keep out bacterial invaders add to the treatment armamentarium and the confusion. Burn units are also maintained at a very high temperature and humidity because patients lack normal skin covering.

The burn unit becomes a cauldron of emotions. In the close and busy environment, staff are challenged to save patients, to salve the dying, and to deal with distraught relatives, police, and insurance investigators. All these interactions contribute to the tensions of relentless hard work, staff guilt, and the staff's concern about the life and death decisions it makes. Individual ambition, special ties between staff members, and differing values all affect the situation. Despite a busy, placid, and professional exterior, these units often experience considerable internal conflict. Because of these tensions, the consultant needs to be sensitive to staff dynamics in order to prevent an adverse consultation outcome.

Stages of Burn Care

The Acute Phase

The psychiatric problems involved in the acute phase of burn care often involve managing agitated patients whose consciousness is clouded. Newly burned patients are often in shock, and after they come out of shock, they may become delirious. Those who become agitated and experience auditory and visual hallucinations are seen by the staff as psychotic rather than delirious. Squirming, twisting patients can tear out intravenous tubing and may require restraints. Patients' agitation can interfere with respirators and other lifesaving equipment. The consultant can be most helpful in this early phase by prescribing neuroleptic medication and by conferring with nurses on how best to handle patients' behavior. Here, the focus is on saving patients' lives. When survival is in doubt, the psychiatrist is often called to deal with families that are upset and often emotionally paralyzed.

The Intermediate Phase

Patients who have sustained major burns undergo numerous surgical procedures under general anesthesia. Patients may undergo 20 or 30 operations in the course of a lengthy first hospitalization. Although some patients accommodate to the operating room, many experience the same desperate terror and fear of dying each time they are taken to surgery. With the tremendous stress and trauma, most of these patients experience clinically diagnosable depression after about six weeks. This depression is manifested by sadness, helplessness, hopelessness, irritability, uncooperativeness, and guilt over causing the injury. Many patients become anorectic and unwilling to eat. They sleep poorly, oversleep, or have interrupted sleep, partly related to the hospital routines that interfere with normal sleep. They may become physically agitated, but hospitalized and immobilized burn patients are more likely to show psychomotor retardation because of their physical illness and the mechanical restriction of their activities. Their guilt about the injury may be quite inappropriate to the actual situation. They often cannot concentrate and have recurring thoughts of death. They do not react to the efforts of people to cheer them up. They lose pleasure in reading the newspaper or hearing the news and complain about their situation. (For further discussion of depression in the medically ill, see Chapter 22).

After patients have been hospitalized for several months, staff usually expect them to become more active. In graduated steps, patients are required to sit up, eat by the bedside, ambulate, and participate more actively in physical therapy. All the while, they are also supposed to be more responsive to relatives or other visitors. At each stage of increasing activation, patients are likely to resist and complain.

Some of the depression seen at this phase is self-limited; some is in reaction to the slow rate of improvement and the fear engendered by each new challenge; some requires active psychiatric treatment. However, none of these depressions responds well to antidepressants. Fortunately, some depressions are terminated by physical improvement and being moved from an isolation room into an area with other patients.

Knowledge of the temporal pattern of the unit greatly aids the consultant in giving practical advice—so as not to go against the scheduling of physical therapy and tubbing. Suggestions about alterations in visitation should not interfere with dressing changes. As on other services, consultations on the burn unit should be clear; recommendations, specific. Nothing should be promised that cannot be executed. "Will follow" must be specifically intended if written on the patient's chart.

The Late Phase

In the late phase, patients have more contact with the outside world and consider going back to work or school. They may deal with insurance companies or litigation related to the accident. They begin to make home visits or go to restaurants. This is also a time to plan continuing physical therapy to loosen up joints and scar tissue or to schedule long-term surgical programs. Burn patients often have difficulty overcoming their earlier passive role in treatment as they are asked to assume more responsibility in their rehabilitation.

Discharge planning involves the difficult task of returning patients to environments where they no longer feel or are accepted because of disfigurement and limited mobility. Adverse responses outside the hospital often depress the patients and in turn engender difficulties in their cooperation with treatment. Disfigured patients are usually unwilling or very reluctant to rejoin their regular social circles. They may become unresponsive to friends, family, or medical care. Family consultation can be vital in preventing or minimizing social withdrawal.

Despair

Burn patients must often mourn the loss of their normal lives. They are frequently able to work and resume generally normal activities, but many no longer have a normal appearance, and some may not be able to have normal lives. Major burns heal with obvious scarring that cannot be completely eliminated; patients often despair over what they perceive as loss of their personal integrity and the fullness of their lives. The evolution of and patients' adaptation to these issues take years. The beginning of the process is illustrated in the following vignette.

> Miss K., a 24-year-old emergency medicine nurse, was admitted after a fire following a gas explosion in her home. Burns covered 30 percent of her body. Her right arm and chest and her right thigh were badly burned; she also sustained burns of both cheeks, her chin, and her nose. It was clear to the staff that she would have extensive scarring. Because she was a nurse in the same age group as most of the staff, she attracted particular attention and strong feelings of sympathy. A psychiatric consultation was requested to help the patient deal with her injuries. The patient consistently disavowed the problems that lay ahead of her. She refused to talk about her damaged appearance with her surgeon, her nurses, or the psychiatric consultant. She was unwilling to examine how scarring would alter her life and maintained a manner of brittle cheerfulness. The issue was dropped because the patient would eventually have to deal with this problem, and there was no reason to prematurely force her to confront such painful issues while she was being severely stressed by immediate hospital procedures.
>
> However, after being seen by the psychiatrist, she was more responsive to the staff's treatment. The staff also felt easier about touching on these issues with her. She went through the usual phase of depression after a month in the hospital, and the nursing staff supported her. They also separated some of their own feelings from her situation. The nurses talked among themselves about their feelings concerning the patient's loss of attractiveness and the change in her life course after the accident. There was much talk about life and death and the uncertainty of human existence, but the nurses kept these issues to themselves and were more consistently supportive with the patient. After she left the hospital, she kept in touch with several of the staff members. She came to visit the ward and burn clinic and corresponded with several of her ward nurses. She also had several of the staff to her home for dinner. She leaned on them emotionally without talking directly about her feelings.

Burn-scarred people often enter a life course of impairment. Some go "into the closet"; others end their lives. Major long-term issues involve encouraging burn patients to continue working in physical therapy, to return for needed surgery, and to continue in counseling. Consultations can be pivotal in these situations.

Dealing with Death

The death of patients raises many complex issues, as seen in the following vignette.

Mr. L., a 34-year-old married Greek immigrant, was burned over 70 percent of his body after setting fire to his restaurant to collect the insurance money. The fire killed his accomplice. The patient was delirious for several days and actively refused treatment. He showed contempt for the nurses, cursed them, demeaned them, and said that he knew what had to be done and that he wanted to be left alone. In spite of his serious condition, he was imperious and demanding of the staff, particularly the nurses. He refused to go to the operating room when advised repeatedly by several different surgeons. When his pregnant teenage girlfriend visited, he treated her with scathing contempt. The patient's wife visited often and he also treated her angrily. The patient's burns eventually became infected and he died after two weeks. The psychiatric consultant who had seen him earlier in his hospitalization was asked to address two issues: the patient's refusal of surgical care and the nurses' intense negative feelings. They were angry, felt guilty about their anger, and felt unable to perform good nursing care.

The patient had been as antagonistic toward the psychiatrist as he had been to other staff members. To the patient, the psychiatrist was just one of the many people advising him to have surgery. The psychiatrist did not fare better than the other staff members in getting him to cooperate. In the course of the patient's hospitalization, the psychiatrist met with the nurses and heard their lamentations. Two nurses broke down and cried—one in rage and frustration that she could not get the patient to do what needed to be done; a second confessed at a nursing meeting that she wished he would die and sobbed about her rage toward this man and feelings of guilt over it. Other nurses acknowledged that he was a patient who was very hard to tolerate, whom they would like to be rid of. There was a general expression of their anger at him as an evil person, a criminal, an arsonist, and a philanderer.

The major part of the psychiatric consultant's work was done with the staff, permitting them to ventilate, to discuss, to share their feelings about this man, and to clarify the mechanisms of their upset feelings. Some of these meetings were also attended by surgical house staff and visiting staff. This reduced the expression of the most intense feelings, but for several weeks after the patient's death, the staff continued to talk about him, to be troubled by him, and to wonder what had happened to his pregnant girlfriend and his wife.

Guilt, shame, and a sense of failure continued to prevail. No one liked hating this man and wishing him dead. Because there was a religious overtone to some of the nurses' guilt feelings, the psychiatrist sought the services of a priest who taught medical ethics and was sophisticated about hospital operations. Together they held a conference on the ward three weeks after the patient's death, with the priest presiding. In this meeting, the priest discussed explicitly the issues of anger at patients and helped the nurses understand their hatred of the patient, whom they felt to be an ignoble person. The priest's expression of his tolerance for the staff's unacceptable feelings greatly enhanced the effectiveness of similar statements made earlier by the psychiatrist.

In most such cases, the consultant alone can help the staff work out their feelings. Occasionally, as in this case, bringing in others to meet with the staff can be helpful.

The Role of the Psychiatrist

Many of the approximately 200 burn units in the United States have psychiatric consultants who render direct care to the patients, and a few units have regular liaison psychiatrists. Some liaison psychiatrists function as consultants in addition to their liaison role, while others do not. Liaison consultants provide indirect care, attending some rounds and leading some groups.

Direct-Care Problems

The psychiatric consultant on a burn unit sees most or many of the patients on the unit. In addition to performing mental status examinations, the consultant usually prescribes medication to relieve pain and treat delirium, to control anxiety and depression. Doses of psychoactive medication are often much lower than on other surgical or medical units because of the patients' debility.

In addition to the general problems of pain and delirium, the consultant must help with problems more specific to individual patients: threats of suicide and other resistance to care that interfere with treatment routines. Occasionally, some individual psychotherapy with burn patients is required. Usually such psychotherapy is of a limited duration and focused on fear of death, failure to comply with medical procedures, or friction with staff members. Patients' fears of the future are best dealt with by staff as discharge planning begins.

Liaison psychiatrists may lead some patient-care groups and may occasionally do psychotherapy of limited duration with burn patients. This type of therapy focuses on fear of death, failure to comply with medical procedures, or friction with staff members.

Pain Management

Pain management is a central issue on the burn unit. Unfortunately, no approach completely removes pain in the course of burn therapy. Although proper narcotic use brings little risk of addiction, surgeons and internists often fear addicting burn patients, and the psychiatric consultant must at times actively advocate narcotics for pain relief when tranquilizers have been used as substitutes for analgesics. Numerous nonpharmacological approaches have been tried for pain management. Hypnosis has been utilized for decades in a number of centers and often with great success in reducing the apprehension about and increasing the tolerance for painful procedures, such as tubbings, dressing changes, and debridement. Self-hypnosis has also been useful. Acupuncture has been tried. Continued intravenous drip of ketamine anesthetic has been used for weeks to reduce the pain levels of children. Patients can be encouraged to summon up pleasant mental pictures in a manner that focuses awareness and helps patients feel detached so they can feel more in control of themselves and their environment.The manipulation of fantasies through imagery can be employed to help patients feel they are escaping from their agonies in the hospital.

In comparing approaches to pain management in which staff keep control and distract patients with approaches in which patients have a better sense of their own control over the dressing change situation, we find greater patient participation and sense of control to be more effective. Every approach attempts to diminish the terror and helplessness of burn patients. In each situation, the morale of the staff is aided by knowing they are trying out new techniques of pain control. Effectiveness in managing pain problems on the burn ward is enhanced by more optimistic approaches to patients using any of these methods. Some burn units attempt to reduce the use of narcotics through intensive and active general nursing attention to patients; nurses negotiate contracts with patients, specifying exactly how painful tubbing or dressing will be executed and what patients can do to signal agony and help control the procedure.

The psychiatrist can help negotiate a rational and systematic pain management plan, because so many different professionals from surgery, anesthesia, pediatrics, and internal medicine all have their own special approaches, and different burn units have used different mixtures of pain medication and types of environmental manipulation to handle pain. Negotiating the simplest drug program and enlisting patients' participation remain the goals in this situation. This requires time and sensitivity to the undercurrents of disagreement about approaches.

Tube Feeding

Tube feeding is often employed to ensure adequate caloric and protein intake. The decision to tube-feed is often made after noting poorly healing wound sites and hearing nurses' complaints that patients refuse food or vomit. Intravenous hyperalimentation is also instituted in these situations. The issue of tube feeding is generally presented as an objective, scientific matter, but it is often related to anger at an uncooperative patient. The consultant's intervention in a discordant situation can frequently help the staff to work with the patient and improve food intake. The critical feature is converting staff irritation into good patient care. Staff frictions need to be worked on discreetly toward this end. Merely exposing the nurses' frustration or dislike for a patient is destructive. Showing how everyone, including the patient, is bothered by eating noncompliance can lead to helping patients to eat better.

The psychiatrist is generally on the side of increasing the human interactions with feeding rather than using a tube. This is more helpful in aiding these regressed and dependent patients to progress psychologically during their recovery. In unusual circumstances, such as when the battle between staff and patient is intractable and detrimental to treatment, the consultant may suggest that an intravenous or nasal tube be used. Experienced nurses see feeding as a universal problem, and eventually become skilled at coaxing their patients to eat. At the same time, they are less likely to convert "eating problems" into a reason for psychiatric consultation.

Indirect Care

Liaison psychiatrists on burn units typically become involved in indirect care by leading nurse training groups, attending psychosocial rounds with the burn team, and performing an educational function.

Liaison psychiatrists are often asked to counsel with families about patients who are dying, to meet with staff members, or to supervise staff members who have difficulty managing a patient. Liaison psychiatrists may also be involved in focused consultations with surgeons, pediatricians, anesthiologists, occupational therapists, chaplains, aides, burn technicians, or nurses.

Tact and Timing in Consulting

Psychiatrists involved in ongoing liaison work become fully immersed in the milieu and more aware of the overt and covert styles of management. They know that certain people are leaders and particular nurses are crucial in facilitating or undermining decisions. It becomes important to read between the lines. Is the consultation being requested as a way for the staff to avoid certain patients and family members? Consultants also become aware of the various surgeons' concerns and involvement with patients; for example, plastic surgeons are more involved with the long-term outcome of burn patients because they will deal with the patients for years, while the trauma surgeons have lifesaving and infection prevention as their main focus. Psychiatrists receive much information not directly related to patient care, and they have to be absolutely discreet about the gossip and personal information communicated by staff members about themselves and their families.

Consultants also have to be clear about their psychiatric beliefs and be ready to assert them forcefully. There is not much time to negotiate an opinion on ward rounds. Clear, terse statements are preferable to the conciliatory evocative style typical of case conferences on the psychiatric unit.

Suggested Readings

American Psychiatric Association (1980). *Biofeedback*. Report of the Task Force on Biofeedback of the American Psychiatric Association, Task Force Report No. 19.

Bernstein, N.R. (1976). *Emotional Problems of the Facially Burned and Disfigured*. Boston: Little, Brown.

Bernstein, N.R. (1979). Chronic illness and impairment. *Psychiatric Clinics of North America* 2:331–346.

Bernstein, N.R. (1982). Psychosocial results of burns: the damaged self-image. *Clinics in Plastic Surgery* 9:337–346.

Dimick, A. (1983). The University of Alabama approach to pain. In *Comprehensive Approaches to the Burned Person*, ed. N.R. Bernstein and M.C. Robson. New York: Medical Examination.

Esmonde-White, M. (1982). Continued intravenous small dose ketamine for burn pain management in South Africa. Personal communication, San Francisco, Sixth International Burn Congress.

Giordano, B. (1981). An alternative approach to nursing care. In *Critical Care Nursing*, ed. C. Kenner, C. Guzzetta, and B. Dossey. Boston: Little, Brown.

Kavanagh, C. (1983). Psychological intervention with the severely burned child: report of an experimental comparison of two approaches and their effects on psychological sequelae. *Journal of the American Academy of Child Psychiatry* 22:145–156.

Kenner, C., and Achterberg, J. (1983). Nonpharmaceutic pain relief for burn patients. Presented at the Annual Meeting of the American Burn Association, New Orleans, La.

Stoddard, F.J. (1982). Body image development in the burned child. *Journal of Child Psychiatry* 21:502–507.

CHAPTER 31

The Renal Transplant/Dialysis Unit

REGE S. STEWART, M.D.

Chronic renal disease and its treatment require an extraordinary life style that can cause or exacerbate psychiatric disorders for many patients. Hemodialysis and renal transplantation each produce or aggravate different sets of psychological predicaments. In order to effectively consult on a renal unit, the psychiatrist needs to understand the phases of renal failure and the ways that it can be medically managed.

Problems of Hemodialysis

Denial and Anger

Most people with end-stage renal disease deny that dialysis is inevitable. This adaptive defense protects the individual from being overwhelmed by anxiety and depression. It also wards off fear of multiple losses and fear of death. The level of denial tends to parallel the level of stress patients experience, with greater stress calling for greater denial. Pathological denial also occurs, for example, when uremic patients refuse dialysis. Cognitive awareness does not always diminish the level of denial. As one young diabetic patient reported to a psychiatric consultant: "I always knew that my kidneys were going to fail, but it didn't seem real until they put the shunt in." Another patient revealed that at first he often skipped dialysis because he didn't believe his kidneys had stopped functioning. Once he discovered that he felt better when he was dialyzed regularly, his compliance became excellent.

Anger is also experienced strongly by dialysis patients. Patients often displace their anger and hostility from their illness onto the dialysis staff. Within reasonable limits, the more support and understanding the dialysis personnel provide, the less angry and demanding patients will be.

Regression and Depression

Good adjustment to dialysis depends in part on patients' ability to regress and accept a dependent role. Partial regression permits effective cooperation with treatment and an independent, gratifying existence outside of treatment. This task is especially difficult for adolescents struggling with developmental issues of dependency and autonomy.

Pathological regression often results from conflicts over dependency. Although it is important for patients to accept dependence on dialysis, excessive dependence on dialysis staff can lead to feelings of helplessness and to lower self-esteem. Passive patients can also stimulate hostile demands by the staff that they assume more responsibility and independence outside of dialysis. For psychologically isolated individuals with poor coping skills, dialysis often becomes a way of life in which they abdicate responsibility for their health and welfare.

Depression is inevitable during dialysis. A quarter to a half of dialysis patients are depressed at any one time. Depression typically emerges as denial diminishes and the patient faces loss of health, job, money, independence, social status, and colleagues and friends. Medical complications or the death of another dialysis patient often precipitates depression, as shown in the following vignette.

Mr. M., a 26-year-old single locksmith on dialysis for three years, had made an excellent adjustment. He had been mildly depressed at the beginning of dialysis but soon recovered and returned to work. When a good friend on dialysis died, he was asked to be a pallbearer. At the funeral, the minister talked about the deceased patient's suffering and suggested that she was better off dead. Immediately, the patient experienced overwhelming anxiety that evolved into a serious depression. Until the funeral, he had been able to repress his fear of death and reasoned that only older patients and those who were poorly adjusted or gravely ill would die. The sermon penetrated his denial and also confronted him with the fact that many viewed his condition with pity and felt that death was preferable to the vicissitudes of dialysis.

The patient's psychotherapist from the renal unit helped him to verbalize his anger at the minister, reaffirmed for the patient that satisfactory living is possible on dialysis, and allowed him to shore up his denial by seeing himself once again as a young, healthy man with a good prognosis.

When evaluating depression in a dialysis patient, the consultant's differential diagnosis should include uremic encephalopathy and conservation-withdrawal. Uremic encephalopathy usually occurs at the initiation of dialysis —these patients are apathetic, withdrawn, nauseated, anorectic, and insomnic. Moreover, they often complain of weakness and lack of energy and have psychomotor retardation. Nevertheless, they deny feelings of depression, helplessness, or hopelessness. Conservation-withdrawal is an adaptive mechanism that allows conservation of emotional and physical energy in the face of overwhelming stress. It resembles depression except that dysphoria and self-accusation are absent.

Staff and family support are often sufficient to help patients without anorexia, insomnia, and severe feelings of hopelessness recover from depression. Those who meet DSM-III criteria for major depressive disorder and those with suicidal ideation benefit from combined antidepressant medication and psychotherapy (for further discussion, see Chapter 22).

Psychopharmacological Agents

Dialysis patients usually require lower doses of antidepressants than healthy adults. Nortriptyline is especially well suited because it is the antidepressant least likely to cause hypotension. One anephric dialysis patient with chronic hypotension and severe depression could not tolerate tricyclic medications; for example, her blood pressure dropped to 50/0 after receiving 25 mg of nortriptyline. Her depression improved when she was given methamphetamine, 5 mg PO, prior to her three-times-a-week dialysis. Manic-depressive patients can be maintained on lithium carbonate as long as their serum lithium is monitored. A dose of 300 to 900 mg of lithium carbonate can be given three times a week following dialysis. The half-life of lithium carbonate is probably more than 100 hours in patients without functioning kidneys.

Noncompliance

One of the most common medical problems for dialysis patients is fluid overload resulting from noncompliance with dietary restrictions. Many dialysis patients dislike severe fluid and salt restrictions and the need to avoid foods rich in potassium and phosphorus. Failure to take medication as directed or refusal to be dialyzed regularly indicates more severe problems of noncompliance. Contributing to noncompliance are:

1. *Characterological problems.* Many patients have a low frustration tolerance and are unable to delay gratification. Most noncompliant

dialysis patients belong to this group. Patients with characterological problems also have a tendency to act out periodically, responding to stress with hostility and aggression. Adolescents striving for independence engage in similar acts of noncompliance.

2. *Denial of illness.* Patients with excessive denial often abuse medications but may function at a reasonably high level because of their denial.

3. *Psychological gain from the sick role.* For these patients, dialysis resolves predialysis conflicts between striving for independence and wishes for continued dependency gratification. These patients fear recovery and resumption of responsibility. Noncompliance with the diet ensures continuation of their disability.

4. *Suicidal behavior.* Attempts at suicide by noncompliance are usually precipitated by a major depressive disorder.

5. *Dysfunctional family.* Families may encourage dietary indiscretion as an expression of conscious or unconscious hostility toward the patient and as a means of perpetuating the family's status quo through the patient's illness.

6. *Irrational prejudices and body-image problems.* Some patients refuse dialysis because of irrational fears or beliefs. One patient felt that once his blood left his body to enter the dialysis machine, he would die or lose his identity.

Compliance with diet is difficult for patients who have used food as their primary solace and gratification. Others feel very deprived by the social and physical restrictions that their illness presents, and for them eating becomes their chief pleasure. Patients are more likely to be compliant if they live with their family, continue to work, and maintain their independence. Age, sex, race, intelligence, and social position do not influence dietary compliance.

Sexual Adjustment

Uremia is associated with impotence in approximately 45 percent of male dialysis patients. An additional 35 percent of patients become impotent after starting dialysis. Kidney transplantation will reverse about 40 percent of such impotence.

Impotence can be caused by several factors. Antihypertensive medication is a well-known cause. Vascular lesions and peripheral neuropathy can be etiological factors in diabetic and elderly males. Low blood zinc and testosterone levels and increased parathormone levels can also lead to impotence. Depression may result in functional impotence. Once the depression is treated, potency may return. The typical impotent dialysis patient is an older, unaggressive man who is not working and has become the dependent partner in his marriage. Young males who work full-time and are active heads of households are less likely to become impotent.

Because impotence can devastate a patient's self-esteem and can result in marital discord, treatment is very important. The psychiatric consultant should rule out depression and medication that can impair sexual functioning should be discontinued if possible. Patients should be carefully evaluated for organic causes of impotence. Younger men with organic impotence may benefit from a penile prosthesis.

Vocational Adjustment

Only about 25 percent of dialysis patients are able to work outside of the home. Most nondiabetic persons and a few diabetic patients are capable of some activity beyond self-care, but diabetic patients often need continuous nursing care; most diabetics on dialysis are blind or have marked visual impairment. Many diabetics also suffer from coronary artery disease and peripheral neuropathy.

Most patients who return to work do so within six months after starting dialysis. The best predictors for continued employment are previous work history, job or vocational satisfaction, and dissatisfaction with the sick role. Those with expectations of quick rehabilitation and good coping skills often return to full-time employment. Individuals whose dependency needs are gratified by their illness frequently do not return to work. If a nondiabetic patient is to return to work, rehabilitation must start soon after dialysis begins.

Family Dynamics

The psychiatric consultant must recognize that hemodialysis places an enormous emotional strain on the marital dyad. In fact, the marital relationship may be more influential in determining the outcome of home hemodialysis than the nature of the illness. Home hemodialysis usually fails if the more dependent partner has to assume responsibility for the formerly dominant spouse. The dominant partner rarely has difficulty caring for the dependent one. Couples whose relationships are mutually rewarding and reciprocal usually do well.

I have observed a high divorce rate among dialysis and transplant patients. The healthy spouse usually experiences enormous hostility, intense guilt, and feelings of helplessness and victimization. Couples with previous marital difficulties and those under age 45 are most likely to divorce. The spouse who is psychologically dependent on the dialysis patient is least likely to seek a divorce. The following case illustrates the difficulties of a couple who experience a role reversal.

> Mrs. N., a 34-year-old airline stewardess, was referred for psychotherapy because of suicidal ideation. She had suddenly developed renal failure two months after her marriage. She was on dialysis for five years before transplantation with a living-related kidney that functioned for only two years. Following rejection, she returned to hemodialysis. Her care was complicated by severe hypotension and chronic hepatitis. In spite of her illness, she worked full-time as a stewardess. During the four preceding years, she had been increasingly upset by her husband's emotional distance. He avoided her by working late at night and on weekends. They had no sexual relations for months. She was a vivacious, outgoing woman who craved attention and love, but the more she demanded attention, the more her husband withdrew.
>
> Her husband described himself as a hard-working loner. He was emotionally exhausted by his wife's chronic illness. Her requests reminded him of his parents' incessant demands and activated his infantile rage. He had married his wife because he admired her beauty and social grace. He had felt socially inept and hoped for social acceptance through her. The marriage was good for the first few years in spite of the wife's renal failure. When her illness advanced to the point that she could not meet her husband's emotional needs, friction developed. The husband felt abandoned and betrayed by her illness. He was enraged by her dependency needs and repulsed by her illness. His rejection precipitated her depression.
>
> Even after two years of psychotherapy, the husband could not accept his wife's dependency needs. He tried to separate but could not tolerate being alone for more than a week. He felt murderous rage and overwhelming guilt. The couple's situation improved markedly when the wife started continuous peritoneal dialysis. Her blood pressure returned to normal levels and she was able to assume a more active role in the marriage. Once she was physically able to meet her husband's needs, the marital relationship became positive again.

Problems of Renal Transplantation

A kidney for transplantation may be obtained from a close blood relative (living-related donor) or from a deceased accident victim (cadaveric donor). Approximately 83 percent of the transplanted living-related kidneys function at the end of one year, while only 50 percent of the cadaveric kidneys do so. At the end of ten years, 55 to 60 percent of the patients with living-related kidneys are still alive, as opposed to 15 to 20 percent of the patients with cadaveric kidneys.

Nephrologists usually present these statistics to their patients and urge them to have their family members (parents, siblings, or adult children) tissue-typed. The relative must have compatible blood and HL-A tissue typing to be acceptable as a donor. Ideally, after the family is typed, the relative with the best tissue match is selected as the donor.

Past and present intrafamilial conflicts often determine the outcome of the family's donor selection process. Families may prevent positively valued members from donating and often pressure deviant, emotionally disturbed members into giving. Spouses usually become the active solicitors for potential recipients. This allows for some psychological distance between prospective recipients and intended donors and may facilitate decision making. Emotional closeness to potential recipients is the best predictor of whether or not relatives will donate. Mothers are most likely to donate. They are overinvested in saving the lives of their children. Fathers and siblings are the next most likely donors. The least likely potential donors are adult children of potential recipients. Children transfer their emotional investment from their parents to their own family. Unresolved adolescent rebellion and hostility to parents may also prevent donation.

Consciously, donors usually feel their wish to donate is purely altruistic. Frequently, however, the motive for donation is a sense of obligation or conscious or unconscious guilt. For example, the biological mother of a diabetic daughter whom she had given up for adoption saw her chance to donate a kidney as a means to expiate her guilt for having given up her infant. A chronic alcoholic man felt that donating his kidney would redeem his wasted life and lead to acceptance by his family.

Donation by siblings often reactivates sibling rivalry. Donors may feel that the recipients are in a favored position, especially since their families' and their physicians' energies are centered around rehabilitating the recipients. Donors may be resentful that their sacrifices are not constantly acknowledged.

Patients undergoing renal transplantation go through several periods of psychological vulnerability. Once a date for transplantation is set, patients anxiously anticipate surgery. Many patients imagine that after transplantation, they will be healthy again. Those with friends who returned to dialysis after a rejection episode are cognizant of the possibility of rejection.

Guilt and feelings of gratitude toward donors often emerge after transplantation. Males view the resumption of urination as evidence of recapturing their masculinity. Impotent men look for restoration of their potency. During this phase, most patients experience a sense of well-being in spite of postoperative pain and discomfort.

In order to obtain informed consent, physicians must overcome unrealistic expectations and lower the level of denial in their patients. Partial denial allows patients to voluntarily undergo life-threatening surgery, and not feel overwhelmed by its potential complications.

Transplant Rejection

Most patients are consciously aware of the possibility of posttransplant rejection. Even patients who are progressing very well look apprehensively for signs of rejection.

If rejection occurs, hope is replaced by despair and depression. Most patients experience sadness, disappointment, and mild depression. Some displace their frustration over the medical complications onto the staff by becoming more demanding and passively aggressive. Approximately a third of the patients experience emotional disturbance during this phase. Kidney rejection is treated with massive doses of corticosteroids, which can trigger depression and delirium. The stress of rejection invariably reactivates repressed intrapsychic conflicts that compound and exacerbate underlying psychopathology. Psychiatrists must understand the interplay between steroid-induced psychological changes and emotional disturbance secondary to intrapsychic and family conflict.

Steroid-induced delirium responds best to low doses of haloperidol (1 to 5 mg PO at bedtime). Patients are often reluctant to complain of hallucinations because they fear that they are becoming mentally ill. Some may become excessively withdrawn and quiet; others may become very anxious and apprehensive. Some may have unusual requests. Others will admit to a brief psychotic episode only after being told that it can occur, that it results from the medication, and that it is readily reversible. For example, a patient requested that his transplanted kidney be removed two weeks after he received it. Although the patient was doing well except for a minor rejection episode, he insisted that the kidney was bad. During a psychiatric interview, the patient revealed that about a week after surgery he noticed that his "mind was not right." After gentle coaxing, he admitted to auditory hallucinations, paranoid ideation, and periodic confusion. His symptoms started one day after he received 1 gm of intravenous Solu-Medrol. He responded well to 5 mg of haloperidol and frank discussion about medication effects.

Psychiatrists can lower the incidence of emotional problems in the transplant population by preparing patients preoperatively for the emotional impact of the surgery and for possible rejection. Weekly group meetings with patients and their families offer a forum in which emotional aspects of transplantation can be openly discussed. Disturbed families may also need periodic psychiatric intervention.

Suggested Readings

Abram, H.S., Hester, L.R., Sheridan, W.F., et al. (1975). Sexual functioning in patients with chronic renal failure. *Journal of Nervous and Mental Disease* 160:220-226.

Gutman, R.A., Stead, W.W., and Robinson, R.R. (1981). Physical activity and employment status of patients on maintenance dialysis. *New England Journal of Medicine* 304:309-312.

Kaplan De-Nour, A., and Czaczkes, J.W. (1972). Personality factors in chronic hemodialysis patients causing noncompliance with medical regimen. *Psychosomatic Medicine* 34:333-344.

Levy, N.B. (1978). Psychological sequelae to hemodialysis. *Psychosomatics* 19:329-331.

Port, F.K., Knoll, P.D., and Rosenzweig, J. (1979). Lithium therapy during maintenance hemodialysis. *Psychosomatics* 20:130-131.

Procci, W.R. (1978). Dietary abuse in maintenance hemodialysis patients. *Psychosomatics* 19:16-24.

Reichsman, F., and Levy, N.B. (1972). Problems in adaptation to maintenance hemodialysis. *Archives of Internal Medicine* 130:859-869.

Stewart, R.S., and Stewart, R.M. (1979). Neuropsychiatric aspects of chronic renal disease. *Psychosomatics* 20:524-531.

Viederman, M. (1974). Adaptive and maladaptive regression in hemodialysis. *Psychiatry* 37:68-77.

Weiner, M.F., and Lovitt, R. (1979). Conservation-withdrawal versus depression. *General Hospital Psychiatry* 1:347-349.

CHAPTER 32

The Spinal Cord Unit

ROLLIN M. GALLAGHER III, M.D.

Coping with spinal cord injury is a long, complex, and difficult process for patients, their families, and health care providers. Each case has its unique problems, but in all cases the patients and relatives wish the problem had never happened, want it to stop, and feel hopelessly inadequate in facing the progression of events they cannot control, as the following case illustrates.

Mr. N., a 40-year-old married craftsman, fell off a roof and sustained a fracture dislocation at the junction of the 5th and 6th cervical vertebrae. He was paralyzed from the neck down. His reaction to spinal cord injury (SCI), was determined by his personality, by his previous personal and family experience with disability, and by his current circumstances. He expressed what the majority of SCI patients feel about this most catastrophic of injuries.

"I've had a kind of horrible fantasy, like a bad dream, that exactly this would happen to me. For a long time, I never thought it would, but I actually did consider it. . . . I mean the possibility actually occurred to me that I would break my neck and end up having no motion from the shoulders down. My father was severely crippled and he died a very slow death. It wasn't a painful death, but it was a very degrading death. I had long ago decided that if I had a severe disability, I would simply try to do away with myself. I don't want to go on with someone else wiping my ass every time my bowels decide to move. I don't like having to ask someone to scratch the side of my nose when it itches. I don't like being totally helpless."

The patient suffered a long and difficult hospitalization. During it he experienced an initial delirium, fear of pain, muscle spasms, acute despair and suicidal intent, and bladder infections. Considerable anger and mistrust arose between him and his wife and between him and the hospital staff. Initially, he was angry that he had been resuscitated from his injury. By the time he was discharged, he was grateful for the opportunity to resolve significant issues in his family, but he continued to express ambivalence about living as a quadriplegic. Two months later, while home on a pass from a rehabilitation center, he developed an upper respiratory problem that rapidly progressed to pneumonia. He refused treatment, and died at home with his family at his bedside.

The Clinical Problem of Spinal Cord Injury

Medical staff often feel overwhelmed by the enormity and complexity of the therapeutic tasks in spinal cord injury (SCI). Mistakes in early management may irreversibly worsen the neurological deficit and increase the incidence of significant psychiatric and medical complications. These problems are likely to prolong hospitalization and impede eventual functional physical, psychological, social, and vocational adjustment.

For several decades, some European centers have provided a coordinated and integrated system of spinal cord injury care that has contrasted, until recently, with a relatively fragmented approach in the United States. Here, highly skilled surgeons cared for the injured tissues during the acute phase but were often unfamiliar with the longer-term management considerations that require a multidisciplinary approach. As a result, rehabilitation centers spent costly time and effort correcting unnecessary complications such as bed sores, contractures, urinary tract infections, and psychiatric problems. In turn, these centers often sent patients home to the community without arranging adequate follow-up care. To develop methods that would achieve both higher-quality and more cost-effective care, the federal government funded several regional spinal cord injury care centers. Over the past decade, their collective experience has greatly enlarged our knowledge base and promoted the development of new medical, surgical, and psychiatric treatment strategies. This chapter describes how these strategies are used in a general medical-surgical hospital.

The Psychiatric Team

The psychiatrist functions as leader of a multidisciplinary psychosocial team that provides comprehensive psychiatric care to patients and their families. Other active team members might include a nurse education specialist, a social worker, a psychologist, an occupational therapist, and primary-care nurses. Leadership tasks for the psychosocial team include developing coordinated strategies for assisting patients, their families, and the health care system to achieve optimal care. Specific therapeutic activities will be delegated differently in every setting—depending on the training, experience, and interests of the various personnel—but roles and responsibilities must be clearly delineated. Opportunities for communicating significant strategies to the rest of the spinal cord injury team (which includes orthopedists, neurosurgeons, physiatrists, urologists, and physical therapists) must be scheduled so that an overall coordinated team effort is provided. Trainees in the setting, be they residents or medical students from any service, must be adequately integrated into the care system and appropriately supervised.

General Principles of Psychiatric Assessment and Management

The many factors within the patient that influence the course and outcome of each SCI should be evaluated. These include personality, coping and adaptation, the impact of significant events and transitions, the development of psychobiological states such as pain, sleep disturbance, anxiety, depression, and delirium, coping and adaptation of the family, and coping of the health care system. A reliable protocol for acquiring this information can be helpful. I use a Chronic Care Protocol form (see Figure 5), that is placed in the patient's chart. The protocol helps the clinician to collate significant data, to communicate these data and therapeutic decisions among various staff, and to remind the team to complete a thorough assessment.

Psychiatric interventions for the complex clinical problems encountered in SCI require the integration of neurobiological, psychodynamic, interpersonal, and behavioral concepts into a pluralistic treatment plan. Therefore, biopsychosocial evaluation is necessary, and because the uncertain medical course can pose new adaptational challenges to patient, family, and health care system, this evaluation must be continuous. Coping strategies are determined by the relationship among several factors—individual and group coping style, the nature of the injury, new events in the medical course, and the meaning of the injury during each significant event.

Phases of Recovery from SCI: Specific Psychiatric Interventions

During the initial hospitalization, several stressful transition points occur. Each creates a new phase with its own set of adaptational challenges that require biopsychosocial reassessment and appropriate treatment modification.

CHRONIC CASE PROTOCOL

A. IDENTIFICATION: name_____chart no._____physician_____

    1) Chronic care problem: (describe - adjustment to: hospital, chronic
       pain or disability, rehab effort, etc.)
    2) Estimated hospital stay:
    3) Orthopedic goals: (briefly)
    4) Significant health care persons: Ortho res -   P.T. -
                                         Social serv -   Chaplain -
                                         Psych -   Nursing -
                                           Family -   O.T. -

B. IMMEDIATE ADJUSTMENT:
   Evaluation (please initial when completed___;   Care Plan
   check ( ) each positive component where indicated).   (management)

    1) Pain: s/o   p/
       a/Somatic ( ), Anxiety ( ), Depression ( ), Learning ( )

    2) Sleep: s/o   p/
       a/Pain ( ), Anxiety ( ), Depression ( )

    3) Delirium: s/o   p/
       a/possible etiologies: drugs/ETOH ( ), withdrawal ( ), toxins ( ),
                                metabolic ( ), neurologic/trauma ( ),
                                cardiopulmonary ( ), stress ( ),
                                other_____

    4) Psychological/Social Trauma: s/o   p/
       a/Situational anxiety/panic ( ), separation anxiety ( ), acute
       grief ( ), depression ( ), vegetative depression ( ), family/couple
       crisis ( ), other _____

    Describe briefly.

C. LONG-TERM ADJUSTMENT
   Evaluation: (please initial when completed;   Care Plan:
             or check ( ) appropriate items).

s/o 1) Patient interview: Interviewer(s)_____

    1.1 Occupational status:
    1.2 Hobbies:
    1.3 Significant others:
    1.4 Responses to stress (coping style-adaptive and maladaptive)

    2) Family interview: Present _____

    2.1 Strengths:
    2.2 Problems:
    2.3 Impact of illness on family (life style, values, roles,
        communication)

a/ 3) Staffing conference: Present _____

    3.1 Coping strategy, patient (intra- and interpersonal)
    3.2 Coping strategy, family (include key roles of individuals)
    3.3 Coping strategy, staff

D. DISPOSITION: Care Plan:

a/ 1) Orthopedic needs:
    2) Financial needs:
    3) Social supports:
    4) Psychological supports:

s = subjective   o = objective   a = assessment   p = plan

Phase I: Injury and Admission to the Intensive Care Unit

An intensive care unit at any major hospital is a place of high work stress for the permanent staff. Nurses must provide vigilant, meticulous care to critically ill patients, care that requires a high level of technical skill. They must also cope with the different demands of the families and the teams of specialist physicians who are constantly auditing their work. (Chapter 26 discusses problems encountered by the nursing staff.) Despite high expectations, outcomes are uncertain and deaths inevitable.

The SCI patient in particular may stress the system. The degree of dysfunction and the suffering of a patient with midcervical spinal cord lesion often creates conflict between technological and humanitarian issues in medical management. For example, heroic short-term lifesaving measures, including resuscitation and respiratory support, often seem pointless when the staff, patient, and family consider the unlikely prospect that a quadriplegic will attain what for each of them would be an acceptable quality of life. In the context of unclear decisions and poor communication, anxious staff or family may project their own values and feelings onto the clinical situation. They may struggle to control the decision-making process. Assertive family members, particularly when their feelings are excluded from decisions, may provoke authoritarian rather than cooperative behaviors from an indecisive or anxious staff.

The psychiatric team has three important roles during this initial phase of care. (1) The psychiatrist diagnoses and advises treatment for the pain, sleep disturbance, delirium, and agitation that frequently result from the many stressors inherent in the setting. These include the severe injuries and their associated complications, the medical interventions themselves (e.g., respiratory support, monitors, medications), and the ICU milieu. (2) The psychiatric team facilitates problem solving for each specialty group while also facilitating effective communication and decision making among all groups. (3) While helping the family plan for their participation in care and their communication with the system, the psychiatric team also develops a comprehensive psychiatric data base and promotes a trusting therapeutic alliance with the family.

Phase II: Transfer to the Orthopedic or the Neurosurgical Unit

The uncomplicated quadriplegic patient generally achieves respiratory independence within three to seven days and is then transferred to an

---

FIGURE 5.
Parts A and B are for identifying significant personnel and guiding assessment and management planning for common problems of immediate adjustment to a trauma service. Parts C and D are for guiding assessment and management planning for problems of long-term adjustment to a trauma service. (see p. 320.)

orthopedic or a neurosurgical floor. Immediate survival is no longer the primary concern. The patient, the family, and the new system must now adapt to each other during the long hospitalization period. Therapeutic alliances developed between family and psychiatric team during the ICU stay greatly facilitate this process. Prior assessment of the impact of the injury on family roles, communication patterns, and coping strategies helps the team to individualize its interventions.

Although psychological mechanisms are usually actively engaged from the moment of injury, the patient may have been a passive participant in care up to this point, particularly if intubated or delirious. The symptoms and signs of this latter delirium may be subtle; and the staff may themselves deny that a blow to the head powerful enough to fracture the spinal column might also have had intracerebral effects with neuropsychological and behavioral sequelae. A careful mental status examination usually identifies a delirium; however, psychological defenses, such as dissociation and extreme denial, may complicate assessment.

Patients may react strongly as they become more aware of the significance of their injury. Serious management problems may occur. Passive suicidal behavior such as starvation, or active attempts by falling off the Stryker frame, must be managed. Angry behaviors, such as refusal to eat, to deep-breathe, or to otherwise comply with nursing care, may complicate the medical course. Patients may complain bitterly and attempt to provoke arguments. These behaviors, which get attention and may provide the patient with a sense of control, can impede rehabilitation. They commonly present in patients who react negatively to dependency or authority, and have particular difficulty trusting professionals on the service. In fact, many adolescent SCI patients do have personality disorders or attention-deficit disorders, and also have difficulty with trust.

The psychiatrist can adopt any or all of several strategies to enhance trust and help the patient gain a healthy sense of control.

First, there is pharmacological intervention for dysphoric psychobiological states such as pain, sleep disturbance, and anxiety. For example, amitriptyline, 25 to 50 mg at bedtime, can help regulate sleep patterns, which become easily disturbed in SCI, and can provide analgesia as well. Symptom relief will produce grateful patients.

Second, empathy can be demonstrated when others react negatively. Angry or suicidal thoughts are often difficult for the staff to tolerate. They feel: "We've given you excellent care. It's been hard work. And now you're going to repay us by wanting to kill yourself?" Or they may identify with the patient, thinking, "If I were a quadriplegic, I believe I would also want to kill myself." These thoughts, which are in conflict with professional goals, often provoke guilt in their thinkers and then rejection of the patient. The psychiatrist can encourage the patient to speak freely to him or her about suicidal or hostile feelings without fearing rejection or retaliation. A simple, effective way to demonstrate empathy is to lie on the floor to interview a patient who is face down on a Stryker frame. This maneuver preserves eye contact and demonstrates awareness of the patient's discomfort in talking to unseen people.

Third, the psychiatrist can enhance the patient's sense of control over the environment, encouraging the patient to participate in scheduling visitors and various therapeutic activities. By teaching psychophysiological techniques such as relaxation and self-hypnosis, the psychiatric consultant can facilitate and enhance the patient's control over emotional responses, pain, disturbed sleep, and muscle spasms.

Phase III: Surgical Stabilization of the Spine

An aggressive surgical approach to fracture dislocations of the spine can minimize morbidity, maximize return to function, and reduce dependence on specialized assistance. Therefore, in most centers, orthopedists and neurosurgeons will surgically stabilize the spines of many patients. Patients and families often hope unrealistically that surgery will change the neurological outcome of the injury. Such denial often seems necessary for maintenance of psychological equilibrium during early hospitalization, particularly when other coping mechanisms are not available. When neurological function does not return after surgery, patients and families are disappointed. Anger or despair may precipitate behaviors that complicate management. For example, patients and families may criticize staff and seek care elsewhere; or they may request more analgesics and sedatives than are usually needed in the postsurgical recovery period.

Surgery usually occurs within ten days after the injury. Afterward, the patient's spine is immobilized by Stryker frame or body jacket. The team can now help the patient begin more active participation in rehabilitation tasks, such as regular physical exercise, self-catheterization, and self-feeding. Difficulty in achieving reasonable goals may indicate pathological denial or may herald a major depressive episode that must be treated aggressively with medications and psychotherapy.

A number of psychotherapeutic techniques are helpful. Supportive psychotherapy can help the patient and family verbalize feelings or beliefs that underlie noncompliance or withdrawal. Behavioral techniques can desensitize patients to fear-laden procedures. Behavioral reinforcement by rewarding successful completion of small tasks of progressively increasing difficulty works well. Relaxation therapy can help to relieve muscle spasm and pain and to control anxiety. Combining these techniques, the psychosocial team can use desensitization to help both patient and family overcome inhibitions about touching the paralyzed part of the body. This work is a crucial precursor to a couple's later discussion of sexual functioning. Peer counseling by carefully selected rehabilitated SCI patients can greatly facilitate patient acceptance of the rehabilitation process. As a general therapeutic strategy, the patient and family should be encouraged to take maximum responsibility for decision making, rehabilitative tasks, and planning for the future.

Phase IV: Removal from Immobilizing Devices

This procedure often has major significance to SCI patients. They may have perceived the immobilization device, particularly the Stryker frame, as partly responsible for their physical limitations. Once they view their immobile and insensate limbs lying helplessly on a bed, the magnitude of their deficit becomes more real. This new or heightened awareness of body image may precipitate anger with acting out, or depression with behavioral withdrawal. In contrast, patients and families who have already accepted the disability usually perceive the removal of the immobilizing device as a milestone toward the goal of regaining control of life in a home environment.

Major tasks in this phase include returning the righting reflexes by use of the tilt table, transferring from bed to chair, and using a wheelchair. Psychotherapeutic strategies include active encouragement and reward for goal setting and achievement, facilitation of grief work for real and anticipated losses, and encouragement of realistic planning.

Phase V: Transfer to Rehabilitation

This transfer is always difficult for the patient, the patient's family, and the health care system. Anticipatory anxiety about entry into new surroundings may be exacerbated by sadness about the loss of intense therapeutic relationships with staff, particularly when the patient is transferred to a distant rehabilitation center. Romantic attachment may have occurred between patient and staff. (For example, a paraplegic from our service married a staff nurse.) The psychosocial team must carefully monitor these relationships, trying not to inhibit their natural evolution when they are beneficial to the patient and trying to minimize their negative impact. The weekly team meeting provides the staff with an opportunity to discuss their relationship with each patient and to develop appropriate strategies to maintain and reinforce psychotherapeutic and rehabilitation achievements. If patients can resolve the loss of these important relationships, they can look forward to helpful new alliances. If not, resentment and the anticipation of future losses may hinder the development of crucial therapeutic relationships in the new setting.

Phase VI: Discharge Home

The patient and the patient's family are generally apprehensive about the return home. The patient's dependence on the staff during the acute phases of recovery must be replaced by independence and self-reliance. A gradual transition, while new skills are integrated into the home environment, facilitates this process. This transition confronts patient and family with the magnitude of their losses. Being unable to turn on the stove, to reach the telephone, or to perform usual household activities or maintenance may have major symbolic significance to the patient. Feelings of helplessness and rage may recur. Team members must be available to provide support and the necessary psychotherapeutic interventions during this difficult adjustment period, which may continue for several years.

The Team Process

It is a difficult task to coordinate the knowledge and skills of many specialists in order to achieve the highly individualized treatment programs required for the exceedingly complex problems of SCI. In fact, perhaps the most difficult challenge for a multidisciplinary, multispecialty SCI team is to reduce territorial behavior among its various members. For example, neurosurgeons may vie with orthopedists for surgical leadership. The group process skills of the consultation-liaison psychiatrist can play a critical role in mediating disputes that might impair effective team functioning. The success of an SCI service ultimately depends on success in this area.

As in many areas of psychiatry, nonmedical mental health professionals may participate on the SCI service. Psychiatrists must provide them with opportunities for professional fulfillment, but they must be certain that their own integrative roles and special skills are complemented, not compromised, by such participation. In the acute-care setting, many educational and counseling roles can be played by nonpsychiatrists; in the rehabilitation setting, psychologists have functioned very effectively as members of the rehabilitation team. However, on our service, the experience has been that only well-trained consultation-liaison psychiatrists can effectively fulfill the functions described in this chapter in the crisis-oriented milieu of the acute medical-surgical hospital.

Suggested Readings

Fordyce, W. (1978). Behavioral methods for engaging the spinal cord injured patient in the rehabilitation process. In *Treatment of the Spinal Cord Injured*, ed. M.G. Eisenberg and J.A. Falconer, pp. 82–100. Springfield, Ill.: Charles C. Thomas.

Gallagher, R.M., McKegney, F.P., and Gladstone, T. (1982). Psychiatric interventions in spinal cord injury. *Psychosomatics* 23:1153-1167.

Guggenheim, F.G., and O'Hara, S. (1976). Peer counseling in a general hospital. *American Journal of Psychiatry* 133:1197-1199.

Gunther, M. (1971). Psychiatric consultation in a rehabilitation hospital: a regression hypothesis. *Comprehensive Psychiatry* 12:572-585.

Hamilton, B.B., Rath, G.J., Meyer, P.R., et al. (1976). A basic evaluation framework for spinal cord injury care systems. *Paraplegia* 14:87-94.

Hohmann, G.W. (1975). Psychological aspects of treatment and rehabilitation of the spinal cord injured person. *Clinical Orthopedics* 112:81-88.

Seligson, D., and Gallagher, R.M. (1982). The psychiatric team on a spinal cord injury service. *Psychosomatics* 23:1152-1159.

Stewart, T.D. (1977). Spinal cord injury: a role for the psychiatrist. *American Journal of Psychiatry* 134:538-541.

Treischmann, R.B. (1978). The psychological, social, and vocational adjustment in spinal cord injury: a strategy for further research. *Publication of the Office of Human Services, HEW*, RSA/13-p-59011/9-01-April.

Young, J.S. (1978). Initial hospitalization and rehabilitation costs of spinal cord injury. *Orthopedic Clinics of North America* 9:263-270.

Specialized Diagnostic
and Management Techniques

In this concluding section, two important means of eliciting information and two important means for managing patients are presented. Drug-augmented interviewing has now reached a high level of technical sophistication. It can be of great help to psychiatrists in differentiating organic from functional disorders and psychotic from nonpsychotic disorders.

Psychological testing is frequently indicated as a potential source of diagnostic information. It not only helps differentiate the organic from the functional components of many disorders, but also sheds light on patients' ability to cooperate, potential management problems, and the type and degree of functional psychopathology and organic mental impairment.

Hypnosis and behavioral control techniques are useful for dealing with patients who are in pain and situations in which emotional reactions to illness greatly aggravate or contribute to symptomatology. These techniques are especially indicated when patients are not manageable with other forms of psychological intervention or with medications. Hypnosis and behavioral control are departures from the traditional psychotherapeutic stance of the office-based psychotherapist—but they are clearly based on traditional physician-patient relationships. Hypnosis follows the traditional doctor-patient relationship in that doctors manipulate processes in patients' bodies—processes that patients are unaware of having conscious control over. Behavioral control measures are also an extension of the traditional doctor-patient relationship in that patients follow doctors' directions instead of doctors being guided by their patients, as in many insight-oriented therapies.

These chapters on specialized techniques indicate the expanding application and refinement of diagnostic and treatment procedures that give psychiatric consultants ever-greater flexibility and scope of function in the general hospital.

M.W.

CHAPTER 33

The Drug-Assisted Interview

JOSEPH A. KWENTUS, M.D.

Judicious use of drug-assisted interviewing can be helpful in distinguishing functional from organic states, for catharsis in posttraumatic states, for treatment of conversion disorders, and for predicting response to antidepressants. But there are two important caveats: Functional and organic disorders can coexist; and material brought forth in drug-assisted interviews is still subject to patients' conscious control and distortion.

The Amytal Interview

Medium-acting barbiturates, used in subanesthetic doses, have a variety of applications in drug-assisted diagnostic interviewing. These agents, such as amobarbital (Amytal) produce generalized cortical depression with resulting changes in behavioral and cognitive functions; patients are rendered more suggestible and less observant. Unfortunately, barbiturates may produce loquaciousness, slurred speech, and sleep. Learning and memory are impaired. Amnesia for significant portions of the interview is common. Titration of drug effect is possible because short- and medium-acting barbiturates are lipophilic and reach maximal brain levels promptly, before being redistributed and metabolized. Shorter-acting agents, such as methohexital, require more rapid titration because narcosis lightens quickly as the drug is rapidly redistributed. For this reason, a medium-acting agent, such as amobarbital, is often preferred. Although sedation is more gradual, the narcosis is more persistent and allows the interviewer to focus attention on the diagnostic interview.

There is no absolute dosage schedule to determine the exact amount of sodium amobarbital to be administered. The individual patient's response to the drug is the best guide. Even when using the drug with mute or apparently stuporous patients, interviewers should thoroughly explain what the procedure entails and that the medication will produce a state of relaxation that will make them feel like talking. If possible, informed consent should be obtained (for a discussion of informed consent, see Chapter 11). Although there should be easy access to respiratory and cardiovascular support systems in case of an unexpected complication, Amytal interviewing is safe.

The interviewer or an assistant should start an intravenous line that will remain patent during the entire procedure. The interviewer can begin to administer 75 mg of a 5-percent solution of sodium amobarbital over 3 to 5 minutes, while observing the patient for slurred speech, yawning, and lateral nystagmus. Administration of the amobarbital solution continues at a rate of 25 to 50 mg per minute—until these effects are noted. The interviewer should continually make the suggestion that soon the patient will feel like talking and should gradually approach affect-laden material. Important areas for exploration can be obtained from a prior interview with friends or relatives. A standard psychiatric interview format, including formal mental status, should be used. Narcosis is maintained at an appropriate level by administering 25- to 50-mg doses of amobarbital, as needed. A rating scale, such as a minimental state or a modification of Weinstein's Amytal Test, can be a helpful adjunct. The rating scale is administered before the Amytal interview and again during narcosis. After the interview, the patient should be closely supervised and vital signs observed. Barbiturates should be used with caution in patients with obstructive pulmonary disease (especially if there is CO_2 retention) and in patients with liver disease, congestive heart failure, or renal failure. Barbiturates are contraindicated in patients with known allergy, porphyria, or concomitant intoxication with other sedatives.

The Amytal interview is useful in the differential diagnosis of the mute or stuporous patient. Since less than 1 percent of patients presenting with stupor have a functional etiology, a medical evaluation needs to be performed first. At a minimum, this includes a physical and a neurological examination, metabolic, toxicological, and hematological laboratory tests, and an electroencephalogram. If there is suggestion of structural neurological damage on the physical exam or in the history, a computerized tomography scan is essential. An elevated temperature, cardiovascular instability, or elevated white count necessitate an evaluation for infection, including lumbar puncture. An electrocardiogram should also be obtained. Finally, all attempts should be made to learn about current medication, drug, and alcohol use. An Amytal interview may be misleading in any condition in which barbiturates may have a therapeutic effect, including subclinical status epilepticus, sedative and alcohol withdrawal, and severe akinesia secondary to phenothiazine administration.

An Amytal interview can temporarily interrupt catatonic stupor. Unfortunately, not all catatonics respond to Amytal. Since the effects of amobarbital on the motor manifestations of organic forms of catatonia have not been definitively studied, interpretation of results should always be based on the patient's verbal performance. Only if the interview reveals a characteristic history of schizophrenic delusions, hallucinations, and prodromal symptoms during the patient's lucid interval can a psychiatrist make a diagnosis of catatonic schizophrenia.

Patients with hysterical stupor may also respond to Amytal interviews. These patients usually do not exhibit waxy flexibility. Nonphysiological neurological signs, such as inconsistency of voluntary muscle control or forced closure of the eyes, suggest the diagnosis of hysterical stupor. A definite event often precedes this form of psychogenic stupor and the patient may reveal that event during the interview. Sometimes it is difficult to distinguish between catatonic and hysterical stupor on the basis of information from an Amytal interview. On a rare occasion, patients with personality disorders of the passive-aggressive or antisocial type feign stupor for secondary gain. In such instances, Amytal interviewing may provide confusing or unreliable results. Sodium amobarbital is not a "truth serum" and should never be presented in that manner. In the following case, evidence of psychosis was elicited by use of a drug-assisted interview.

Miss P., a 28-year-old unemployed white woman, was admitted to the medical service in a stuporous condition following a three-day fast. She had normal blood chemistries, including glucose, and a normal EEG. Her neurological exam was normal, except for altered mental status. Inconsistencies of motor tone and an almost deliberate uncooperativeness were noted. Waxy flexibility was absent. The family described the patient as overly dramatic, overly dependent, and demanding.

The psychiatric consultant performed a drug-assisted interview with amobarbital. Shortly after the induction of nystagmus, the patient responded to the interviewer's suggestion that she would feel like talking. She revealed that she had been commanded by God to fast after she learned that an acquaintance had become seriously ill. She spoke passionately about her religious beliefs and about her concerns for her own health. Her affect was inappropriate and her language idiosyncratic. After the interview, the patient was transferred to the psychiatric service where she responded to a low dose of a neuroleptic.

The next case demonstrates the dangers of overinterpreting motor effects of Amytal on a stuporous patient.

Mrs. Q., a 50-year-old white married housewife with previously diagnosed diabetes and schizophrenia was brought to the emergency room in a stuporous condition. Her neurological exam was normal except for altered mental status. Her husband said that she might have taken an insulin overdose before going to bed the night before. He had not become alarmed until the next afternoon when she did not waken.

In the emergency room, Mrs. Q.'s blood glucose was normal. Extensive evaluation on the neurological service was unrevealing. She remained stuporous. Psychiatric consultation was requested two weeks after admission. An Amytal interview was performed by the psychiatric resident, who reported that her affect had brightened and that she seemed to follow him with her eyes. She did not speak. Based on these observations, he made the diagnosis of catatonic schizophrenia and transferred the patient to a psychiatric unit. Six months later, she still remained in a stupor despite vigorous attempts at psychiatric treatment. At that point, her physicians reluctantly concluded that her stupor was the result of structural damage from the insulin overdose.

Properly performed Amytal interviewing can be very helpful in diagnosing delirium and stupor. Patients with organic brain syndromes usually demonstrate increased disorientation, confabulation, and denial of illness during an Amytal interview. Diagnosis should always be based on analysis of the patient's verbal production during the interview. If a stuporous patient clears completely and then acknowledges previously undisclosed psychiatric symptoms, a functional etiology can be safely presumed. Motor responses and equivocal changes in affect or behavior should be entirely discounted.

The tendency for amobarbital to exacerbate organic brain syndromes has diagnostic implications in elderly patients. Amytal interviews can be used to differentiate depression-related pseudodementia from true dementia. Depression in the elderly may present as delirium, stupor, or dementia and may be difficult to distinguish from those organic syndromes. While some depressed patients change little under amobarbital, other depressed patients may appear less confused and less nonproductive. If an elderly patient's cognitive performance improves substantially during an Amytal interview, the diagnosis of depression should be vigorously pursued. If the patient becomes more confused, has increased denial of illness, or exhibits confabulation, an organic process is more likely.

Drug-Assisted Interviewing in Conversion, Dissociation, and Amnesia

Some psychiatric centers have advocated Amytal interviews to elicit historical data from withdrawn patients for differential diagnosis. With the notable exception of catatonic patients, patients tend to reveal new information whether amobarbital or placebo is used. Although amobarbital does not appear to exert a specific effect in the elaboration of data important for differential diagnosis other than in the evaluation of catatonia or organic brain syndrome, it may occasionally be useful to clinicians dealing with an extremely inhibited patient or with a fully alert, mute patient. An Amytal interview of a patient with conversion aphonia or other forms of unexplained muteness may allow the interviewer to obtain important information regarding the need for psychiatric hospitalization, as seen in the following example.

> Miss R., a 23-year-old black mother of two, was brought into the emergency room, fully alert but unable to speak. Neurological and ENT consultations were unrevealing. A psychiatric consultant was called. After several suggestions that the patient would soon feel like speaking were unsuccessful, the patient agreed in writing to an Amytal interview. After the induction of nystagmus and slurred speech, the interviewer noted that the patient appeared sad. She suddenly broke into tears. In a whisper, she told the interviewer that while singing in the church choir, she peered out of a window and saw her fiancé kissing her best friend. From that moment on, she could neither sing nor speak. As the interview proceeded, the patient's voice rose in anger as she shared her sense of betrayal. The patient was discharged to outpatient follow-up.

Amytal interviewing also has dramatic diagnostic and therapeutic use in more intractable chronic conversion symptoms than the one just presented (for a discussion of the somatoform disorders, see Chapter 14). For clinicians to use this approach, they should build a positive, somewhat authoritarian relationship with patients in a series of predrug sessions. Symptom amelioration through hypnosis prior to the Amytal interview can be attempted. Hypnotic induction techniques (discussed in Chapter 35) can be used during the early phases of the Amytal interview to augment the suggestibility produced by the drug-related alteration in consciousness. Since patients with conversion often elicit hostility from therapists, care must be taken to phrase suggestions in a supportive, nonjudgmental manner. Direct suggestion is usually more effective than attempts at abreaction. However, a successful outcome may lead to some display of emotions. Drug-assisted interviewing has the advantage over hypnosis that it does not depend on maintaining a hypnotic trance. Nonetheless, if the patient wishes to defeat the interviewer, symptoms may not change or may even worsen during the interview. As with any technique that relies on suggestion, some patients later experience a return of symptoms. Other patients, who have used a particular somatic symptom for defensive purposes, may become acutely dysphoric after "cure." This technique is most useful with motor conversions and with mutism or blindness. It is not as useful with more subjective symptoms such as pain. If the patient is malingering, the chances of success are remote, but many patients with true conversion symptoms will respond positively, as the next case illustrates.

> Mr. S., a 22-year-old single unemployed man, had a brachial neuritis that removed him from active military service. In the physical therapy department, the patient behaved in a passive-aggressive manner. The

attending neurologist felt that his inability to raise his arm was a conversion phenomenon and requested a psychiatric consultation. The psychiatrist conducted an Amytal interview during which he elevated the patient's arm and suggested that he would feel stronger. After several minutes of passive movement, the patient began to actively move his arm in the previously neglected range of motion. He then responded to suggestions to show his strength. In subsequent psychiatric interviews, the patient openly vented his anger at his immediate superiors for not allowing him to go to sick call during the early phases of his illness. The physical therapy department reported that he had become more cooperative.

Amytal interviewing can aid memory retrieval in patients with functional amnestic syndromes. The interview may be preceded by a 15-mg oral dose of amphetamine to produce greater vigilance. Although drug-assisted memory retrieval has been applied to battle casualties, accident victims, and patients with various dissociative states, it tends to be helpful only with cooperative, eager patients. Although patients generally report new information during such interventions, there is no guarantee that this information is more correct than that obtained during more standard forms of interviewing. Subjects who wish to cover up information in a drug-assisted interview do so with ease, while some guilt-ridden subjects may report unflattering fantasy as fact.

In some instances, memory retrieval may be facilitated by a mood state similar to that present at the time the memories were encoded. A skilled interviewer may be better able to facilitate the emergence of appropriate affective states when the patient is provided with a chemical protection against the most frightening aspects of the experience. Because drug-assisted interviewing may even promote the emergence of memories in some organic amnestic states, it is important not to rely solely on this technique to differentiate psychogenic from organic amnestic states.

The quick recovery of memory for amnestic episodes is often extremely important in the treatment of posttraumatic stress disorder, and Amytal interviewing may play a crucial role in the early management of these cases. The technique elaborated by Grinker remains among the most effective. Prior to the induction of narcosis, the interviewer establishes a trusting relationship with the patient and obtains as much material as possible using standard psychiatric techniques. After an appropriate amount of amobarbital is administered, a crucial verbal stimulus is given and the patient is encouraged to free-associate. When there is hesitation, the interviewer encourages the patient to continue and gives additional cues. Success depends on a supportive, nonjudgmental interview and on avoiding oversedation while maintaining an appropriate level of narcosis by slow titration of the barbiturate. The procedure should be continued for a sufficient length of time to explore all the areas of suggested conflict. Patients with coexisting major psychiatric disorders and malingerers tend to be refractory.

One of the most useful, and often neglected, indications for drug-assisted memory retrieval is diagnosis of suspected suicide attempts. A patient may make a suicide attempt and, after medical treatment, deny that the attempt was intentional. For a number of psychological and even physiological reasons, some of these patients may actually be amnestic for the event. Data supporting a diagnosis of depression may be difficult to obtain, even from friends and relatives. A well-timed drug-assisted interview may facilitate an accurate recall of the event.

Physostigmine

Physostigmine has recently come into clinical use for specific diagnostic tasks because of its ability to inhibit acetylcholinesterase and to reverse cholinergic blockade. Although a variety of central anticholinergic syndromes may be successfully diagnosed with physostigmine, psychiatrists are most likely to use this agent in diagnosing toxic psychosis secondary to accumulated anticholinergic effects of antipsychotic, antidepressant, and antiparkinsonian drugs. Physostigmine does not interfere with the patient's ability to communicate. It can be particularly useful in acutely psychotic patients whose disorganized thinking worsens after the initiation of therapy. Although deterioration and impairment of recent memory are the hallmarks of anticholinergic delirium, mental status testing may be difficult in an agitated psychotic patient with active psychiatric illness. Signs of peripheral anticholinergic activity will be present, but they are difficult to quantitate when the patient's therapy includes anticholinergic medication. If the patient's mental state clears after the injection of physostigmine, anticholinergic medication should be withdrawn and the test repeated after an appropriate interval. Anticholinergic drugs should then be kept to a minimum.

Physostigmine may be useful in other forms of anticholinergic psychosis presenting to the psychiatrist, including cases of deliberate or accidental overdose of adulterated street drugs or over-the-counter sleeping pills.

Physostigmine inhibits both central and peripheral acetylcholinesterase, producing cholinomimetic actions. The onset of action is extremely swift, usually within 5 minutes after intravenous administration. The usual dose is 1 to 2 mg administered at a rate no faster than 1 mg per minute. A second trial can be performed in 15 minutes, up to a maximum of 4 mg. Physostigmine can cause bronchospasm, increased secretions, muscle weakness, bradycardia, hypotension, heart block, vomiting, and seizures. Most physostigmine toxicity is due to excessive cholinergic-parasympathetic stimulation; 0.5 mg of atropine sulfate per milligram of physostigmine is an effective antidote.

Physostigmine should be used with extreme caution in patients with gangrene, coronary artery disease, heart block, peptic ulcer, hypothyroidism, asthma, ulcerative colitis, bowel and bladder obstruction, glaucoma, pregnancy, and myotonia.

Although the diagnostic uses of physostigmine are well established, the use of these drugs in the *treatment* of anticholinergic delirium is controversial because of the risk of complications. False positives are sometimes observed because physostigmine may have a nonspecific arousal effect in some forms of toxic psychosis.

The use of physostigmine in differentiating some forms of active disorder from schizophrenia is still in the investigational stage. Physostigmine has also been used recently for differential diagnosis of drug-related movement disorders because it tends to exacerbate parkinsonian movements and to ameliorate movements related to tardive dyskinesias.

Amphetamines

Amphetamine and related stimulants have also been used for diagnostic interviewing. The amphetamine challenge test can help differentiate depressions that may respond to noradrenergic types of antidepressants from depressions that will respond to agents with more pronounced effects on serotonergic symptoms (for a fuller discussion of the treatment of depression, see Chapter 6). In this test, a baseline interview is performed to rate the patient's depressive symptoms. Amphetamine in a dose of 15 mg is administered orally, and the patient's symptomatology is recorded at set intervals following the test dose. An additional dose is administered several hours later and is followed by a structured interview. If the patient reports a remission of depressive symptoms, a noradrenergic drug may be more helpful. If the patient becomes more irritable, a serotonergic drug can be tried first. This test has not been subjected to vigorous scientific study with large numbers of patients. In addition, results can be confounded by daily variation in mood. As a result, amphetamine challenge should always be used in combination with other data such as previous drug response, cortisol suppression by dexamethasone, and current symptomatology. Occasionally, a patient with profound psychomotor retardation and sufficient impairment of attention and concentration to mimic delirium (assuming organic etiology of delirium has been ruled out) may respond to amphetamine challenge with sufficient symptomatic improvement to both suggest a therapy and help confirm the diagnosis of depression. In order to obtain the most useful data from an amphetamine challenge, careful structured interviews using a symptom checklist are essential.

When acute and partially treated schizophrenics are treated with intra-venous amphetamine, a dramatic increase in psychotic symptoms often follows. Normals, depressives, and schizophrenics in remission do not show this effect. The effect of amphetamine on acute schizophrenics can be partially blocked by administration of physostigmine. Although stimulant-assisted interviews would not be expected to be of diagnostic value in most cases of schizophrenia, this effect should be kept in mind when amphetamines are used in conjunction with barbiturates in other forms of diagnostic inter-viewing.

Summary

Drug-assisted interviewing is of value in differentiating organic from functional delirious states. Its role in the differential diagnosis of major mental illness is becoming more defined. Drug-assisted interviewing may facilitate retrieval of unavailable memories, leading to a number of diagnostic and therapeutic applications. The use of drug interviews, in a manner similar to hypnosis, to facilitate the treatment of intractable conversions has long been known in clinical practice. The use of intravenous drugs in psycho-therapy has generated encouraging reports that have never been subjected to controlled study and therefore must be viewed with some skepticism. Drug-assisted desensitization may be an exception to this. As newer agents and applications are introduced, drug-assisted interviewing may become even more useful in a range of diagnostic and therapeutic situations.

Suggested Readings

Dysken, M.W., Chang, S.S., Casper, R.C., and Davis, J.M. (1979). Barbiturate facilitated interviewing. *Biological Psychiatry* 14:421–432.

Granacher, R.P., and Baldessarini, R.J. (1975). Physostigmine: its use in acute anticholinergic syndrome with antidepressant and antiparkinsonian drugs. *Archives of General Psychiatry* 32:375–379.

Grinker, R., and Spiegel, J.B. (1945). *War Neurosis*. Philadelphia: Blakiston.

Lindemann, E. (1932). Psychological changes in normal and abnormal individuals under the influence of sodium amytal. *American Journal of Psychiatry* 88: 1083–1091.

Mawson, A.B. (1970). Methohexitone-assisted desensitization in the treatment of phobias. *Lancet* 1:1084–1086.

Perry, J.C., and Jacobs, D. (1982). Overview: clinical applications of the amytal interview in psychiatric emergency settings. *American Journal of Psychiatry* 139:552–559.

Stevens, H. (1963). Conversion hysteria: a neurologic emergency period. *Mayo Clinic Proceedings* 43:54–64.

Stevenson, I., Buckman, J., Smith, B.M., and Hain, J.D. (1974). The use of drugs in psychiatric interviews: some interpretations based on controlled experiments. *American Journal of Psychiatry* 131:707–710.

Weinstein, E.A., Kahn, R.L., Sugerman, L.A., and Malitz, S. (1954). Serial administration of the "Amytal Test" for brain disease. *Archives of Neurology and Psychiatry* 71:217–226.

Woodruff, R. (1966). The diagnostic use of the amylobarbitone interview among patients with psychotic illness. *British Journal of Psychiatry* 112:727–732.

CHAPTER 34

Psychological Testing in the General Hospital

ROBERT LOVITT, Ph.D.

In certain difficult clinical situations, psychological testing is helpful to psychiatric consultants. It provides objective data to supplement clinical examinations, and it facilitates accurate diagnosis and management. Far too often, however, psychiatrists ask for "a Rorschach" or "testing" instead of conceptualizing the patient's problem and asking, for example, "How does the patient handle aggressive impulses?" or "Is there a psychogenic component to the patient's complaints of pain?"

To secure appropriate testing, two critical questions must be addressed by physicians and psychologists: (1) What specific personality factors may impact on the clinical situation in question? (2) What tests and what specific test patterns measure the personality processes being evaluated?

A referral for testing is indicated when there is a relationship between personality processes, the clinical condition being evaluated, and specific psychological tests. For example, a 24-year-old man who may have stopped taking his insulin is hospitalized for diabetic ketoacidosis. He has average intellect and a normal mental status examination, but the psychiatrist suspects that subtle reasoning difficulties may interfere with the patient's taking his insulin. Psychological testing might help in the following fashion.

A specific personality attribute that may partially account for poor compliance is reasoning dysfunction, particularly in relation to physical health. Tests and test patterns that assess reasoning dysfunction are the Similarities and Comprehension Subtests of the Wechsler Adult Intelligence Scale (WAIS); scales 6, 7, and 8 of the Minnesota Multiphasic Personality Inventory (MMPI); and the F+% and special scoring categories of the

Rorschach test. Testing would therefore be potentially helpful to assess this patient's reasoning processes.

The following discussion describes clinical situations in which testing may be helpful when conceptualized according to the two critical questions presented earlier.

Noncompliance

Psychiatrists are often asked to assess patient's potential compliance with complex and expensive medical procedures such as renal transplantation. Dimensions of personality functioning related to potential compliance are limited intellect, cognitive dysfunction, and patients' illness behavior.

Limited Intellect

Patients who do not understand their physicians have difficulty following directions. Although poor compliance due to limited intellect is most often found in patients in facilities serving the medically indigent, limited intellectual functioning is misdiagnosed and neglected in many settings, as illustrated in the following vignette.

> Mrs. T., a 29-year-old housewife with a history of bronchial asthma, was uncooperative and antagonistic during hospitalization. She was referred for psychiatric evaluation because she refused to talk and to take medication and spent her time staring out the window. When interviewed, she was sullen and made poor eye contact, and her associations were difficult to follow, leading her physicians to suspect a schizophrenic disorder. Wechsler testing showed a Full Scale IQ of 57; she had a fund of information more developed than her other areas of intellectual functioning that allowed her to present a "front" of adequate intellectual functioning. She developed a series of behavioral tactics to evade and distract when confronted with problems with which she was unable to cope. In this situation the diagnosis of mental retardation was missed clinically and a functional psychosis was suspected as a cause of her poor compliance.

There are three highly validated, clinically useful techniques for assessing intellectual functioning. The Wechsler Adult Intelligence Scale (Revised) (WAIS-R), which takes about an hour to complete, is the most thoroughly researched test of intellectual functioning, and is composed of 11 subtests and generates three IQ scores. In Figure 6, we see three types of intellectual patterns related to compliance difficulties.

Pattern A indicates a mentally retarded level of functioning with an approximate IQ score of 57. It shows diffuse impairment of intellectual

TABLE OF SCALED SCORE EQUIVALENTS

Scaled Score	RAW SCORE: VERBAL TESTS: Information	Digit Span	Vocabulary	Arithmetic	Comprehension	Similarities	PERFORMANCE TESTS: Picture Completion	Picture Arrangement	Block Design	Object Assembly	Digit Symbol	Scaled Score
19	—	28	70	—	32	—	—	—	51	—	93	19
18	29	27	69	—	31	28	—	—	—	41	91-92	18
17	—	26	68	19	—	—	20	20	50	—	89-90	17
16	28	25	66-67	—	30	27	—	—	49	40	84-88	16
15	27	24	65	18	29	26	—	19	47-48	39	79-83	15
14	26	22-23	63-64	17	27-28	25	19	—	44-46	38	75-78	14
13	25	20-21	60-62	16	26	24	—	18	42-43	37	70-74	13
12	23-24	18-19	55-59	15	25	23	18	17	38-41	35-36	66-69	12
11	22	17	52-54	13-14	23-24	22	17	15-16	35-37	34	62-65	11
10	19-21	15-16	47-51	12	21-22	20-21	16	14	31-34	32-33	57-61	10
9	17-18	14	43-46	11	19-20	18-19	15	13	27-30	30-31	53-56	9
8	15-16	12-13	37-42	10	17-18	16-17	14	11-12	23-26	28-29	48-52	8
7	13-14	11	29-36	8-9	14-16	14-15	13	8-10	20-22	24-27	44-47	7
6	9-12	9-10	20-28	6-7	11-13	11-13	11-12	5-7	14-19	21-23	37-43	6
5	6-8	8	14-19	5	8-10	7-10	8-10	3-4	8-13	16-20	30-36	5
4	5	7	11-13	4	6-7	5-6	5-7	2	3-7	13-15	23-29	4
3	4	6	9-10	3	4-5	2-4	3-4	—	2	9-12	16-22	3
2	3	3-5	6-8	1-2	2-3	1	2	1	1	6-8	8-15	2
1	0-2	0-2	0-5	0	0-1	0	0-1	0	0	0-5	0-7	1

----Pattern A

TABLE OF SCALED SCORE EQUIVALENTS

Scaled Score	RAW SCORE: VERBAL TESTS: Information	Digit Span	Vocabulary	Arithmetic	Comprehension	Similarities	PERFORMANCE TESTS: Picture Completion	Picture Arrangement	Block Design	Object Assembly	Digit Symbol	Scaled Score
19	—	28	70	—	32	—	—	—	51	—	93	19
18	29	27	69	—	31	28	—	—	—	41	91-92	18
17	—	26	68	19	—	—	20	20	50	—	89-90	17
16	28	25	66-67	—	30	27	—	—	49	40	84-88	16
15	27	24	65	18	29	26	—	19	47-48	39	79-83	15
14	26	22-23	63-64	17	27-28	25	19	—	44-46	38	75-78	14
13	25	20-21	60-62	16	26	24	—	18	42-43	37	70-74	13
12	23-24	18-19	55-59	15	25	23	18	17	38-41	35-36	66-69	12
11	22	17	52-54	13-14	23-24	22	17	15-16	35-37	34	62-65	11
10	19-21	15-16	47-51	12	21-22	20-21	16	14	31-34	32-33	57-61	10
9	17-18	14	43-46	11	19-20	18-19	15	13	27-30	30-31	53-56	9
8	15-16	12-13	37-42	10	17-18	16-17	14	11-12	23-26	28-29	48-52	8
7	13-14	11	29-36	8-9	14-16	14-15	13	8-10	20-22	24-27	44-47	7
6	9-12	9-10	20-28	6-7	11-13	11-13	11-12	5-7	14-19	21-23	37-43	6
5	6-8	8	14-19	5	8-10	7-10	8-10	3-4	8-13	16-20	30-36	5
4	5	7	11-13	4	6-7	5-6	5-7	2	3-7	13-15	23-29	4
3	4	6	9-10	3	4-5	2-4	3-4	—	2	9-12	16-22	3
2	3	3-5	6-8	1-2	2-3	1	2	1	1	6-8	8-15	2
1	0-2	0-2	0-5	0	0-1	0	0-1	0	0	0-5	0-7	1

......Pattern B
—Pattern C

FIGURE 6.
Intellectual deficits associated with compliance difficulties.

ability. These individuals will have difficulty understanding and following medical directions because of an inability to understand novel and complex information and an inability to organize and order their lives to adhere to a treatment program.

Pattern B suggests superficially intact verbal abilities and the ability to express a narrow range of ideas in an articulate, but superficial, fashion. These skills mask deficits in broad areas of perceptual functioning and verbal comprehension. Clinicians tend to see these individuals as brighter than they actually are.

Pattern C shows adequate verbal skills but poor perceptual skills. These individuals are better able to understand the nature of their illness but have difficulty handling medications, diet, and self-care when they have to organize and integrate these activities into the ongoing pattern of their lives.

When a qualified psychologist is unavailable, approximate IQ scores may be obtained through the use of screening instruments such as the Shipley Institute of Living Scale and the Peabody Vocabulary Test. The major disadvantages of these instruments are the likelihood of obtaining inaccurate IQ scores from uncooperative individuals and the decreased precision and the oversimplification of data. People with suspected severe intellectual limitations should be more fully evaluated with the WAIS-R.

The Shipley Institute of Living Scale was constructed to detect mild degrees of intellectual impairment in people of normal intellectual functioning. Studies have revealed a high correlation between Shipley scores and WAIS Full Scale IQ scores in the middle range of intelligence. The test does not discriminate well within superior and retarded levels of functioning. However, it does detect individuals of below-average intellect. The test has a vocabulary section and a section that assesses abstract reasoning. Total testing time is about 20 minutes; the test can be administered and scored by a clerical person.

The Peabody Picture Vocabulary Test takes about 15 minutes to administer and score. It too can be administered by a trained clerk. Patients are shown pictures and are required to select from four choices the word that most accurately describes the picture presented. The IQ scores obtained correlate well with established measures of intellectual functioning. The test has been standardized on a population between 2 and 18 years of age, so generalization to adult populations must be made cautiously.

Cognitive Dysfunction

Individuals with average levels of intellect who have difficulties with attention/concentration or with organizing and regulating their lives may have difficulties following physicians' orders. These symptoms occur in a variety of pathological conditions, including affective disorders, schizophrenia, borderline conditions, and organic conditions. As the cognitive dysfunction becomes more severe, patients have greater difficulty retaining, processing, and acting on medical information.

Illness Behavior

Patients' styles of coping with disease may predispose them to maladaptive and self-destructive patterns in which medical advice is dealt with poorly. This may occur because of transference, character problems, excessive denial, or distortion in the experiencing of symptoms.

Patients with serious problems concerning authority figures and physicians may have difficulty identifying with and incorporating information from physicians. They have a negative affective and cognitive set toward authorities in general and react with skepticism toward certain types of medical advice, particularly if they do not see a concrete and immediate consequence of negligence or positive compliance. Selected MMPI patterns are helpful in identifying these individuals.

The MMPI, which takes about 1½ hours to complete, is an objective, extensively validated personality inventory that most patients are able to complete without undue stress. Figure 7 shows several maladaptive profiles.

Profile A is called a "4-9." These individuals may have deeply ingrained negative feelings about being helped, counseled, and guided by authorities. They have a limited frustration tolerance and a tendency to engage in abrupt action to reduce anxiety. Treatment programs requiring dietary restrictions, rigid adherence to schedules and appointments, and sustained effort are difficult for such persons when they interfere with anxiety-reducing behaviors.

Profile B, the "6-8" profile, suggests suspicious people who have difficulty in organizing and regulating their lives, often because of their chaotic and disorganized sense of self. Such individuals may distort the instructions of physicians and invest them with overelaborated and highly personalized meaning and may have problems in acting on information in a clear and consistent fashion.

Profile C, the "1-3" profile, is that of people who react to chronic disease with severe denial and repression of appropriate sadness, unhappiness, and depression. These individuals overreact to minimal frustrations and may circumvent and sabotage a carefully developed treatment program.

Psychological Factors Affecting Physical Condition

Patients with a sizable emotional component to their organic symptoms are often seen in psychiatric consultation. The questions that psychological testing can address are:

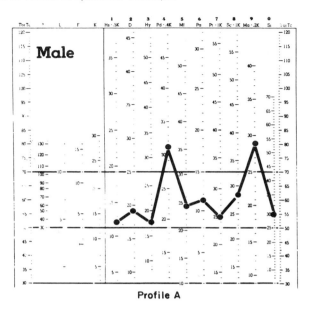

Profile A

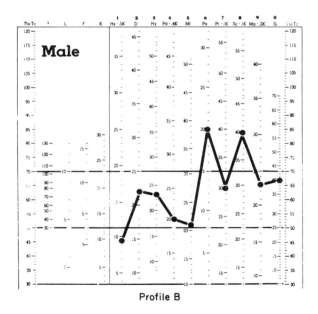

Profile B

FIGURE 7.
MMPI profiles of personality patterns with maladaptive illness behavior.

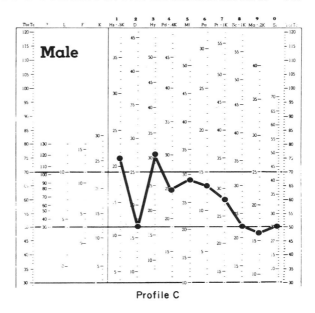

Profile C

1. Is there a pathological relationship between psychological functioning and physical functioning? If so, what are the degree and nature of that relationship?
2. If the patient is predisposed to somatization, at what level of psychological development does it occur?
3. If the patient has a chronic illness such as diabetes or renal failure, what is the extent and nature of the psychological regression accompanying the illness?

The test instruments useful in assessing these dimensions are the MMPI, the Rorschach, and the SCL-90 (see p. 349).

Figure 8 shows a group of profiles associated with people who partially substitute bodily preoccupation and concern for psychological processes. Three MMPI profiles representing somatization at three levels of psychosexual development are shown. Profile A, with elevations on scales 1 and 3, and other scales at an average level, shows a conversion disorder occurring at a psychoneurotic level. In Figure B, additional elevations on scales 4 and 6 reflect significant character pathology. This is typical of a conversion disorder occurring in a severe passive-aggressive personality disorder. Profile C, with elevated 6, 7, and 8 scales, reflects the use of a conversion mechanism as a last-ditch defense against a decompensating personality and incipient psychosis.

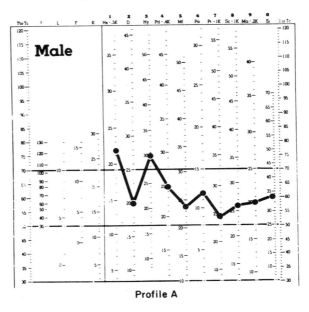

Profile A

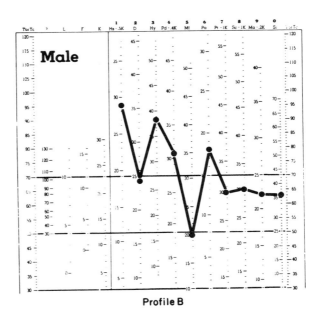

Profile B

FIGURE 8.

MMPI profiles of somatization disorders at their levels of psychosexual functioning.

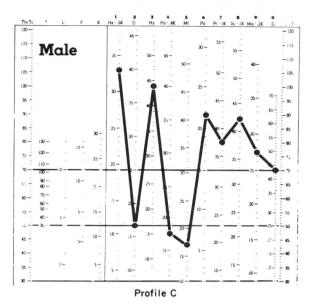

Profile C

Psychiatrists dealing with the chronically ill are often asked the degree and complexity of rehabilitation effort that patients can tolerate. In order to answer this question, it is critical to understand the amount of regression accompanying chronic illness and the debilitating effect of that regression. Figure 9 shows MMPI profiles of individuals adjusting differently to renal failure. Profile A shows appropriate bodily concern and depression. Profile B reflects broad ego deterioration encompassing the ability to organize and direct one's life. Patient B will probably have difficulty with sustained rehabilitation efforts and is subject to the debilitating effects of severe emotional dysfunction.

Patients who cooperate marginally because of compromised ego functioning are often unwilling to complete an MMPI and circumvent it by complaining of fatigue or pain. We have much better success with completing a valid Rorschach examination (about 45 minutes for test administration) in those cases because a skilled examiner can support the patient's efforts. Although determining the reaction to chronic illness from the Rorschach depends more on the individual examiner's skill than on highly validated and standardized research, Rorschach testing can add significantly to the psychologists' armamentarium. Helpful Rorschach interpretation involves a close integration of Rorschach psychology, psychodynamic theory, and ego psychology and an understanding of behavioral reactions to illness. Cogni-

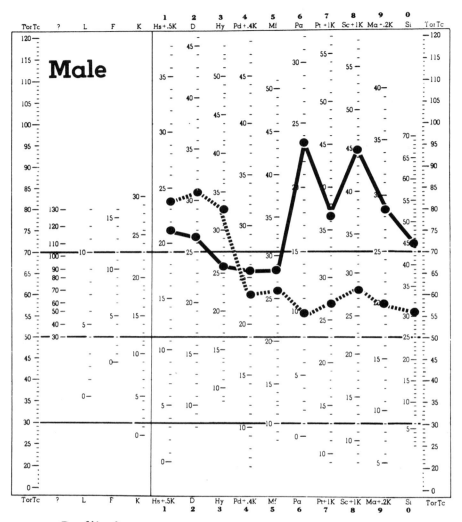

.... **Profile A**
——— **Profile B**

FIGURE 9.
Adaptive and pathological responses to renal failure.

tive decompensation can be partially evaluated by determining the percentage of accurately perceived forms reported by patients. For example, the perception of a butterfly in the circled section of Figure 10 is scored F+, indicating that individuals with intact reality testing perceive that particular area as a butterfly. The perception of a buffalo in that area is scored F−, indicating that well-functioning individuals do not report this area as a butterfly. Each response is scored F+ or F−. Individuals with intact and reality-based cognition tend to score F+ percent between 70 percent and 90 percent; individuals with impaired cognitive contact secondary to repression tend to score F+ below 65.

The Symptom Check List-90 (SCL-90) is a relatively new alternative to MMPI evaluation of behavioral reaction to disease. It is a 90-item, self-report inventory requiring about 25 minutes for completion and scoring. It therefore has the advantage of being much briefer than the 1½- or 2-hour MMPI evaluation. The SCL-90 generates scores along nine primary symptom dimensions and produces three global indexes of distress in areas significant to understanding the psychological reaction to illness. Sound reliability data, extensive norms, and comprehensive validity studies have been reported. The SCL-90 can measure behavioral reactions to psychopharmacological interventions and can also serve as a screening device for detecting individuals with severe behavioral reactions in conjunction with organic

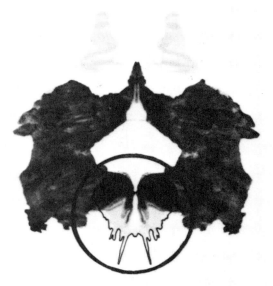

FIGURE 10.
Accurate and impaired perceptual functioning on the Rorschach.

disease. It promises to be an important addition to the testing techniques available to psychologists. It is not as powerful a test as the MMPI because it is easier for patients to consciously misrepresent themselves.

Neuropsychological Evaluation

Neuropsychological testing has undergone many advances in the past 20 years and is based on extensive, highly sophisticated research studies. It may be used to answer the following questions:

Is there evidence of an organic brain syndrome interfering with behavioral adaptation?

The WAIS-R is the cornerstone for determining the answer to this question. Divided into 11 subtests and producing 14 quantified measures of functioning (three IQ scores plus a score on each of the 11 tests), it permits qualitative and quantitative analysis of higher-level forms of thinking. Because norms exist for ages 16 through 75, the effects of higher cortical dysfunction can be separated from the effects of normal biological decline. The quality and effectiveness of various language and perceptual modes of functioning are evaluated.

Briefer tests of neuropsychological functioning measuring more limited areas also evaluate cortical dysfunction. However, to be used accurately, these tests must *always* be integrated with the WAIS for accurate interpretation because of the positive correlation between performance on these tests and the WAIS Full Scale IQ.

The Bender Gestalt and the Cantor Interference Bender (5 to 10 minutes to administer) are powerful discriminating instruments. They evaluate complex visual-spatial drawing and are sensitive to cortically induced deficits in this area. The Cantor procedure compares Bender drawings made on blank sheets of paper with drawings made on paper with distorting background lines. Patients with cortical dysfunction show greater disruptions on lined paper than do patients with functional disorders.

The Trailmaking Test (5 minutes to administer) evaluates the ability to rapidly shift from one conceptual system (letters and numbers) to another in a serial fashion. The patient must draw lines connecting numbers and letters, and is timed on the ability to do this. The test is highly sensitive to both functional and organic impairments.

Are specific deficits important in terms of patient management?

The Halstead-Reitan Battery is an extensively validated set of measures for evaluating the impact of impaired brain functioning on a broad range of human abilities. The adult battery includes 14 separate tests, producing 26 variables, plus an aphasia and a constructional praxis test of 31 items. The battery is used in conjunction with the appropriate Wechsler Intelligence Scale and typically requires 4 to 5 hours to administer. More impaired persons require much more time to complete the battery.

A broad range of neuropsychological functioning is measured, including sensory, perceptual, and motor tasks, psychomotor problem solving, and higher-level psychological functioning relating to symbolic and communicational aspects of language, the ability to deal effectively with visual-spatial relations in manipulatory problems, and abstraction and concept-formation abilities. The test data are evaluated by comparing performance on the right and left sides of the body, evaluating pathognomonic signs (such as construction apraxias and aphasias), interpreting scatter between various tests, and evaluating the level of performance in conjunction with the patient's occupational and cultural levels. Rehabilitation programs are being developed to remedy deficits in these specific areas. This is one of the most powerful and discriminating batteries of tests available for obtaining an understanding of human brain functioning as it affects behavior.

The Luria-Nebraska Battery is a 266-item exam that takes 3 to 4 hours to administer and offers a number of appealing features to the clinician. It too permits a comprehensive assessment of brain functioning, generating scores in 13 separate areas of neuropsychological functioning. The technique offers much promise for rehabilitation. The research underpinning for the Luria-Nebraska is considerable; however, it does not enjoy the time-tested and broad acceptance of the Halstead-Reitan Battery.

Suggested Readings

Exner, J. (1974). *The Rorschach: A Comprehensive System*, vol. 1. New York: Wiley.

Filskore, S., and Ball, T. (eds.) (1981). *Handbook of Clinical Neuropsychology.* New York: Wiley.

Golden, C. (1982). *Diagnosis and Rehabilitation in Clinical Neuropsychology.* Springfield, Ill.: Charles C. Thomas.

Graham, J. (1977). *The M.M.P.I.: A Practical Guide.* New York: Oxford University Press.

Lovitt, R. (1982). Psychological Testing and Consultation–Liaison Psychiatry. *General Hospital Psychiatry* 4:233–240.

—— (1984). Rorschach interpretation in a multi-disciplinary hospital setting. *Professional Psychology Research and Practice* 15:244–250.

Maloney, M., and Ward, M. (1976). *Psychological Assessment: A Conceptual Approach.* New York: Oxford University Press.

CHAPTER 35

Hypnosis on the Medical Wards

HAROLD B. CRASILNECK, Ph.D.

In the past 30 years, hypnosis has become part of the armamentarium of many general-hospital psychiatrists. Hypnosis has many uses in the hospital environment. It can spark the motivation and speed the progress of hitherto negativistic, hostile, and uncooperative patients. The pain and discomfort of many medical procedures may be entirely eliminated with hypnoanesthesia. Patients' fear of and negative attitudes toward their illness, their physicians, and their discomfort are often replaced by a positive disposition toward the entire treatment course and all people involved.

Hypnosis can divert patients' minds from maladaptive or self-destructive fantasies and encourage them toward more productive thoughts and actions. When chronically ill patients have lost the will to live, hypnotic suggestions may inspire them to keep up the struggle. This shift in attitude may be the difference between life and death. Thus hypnosis may act as a catalytic agent for motivating patients to cope, adjust, and realistically accept illness and treatment.

Hypnosis has been helpful in the treatment of hyperemesis gravidarum, insomnia, anorexia nervosa accompanied by bulimia, exogenous obesity, tobacco habituation with chronic cough, chronic and acute asthma, musculoskeletal pain, addiction to medication, poststroke rehabilitation, headaches, trigeminal neuralgia, herpes zoster, and cancer pain. Hypnosis may be requested by terminally ill patients to reduce pain and dependence on

I wish to thank Ms. Sherry Knopf for her assistance in the preparation and editing of this article.

sensorium-clouding analgesics, enabling them to live with dignity until the moment of death.

The Process of Hypnosis

The process of hypnosis requires the establishment of rapport, induction, and determination of level of trance.

Establishing Rapport

In establishing rapport, one should remember that patients are usually apprehensive about hypnosis. It is judicious to explain what it feels like to be hypnotized, what is to be accomplished, the advantages of hypnosis, and the fact that patients do not lose control over themselves; patients completely govern the depth of trance.

Hypnosis is best explained as a tranquilizing experience in which there is an altered state of consciousness that allows patients to use unconscious processes that were formerly unavailable to their conscious minds. Patients need to be told that in the early stages of trance they will be aware of physical and psychological perceptions. It is only in deep trance that an amnestic state occurs, that is a sleeplike state that is usually associated with levels of tranquility.

Induction

The method of hypnotic induction is determined by patients' personalities. If, for example, the patient has an authoritarian personality, a hand-levitation method is preferable because that approach allows the patient to control the induction and maintain the level of trance achieved. When inducing hypnosis in a passive patient with a strong parental attachment, an eye fixation induction with an assertive approach is usually successful. Other methods of induction include theater, television, coin, nonverbal, and Chiasson's relaxation techniques.

Level of Trance

Some patients are not capable of entering hypnosis deeply during the initial induction. Since deep hypnosis is not necessary to treat most ailments in a hospital setting, patients should not be concerned about depth of trance. Many of the goals are accomplished in the medium-trance levels. However, deeper levels are required for treating severe pain problems. If patients are incapable of entering deep levels of trance, hypnotherapists may continue suggestions of pain relief in a lighter level and hope that in subsequent inductions patients will feel more secure and will reach deeper levels of trance. If this does not occur, hypnotherapy should be discontinued.

There are four major levels of trance: hypnoidal, light, medium, and somnambulism. Each of these levels has substages, and as the hypnotherapy proceeds, the therapist may check to determine which level is in effect.

The hypnoidal state is indicated by fluttering of eyelids, physical relaxation, closing of eyes, and slowness of movement. A stage of light trance is indicated by the patient's inability to open his eyes, by deep slow respiration, and by progressive deepening of lethargy. The level of medium trance has been reached when induction of glove anesthesia is possible, when there is development of partial amnesia, and when hallucinations can be induced. The somnambulistic stage is indicated by the patient's ability to open eyes without affecting the trance, pallor of the lips, by the ability to induce extensive anesthesia, extensive amnesia, and posthypnotic anesthesia and analgesia. The ability to undergo age regression is also part of this stage, as are the acceptance of positive and negative posthypnotic suggestions.

Precautions

Hypnosis is undertaken with certain definite precautions. In establishing rapport with the patient, the hypnotherapist should explain that hypnosis is not magic, that the patient must cooperate or hypnosis will not be successful. In giving hypnotic suggestions, organic pain is not removed completely, either by heterohypnosis or by self-hypnosis, except during obstetrical anesthesia, during surgery, in treating a terminal disease, and in extreme chronic pain, such as the pain of chronic herpes zoster.

Individuals with strong sadomasochistic tendencies, severe depression, conversion reaction, or paranoid ideation should be hypnotized with considerable caution. Psychological symptoms should not be ruptured or completely removed; they may be substituted or reduced. Patients treated by hypnosis can be helped to gain intellectual and emotional insight into their problems, and secondary gain is always investigated and dealt with. Almost all patients can be taught self-hypnosis from the first session. With self-hypnosis, the patient repeats the suggestions (heretofore given by the hypnotherapist) in the first person. The patient repeats silently: "I am relaxed and at ease, free from most of my discomfort, free from most of my pain." Traditionally, the response is the same as perceived in heterohypnosis. Patients are cautioned not to use self-hypnosis with unrealistic suggestions that may endanger health, such as eliminating fatigue after strenuous exercise.

Hypnosis in Differential Diagnosis

Occasionally, patients admitted to a medical or surgical service present physicians with the problem of distinguishing between organic and functional complaints. At times, hypnosis can be used to help differentiate functional from organic problems, as illustrated here.

Mr. U., a 30-year-old single attorney injured in an automobile accident, was admitted to the hospital in a semiconscious condition with abrasions and contusions of the head and face. He complained of "no feeling in my feet and legs." During the first 24 hours of hospitalization, no demonstrable organic pathology was found. In spite of that, the patient was unable to move his toes, feet, or legs and could neither stand nor walk. He kept referring to his condition as "my paralysis." When hypnosis was suggested as an additional diagnostic procedure, the patient agreed.

After establishing rapport, induction was initiated, and the patient entered a very deep state of trance. The hypnotherapist then established anesthesia of the patient's right hand by using the following suggestions: "Your hand feels as though you are wearing a thick electrician's glove . . . absolutely no feeling. Now, open your eyes. I touch your fingers with this file [a blunt nail file]; now, the inside of your hand. The back of your hand up to and including the wrist of this hand will also lose feeling. There is no perception of pain. The hand feels like you are wearing a thick electrician's glove. No feeling. No pain. Now watch as I jab your middle finger fast and hard. Pressure. No pain. Pressure. No pain."

"Now normal sensation returns to your hand." The therapist touched the identical areas of the patient's hand with the file, stating: "You have removed the glove. Glove anesthesia is gone. All normal sensations return. As you feel me jab the middle finger, pull your hand away. Good. Now close your eyes."

Verbal reinforcement of body control was repeated. "If you can control the awareness of pain with your unconscious mind in one part of your body, then you can control feeling and movement in other parts of your body."

At that point, the therapist deepened the level of trance and induced olfactory and auditory hallucinations. Then he said, "Normal sensations are returning to your feet and legs. Because of the strength of your unconscious mind, you are in control of all sensations in your feet and legs. You are now experiencing warmth and the return of function. Nod your head as you become aware of this immediate change arousing warmth in your feet and legs. Good." These suggestions were repeated several times.

The therapist asked the patient to move the toes of his left foot. When that was accomplished, he was asked to move the toes of his right foot. Calmly and diligently, each progressive suggestion was introduced into the awareness of the patient's lower extremities, and the association of the hypnotic verbalization was manifested as the patient confirmed the connection between the suggestion and the stimuli by moving his feet and legs. During the trance state, the patient was brought to his feet. He took a few steps holding the therapist's hands and then was returned to bed. A suggestion for amnesia was given the patient before awakening him. Over the next week, the patient was treated with hypnotherapy, and his conversion symptoms were gradually reduced. Shortly thereafter, the patient was discharged from the hospital. He returned weekly for combined individual psychotherapy and hypnotherapy as an outpatient for the next six months.

His conversion reaction stemmed from his anger with his parents over forcing him to support his sociopathic younger brother. During the first weeks of treatment, the patient repeated, "I cannot support myself and take care of my brother, too. I can't stand the fact that my parents are forcing me to do this."

As the patient's symptoms resolved and he gained intellectual and emotional insight into his affliction, his changed attitude was indicated by his statement that "if I can stand on my own two feet, my brother will have to learn to do the same." The patient recovered completely.

Pain Problems

Acute or chronic pain problems of all age groups may be treated with hypnosis. Many pain problems can be controlled with hypnosis alone, but if necessary, hypnosis can be combined with biofeedback, acupuncture, and/or medication (for further discussion of treatment of pain problems, see Chapter 24). Since deep levels of trance are necessary to achieve complete control over pain, the patient must be highly motivated in order for hypnosis to be successful. The following patient had the needed high level of motivation.

Mr. W., a 42-year-old happily married man with one child, held a responsible position as an economist. He had suffered from migraine headaches for 20 years and had consulted many physicians but had little positive result from medication.

The headaches occurred daily and had become so severe that the patient had to be hospitalized. He was habituated to codeine, suffered from insomnia, vomited frequently, and had become extremely depressed. The patient was referred for hypnotherapy after a thorough neurological examination proved negative.

While establishing rapport, the therapist explained the benefits of hypnotherapy. The patient agreed eagerly to accept this approach and soon entered a deep level of trance. Glove anesthesia was established. The therapist suggested that the patient touch the back of his hypno-anesthetized hand to his forehead and that he would be free of headaches most of the time, awake or asleep. Whenever he felt a headache starting, he would abort it immediately by inducing self-hypnosis, creating the hypnoanesthetic condition in his hand and touching his head with his hand. Even if a headache occurred during sleep, his unconscious mind would undergo the process of hypnotically controlling the pain.

The patient was told, "Because of the omnipotence of your mind over your body, you will control most of the pain of your migraine headaches." When asked to estimate the relief of pain, the patient stated, "Eighty-five percent of the pain is under control."

The patient was seen daily for the next two weeks, during which time his physician withdrew him from codeine. The patient's fears concerning the impact of his headaches on his life situation were discussed. Secondary gains were investigated, and the patient was allowed to abreact and deal with the emotional meaning of his discomfort. The acute pain was substantially reduced, and he was anxious to be discharged from the hospital so he could put what he had learned to the test outside the hospital.

The patient later reported a weekly slight headache that was controlled by self-hypnosis. He continued to respond well during weekly sessions for the next six months. The hypnotherapist made a tape recording for the patient to use as an aid to induce the self-hypnotic trance. He was discharged from treatment shortly thereafter.

Hypnosis is also used with cancer patients to help control pain, nausea, and vomiting during various stages of chemotherapy and in the terminal stages of life.

Many terminally ill patients, especially physicians, request hypnotherapy. In most cases, there is no drug addiction, pain is minimal, thinking becomes normal, and death comes with grace and dignity.

Many children and adults must endure painful and unpleasant therapeutic procedures during chronic illness. Hypnosis, used prior to these procedures, can make them easier to endure. After the hypnotherapist establishes rapport and glove anesthesia, the patient is told to place the anesthetized hand on the area to be hypnotically anesthetized and the anesthesia is transferred to that area. This technique has been used to prepare patients for bone marrow aspirations and other painful procedures. Suggestions include a complete obliteration of pain and no discomfort whatsoever, thereby minimizing anxiety and producing a cooperative patient in an otherwise intolerable situation.

Sometimes, as in the following case, pain is part of a larger maladaptive syndrome.

Ms. X., who weighed approximately 450 pounds, was hospitalized on a general medical service for several medical problems. She had severe back pain and frequent excruciating headaches, and she ate compulsively. She was placed on a diet of 300 calories per day. One week later she was discovered bribing certain staff members to buy candy bars and sandwiches for her. She stated, "I simply will die if I am not allowed more food." She was, however, willing to try hypnotherapy.

The therapist and the patient entered an alliance of harmony and close agreement. The patient entered a very deep level of trance on the first session. During the next 12 weeks, hypnotherapy was used and the patient kept to her limited diet and freely discussed her conflicts. She lost an average of 9 pounds per week while hospitalized and weighed 340 pounds on discharge. Her backaches and headaches abated drastically. Hypnotic treatment continued on a weekly basis, and she never missed a session. Six months later she weighed 230 pounds. When her weight had gotten down to 180 pounds, her sessions were reduced to twice a month until she reached her final goal of 140 pounds.

During the entire hypnotherapeutic series, she saw her internist frequently for follow-up studies. The patient was discharged with the knowledge that she could return whenever necessary.

Hypnosis is useful in pulmonary medicine for smoking habituation, asthma, and severe cough. Asthmatics can achieve partial relief with hypnotherapy, especially from that portion of their symptoms due to overbreathing.

For the asthmatic who is hyperventilating, hypnotic suggestions are best offered along with the rhythm of the patient's breathing. If breathing is very rapid, the induction method is very rapid, and as the breathing slows, the suggestions are made with a decrease in verbal tempo. The rate of speech should be slowed to metronome timing, and the patient's breathing soon slows to normal. Self-hypnosis can be taught to the asthmatic patient. The following case illustrates the use of hypnosis with a habituated smoker.

Dr. Y., a physician who had had coronary bypass surgery three days earlier, demanded that his wife buy cigarettes. He was seen by the therapist on the next day, and hypnosis was suggested. The patient was uncertain about hypnosis but stated that he would do the best he could. He was seen daily, given the suggestion to not continue a life-destroying habit, and told to substitute cinnamon sticks, chewing gum, and low-calorie drinks when he had the desire to smoke. By the end of the first week, he felt secure that he would never smoke again. Thirty days later his chronic cough was almost gone, and he was pleased at having conquered a life-threatening habit.

Hypnosis can be used as an emergency therapeutic procedure. For example, patients with hyperemesis gravidarum are frequently referred for hypnotherapy. After establishing rapport, induction, and glove anesthesia, and then allowing the patient to see the control she has over the pain of pin pricks while in the trance state, the hypnotherapist requests that the patient close her eyes, deepens the trance, and says, "You witnessed the control you had over your body. And you will be relaxed and at ease. The nausea and discomfort will grow less. You are going to be much more calm and relaxed.

The nausea and vomiting will come under control. As you are aware that the nausea has come under control, move the index finger of your right hand. Good." The patient is taught self-hypnosis and given a tape recording when appropriate. Seventy-five percent of such individuals' hyperemesis can be brought under control through the use of hypnotherapy.

Hypnotherapy was recently used with a patient who had developed hiccoughs while hospitalized with coronary heart disease. He had been hiccoughing for three days and had not responded to other therapeutic procedures. Following induction and customary deepening procedures and tests for depth of trance, the patient was given the suggestion that his breathing would be normal, that he would be able to control his body functions with his unconscious mind, and that the hiccoughing would discontinue.

After obtaining positive results during three consecutive 40-minute sessions, a tape was made for the patient to use on his own.

Dissociative Episodes

Hypnosis is used with dramatic results in dealing with the amnestic patient brought to the emergency room. In addition to gaining information concerning the causative trauma or conflict through age regression, the patient is allowed to resume the amnestic state and the precipitating trauma or conflict is treated hypnotherapeutically while the patient's memory is gradually recovered.

> Ms. Z., age 24, was seen in an emergency room following a rape. She did not know her name, the city she lived in, or what had happened.
>
> She was age-regressed under hypnosis to the beginning of the rape. She abreacted violently as she experienced the memory of the attack in minute detail. She was made amnestic prior to terminating the trance. She remained in the hospital for three weeks while being treated with combined hypnotherapy and psychotherapy.

A Final Word

Although hypnosis can provide much benefit to inducible patients, many patients do not respond to hypnosis. Some individuals will respond positively at the beginning of treatment and then reject further hypnosis. There are some who cannot enter the depth of trance necessary for certain goals, such as pain relief, to be accomplished.

In summary, hypnosis is a useful tool for helping many hospitalized patients with organic and functional medical problems. It is applicable to all age levels. Its dangers are reduced if therapists not only treat the symptoms but also help patients deal with the psychological problem causing or aggravating their symptoms.

Suggested Readings

Cangello, V.W. (1961). The use of hypnotic suggestion for pain relief of malignant disease. *International Journal of Clinical and Experimental Hypnosis* 9:17–22.

Chiasson, S.W. (1973). *A Syllabus on Hypnosis*. Des Plaines, Ill. American Society of Clinical Hypnosis Education and Research Foundation.

Collison, D.R. (1975). Which asthmatic patients should be treated by hypnotherapy? *Medical Journal of Australia* 1:776–781.

Crasilneck, H.B. (1980). Clinical assessment and preparation of the patient. In *Handbook of Hypnosis and Psychosomatic Medicine*, ed. G.D. Burrows and L. Dennerstein, pp. 106–118. New York: Elsevier/North Holland Biomedical Press.

Crasilneck, H.B., and Hall, J. (1975). *Clinical Hypnosis: Principles and Applications*. New York: Grune & Stratton.

Crasilneck, H.B., McCranie, E.J., and Jenkins, M.T. (1958). Special indications for hypnosis as a method of anesthesia. *Journal of the American Medical Association* 162:1606–1608.

Hilgard, E.R., and Hilgard, J.R. (1975). *Hypnosis in the Relief of Pain*. Los Angeles: William Kaufman.

Horne, D., and Powlett, V. (1980). Hypnotizability and rating scales. In *Handbook of Hypnosis and Psychosomatic Medicine*, ed. G.D. Burrows and L. Dennerstein, pp. 119–129. New York: Elsevier/North Holland Biomedical Press.

Spiegel, H., and Spiegel, D. (1978). *Trance and Treatment*. New York: Basic Books.

Wolberg, L.K. (1948). *Medical Hypnosis*, vol. I. New York: Grune & Stratton.

CHAPTER 36

Behavioral Treatment
Techniques in Medical Settings

ROBERT J. GATCHEL, Ph.D.

In recent years, a number of effective cognitive/behavioral treatment techniques have been developed to deal with a variety of psychological/behavioral problems. Many of these techniques help with problem behaviors seen in medical settings. Before describing these techniques, the general learning principles on which they are based will be briefly reviewed.

Basic Principles of Behavioral Techniques

Classical Conditioning

Ivan Pavlov (1849–1936) first described the process of classical conditioning in his work on the conditioned reflex. Reflexes are specific, automatic, unlearned reactions elicited by a specific stimulus. If, for example, a piece of dust suddenly enters the eye, the lids automatically blink and the lacrimal glands secrete tears. Such unconditioned reflexes are automatic and have survival value. Pavlov demonstrated that such unconditioned reflexes could be conditioned or learned. Pavlov found that when a neutral stimulus or event such as ringing a bell is presented repeatedly to a dog just prior to presenting food (which normally elicits an unconditioned reflex of salivation), eventually, ringing the bell (now a conditioned stimulus) elicits a conditioned or learned salivation response when presented in the absence of food. This is the process of classical conditioning. It is based on a learned association or connection between two stimuli, such as the bell's ring and food, that have occurred at approximately the same time. An association is learned between a weak stimulus (such as the bell ringing) and a strong stimulus (such as the sight of food), so that the weak stimulus comes to elicit the same response of salivation originally elicited only by the stronger one. Pavlov called this tendency to respond to the neutral conditioned stimulus (CS) as though it were the unconditioned stimulus (UCS) stimulus substitution. Conditioned reflexes are automatic responses to an eliciting stimulus or event. Such behavior is termed *respondent* because it responds to some event in the environment. Classical conditioning is often called respondent conditioning. When the organism responds voluntarily and operates on the environment to produce some effect, the term *operant behavior* is used.

Many behavioral treatment techniques are based on classical conditioning principles. One of the most widely used—systematic desensitization and its variants—will be discussed later in this chapter.

Operant Conditioning

Unlike classical conditioning, operant or instrumental conditioning develops new behaviors that bring about positive consequences or remove negative events. In classical conditioning, a new stimulus (such as a ringing bell) is conditioned to elicit the same response that had previously been elicited by the unconditioned stimulus, whereas in operant conditioning, a new response is learned. Behavior that produces food, social approval, or other positive consequences or that reduces damaging or aversive events is operant behavior.

The toilet training of young children involves basic principles of operant conditioning. The key stimulus in operant conditioning is reinforcement. Reinforcement is any consequence that increases the likelihood that a particular behavior will be repeated or that strengthens that behavior. Extinction involves the gradual decrease in the strength of, or tendency to perform, a response because of the elimination of reinforcement.

Numerous behavioral treatment programs employ operant conditioning procedures. A number of these—biofeedback, contingency management, and stimulus control procedures—will be discussed here.

Observational Learning

Many complex forms of behavior are learned without the apparent direct external reinforcement vital to classical and operant conditioning procedures. Indeed, recent research indicates that much learning comes through simple observation without any tangible direct reinforcement. Such observational learning is also called imitation learning, cognitive learning, vicarious learning, or modeling.

Examples abound of behavior acquired by observational learning. Aggressive responses, learning to fear particular objects or situations, as well as other complex adaptive and maladaptive behaviors, can be developed through modeling. Also, observational learning may be used to increase desired behaviors or to lessen undesired behaviors by presenting a model that performs appropriate responses. Thus learning can occur in people without their ever having made a particular response themselves, and without their ever having received any type of tangible external reinforcement for the behavior. The capacity of individuals to perform such novel behavior underscores the importance of the internalizing and cognitive abilities that allow people to transform observations into a number of new patterns of behavior. This highlights the importance of such cognitive factors and explains why such variables are considered in currently developing learning approaches.

Behavioral Therapy Approaches Based on Classical Conditioning

Systematic Desensitization

Systematic desensitization is a technique developed to alleviate anxiety or specific fears. It is based on the principle of counterconditioning, in which, through learning, relaxation (an adaptive behavior) is substituted for anxiety or fear (the deviant or maladaptive behavior) in response to a particular object or situation. The procedure typically involves pairing deep muscle relaxation, taught using a progressive muscle relaxation technique developed by Jacobson in 1938, with imagined scenes depicting situations or objects associated with anxiety or fear. Patients are often asked to imagine fear-provoking objects or situations because of the abstract nature of many fears (e.g., fear of rejection by a loved one) and therefore cannot easily be presented in vivo. However, when objects, such as hypodermic needles, or places, such as hospitals, can be presented, in vivo desensitization is often employed.

A graded hierarchy of scenes is constructed in this treatment procedure. The hierarchy consists of items ranging from low-anxiety provocation to high-anxiety provocation. The individual gradually "works up" this hierarchy, learning to tolerate more and more anxiety-producing scenes as he or she relaxes. The relaxation response inhibits anxiety or fear in response to the imagined scenes. The ability to tolerate fear-provoking images of objects or situations decreases anxiety in related real-life situations. This therapeutic procedure has been effective with many anxiety-related disorders, such as injection phobias and hemodialysis phobias, insomnia, and stress-related disorders.

Progressive Muscle Relaxation

Progressive muscle relaxation, an important component of systematic desensitization, is a powerful therapeutic technique in its own right. Clinicians often use it to treat generalized anxiety, insomnia, headaches, neck tension, and mild forms of agitated depression. Its use is based on the premise that muscle tension is closely related to anxiety and that an individual will experience significantly less anxiety if tense muscles can be relaxed. Other techniques, such as biofeedback, transcendental meditation, yoga, and Schultz and Luthe's autogenic training, are also commonly used to reduce physiological activation, which is also assumed to be closely tied to anxiety.

Flooding Techniques

In contrast to systematic desensitization, in which anxiety arousal is diminished, flooding is rapid exposure to fear-provoking stimuli with no attempt to minimize arousal. It is based on the classical and operant conditioning principle that repeated exposure to a fear stimulus without any traumatic consequences will lead to fear extinction.

Flooding techniques effectively treat focused fears and may be more effective than systematic desensitization in treating phobias. However, the danger of untoward reactions during treatment because of the direct exposure to the feared stimulus demands that only therapists experienced in using flooding administer the technique.

Behavioral Therapy Approaches Based on Observational Learning

Modeling

Fear can be reduced by having fearful individuals repeatedly observe persons effectively engaging in the feared activities. Repeated observation that feared performance does not lead to unfavorable or negative consequences leads to extinction or elimination of anxiety responses and fear-arousing thoughts. This principle and modeling procedure is often called vicarious extinction. It should be noted that even when using models, it is usually beneficial to employ a graduated hierarchy: Models perform a sequence of activities beginning with those that are least feared and progress to those that are most feared.

An example of a modeling procedure effectively employed to reduce hospital- and surgery-related anxieties in children is the use of a movie shown to children about to undergo herniorrhaphy, tonsillectomy, and genitourinary surgery. One movie depicts a 7-year-old child hospitalized for a herniorrhaphy. The film shows events that most children encounter when hospitalized for elective surgery. It includes the child's orientation to the hospital, the surgeon, and the anesthesiologist; having a blood test; exposure to standard hospital equipment; separation from the mother; and scenes in the operating and recovery rooms. In addition to receiving explanations of the hospital procedures provided by the medical staff, the child describes the feelings and concerns that he has at each stage of the hospital experience. The child's behavior and verbal remarks exemplify adequate coping. Although he exhibits some anxiety and apprehension, he is able to overcome his initial fears and complete each event in a successful and non-anxious manner. (Film models who are anxious initially and overcome their anxiety reduce the viewers' anxiety more than models who exhibit no fear.)

This peer-modeling film has an effect on reducing anxiety in children above and beyond that produced by standard hospital preoperative procedures. Such peer modeling is probably especially important for young children because it is often easier for a child to understand another child's behavior than it is for the child to understand an adult explanation.

Behavioral Rehearsal

Acting out or role playing interpersonal problems and one's usual manner of behaving is a method used in many different forms of psychotherapy. In behavior therapy, role playing or behavioral rehearsal methods that simulate real-life situations have been developed and formalized to train individuals to perform new behaviors. Therapists often model or coach the behavior that patients lack. Patients lacking self-care skills, for instance, would be taught appropriate skills through behavioral rehearsal.

Related to these procedures are *assertion training* techniques, which are used with individuals who experience intense anxiety because of problems in asserting themselves. Assertion training may be valuable adjunctive treatment in dealing with physical disorders aggravated by emotional tension. Often, because of a lack of adequate interpersonal social skills, individuals cannot cope effectively with stressors that cause and/or exacerbate physical symptoms. For example, an overly demanding boss or spouse may be causing a great deal of inner tension in a patient. By providing means to deal more effectively with those demands through assertion training, one can help the patient to reduce environmental stress.

Behavioral Therapy Approaches Based on Operant Conditioning

Contingency Management

Contingency management is the process of changing the frequency of a behavior by controlling the consequences of that behavior. We all use contingency management procedures in everyday life, for example, in rewarding or punishing a child for some behavior or in giving a bonus to an employee for an outstanding work performance. These are attempts to encourage or discourage particular behaviors by associating a desirable or undesirable consequence with them. Behavior therapists have developed systematic contingency management programs to increase compliance with medical regimens and to treat chronic pain.

An example of such a program is Fordyce and Steger's chronic pain treatment procedure at the University of Washington. It involves a 4- to 8-week inpatient period designed to gradually increase the general activity level and socialization of the patient and to decrease medication usage. The program is based on the assumption that although pain may initially stem from organic pathology, environmental consequences (such as attention of the patient's family and the rehabilitation staff) can modify and further maintain various aspects of "pain behavior" such as complaining, grimacing, slow and cautious body movement, and requesting pain medication. In viewing pain as an operant behavior, it is assumed that the potentially reinforcing consequences, such as the concern and attention from others, rest, medication, avoiding unpleasant responsibilities and duties and other events, frequently follow and reinforce the maladaptive pain behavior and, as a consequence, hinder the patient's progress. In this treatment program, the major goal is to increase adaptive behavior, such as participation in therapy and activity, through reinforcement (staff attention, rest, etc.), while concurrently decreasing or eliminating pain behavior by withholding reinforcement. Such a program has been shown to produce decreases in patients' complaints of pain and their use of analgesic medication.

Stimulus Control

The concept of a discriminative stimulus or cue is important in operant conditioning. During cold weather, asthmatics often cover their noses and mouths. They are aware of the importance of performing such a behavior to avoid stimulating bronchospasm or, even worse, a full-fledged asthmatic attack. The cold air is a discriminative cue or stimulus for the behavior of covering nose and mouth. As another example, dizziness is a discriminative stimulus to reduce the dose of antihypertensive medication. Thus it tells when and where it is appropriate to emit a certain behavior in order to receive reinforcement or, in this case, to avoid the aversive consequence of postural hypertension. Strictly defined, a discriminative stimulus is an environmental cue that informs us when it is likely that a response or behavior will be reinforced. Discriminative stimuli provide an occasion for the potential occurrence of an operant response. Behavior prompted by a discriminative cue or stimulus is said to be under stimulus control. Many problem behaviors are under stimulus control and occur more frequently in some situations than in others. As a consequence, treatment programs have been developed that take into account this principle of stimulus control.

Stimulus control has been employed in an obesity treatment program of gradually restricting and eliminating stimuli that elicit eating behavior. The program involves restricting eating to specific times and places, not eating while engaged in other enjoyable activities such as watching television or listening to the radio, ridding the house of fattening foods, and avoiding passing a restaurant or going grocery shopping when hungry. Thus "stimulus control" is achieved by restricting eating to specific times and places and eliminating eating cues from the environment.

Stimulus control procedures are effective with a variety of other problem behaviors, such as insomnia.

Biofeedback

Before Harry Houdini performed one of his famous escapes, a skeptical committee would search his clothes and body. When the members of the committee were satisfied that Houdini was concealing no keys, they would chain, padlock, and handcuff him. Houdini, of course, could not open a padlock without a key. When he was safely behind the curtain, he would cough one up. He could hold a key suspended in his throat and regurgitate it later, when unobserved. Houdini had learned to control his gag reflex by practicing for hours with a small piece of potato tied to a string.

Such acts of bodily control have traditionally been viewed as rare feats that only extraordinarily gifted people can accomplish. However, behavioral scientists have demonstrated that the average person can learn a degree of control over physiological responses through the use of biofeedback. Biofeedback is based on the fundamental principle that we learn to perform a particular response when we receive feedback or information about the consequences of the response we have just made and can make appropriate adjustments. That is how we learn to perform the wide variety of skills and behaviors we use in everyday activities. The availability of feedback is also important in learning how to control internal physiological responses. Since we normally do not receive feedback from those internal events in day-to-day life, we cannot control them. However, if patients are provided feedback of muscle tension by a visual-display monitor, they become aware of the consequences of muscle tension changes and of how adjustments can be made to modify and eventually control muscle tension. The recent development of sensitive physiological recording devices and digital logic circuitry has made it possible to detect small changes in visceral events and provide subjects with immediate biofeedback of these events.

Broad-Spectrum Behavioral Therapy

The term *broad-spectrum behavioral therapy* emphasizes the fact that most behavioral therapists employ several different treatment procedures for a specific disorder to deal effectively with all the important controlling or causal variables. Just as traditional psychoanalytic therapy attempts to determine the underlying unconscious causes of a behavior disorder, behavioral therapy also seeks to assess the major causes of such behavior. However, the search is not for underlying unconscious causes, which are difficult to assess reliably, but for the learned and environmental determinants or causes. In that sense, the goal and task of traditional psychotherapists and behavioral therapists are the same. The chief difference is that behavioral therapists assume that the most feasible and effective approach is to search for environmental determinants and directly modify behavior, while psychoanalytically oriented psychotherapists assume that it is more important to uncover and deal with unconscious motivations for behavior.

Most behavioral therapists therefore use several different treatment procedures for a specific disorder in order to deal effectively with all the important controlling or causal variables—systematic desensitization and its variants, progressive relaxation training, behavioral rehearsal and assertion training, contingency management methods, biofeedback, to name a few.

The treatment of tension in asthmatics can be used as an example of the broad-spectrum or multimodal approach to treatment. In training asthmatics to relax, the therapist might begin with progressive muscle relaxation training as a means of teaching patients to decrease their arousal level. Then, biofeedback training for the specific purpose of reducing tension in the frontalis muscles could be administered. Concurrently, treatment directed at dealing with the situational factors contributing to general emotional tensions such as job or marital problems could also be provided. The goal is to deal with all the important controlling or causal variables involved in provoking the disorder.

The following case study demonstrates the use of such a multimodal approach with the problem of headache.

Mrs. A., a 45-year-old housewife with two young children, sought help in an outpatient clinic for tension headaches. She had suffered from headaches almost daily for the preceding year and a half. The patient was initially instructed to carefully monitor her headaches on a daily basis, noting where, when, and for how long each headache occurred, as well as what was happening at the time. On the basis of these self-monitoring data, the therapist and the patient were able to isolate the fact that the headaches usually occurred upon awakening in the morning, after lunch, and in the evening after dinner.

Further evaluation revealed that during these times she was either angry at her husband for not helping with the children and household tasks and for being overly critical of her, or she was experiencing guilt for wanting to relax and "get away" from the children and the house. With some of the important cues that appeared to trigger the headaches identified, the therapist was able to teach the patient more effective ways of dealing with these cues—learning to be assertive and to express her needs to her husband. She was also administered muscle relaxation and biofeedback training to deal with the somatic, headache symptoms. Finally, since the patient's husband played an active role in contributing to her headaches by being overly critical of her, couples therapy was also initiated so that he would become aware of the nature of his behavior and the effect it had on his wife. The therapist also provided help in ways in which patient and spouse could assist one another, and ways of giving additional attention and affection to one another.

This multimodal treatment program almost totally eliminated the patient's headaches.

In conclusion, sensitive application of behavioral treatment techniques can augment the medical treatment of many patients, especially patients who are concerned with the control of symptoms mediated by autonomy or voluntary motor systems.

Suggested Readings

Bandura, A. (1971). Psychotherapy based upon modeling principles. In *Handbook of Psychotherapy and Behavior Change: An Empirical Analysis*, ed. A.E. Bergin and S.L. Garfield, pp. 653–708. New York: Wiley.

Barlow, D.H., and Wolfe, B.E. (1981). Behavioral approaches to anxiety disorders: A report on the NIMH-SUNY, Albany, research conference. *Journal of Consulting and Clinical Psychology* 49:448–454.

Fordyce, W.E., and Steger, J.C. (1979). Chronic pain. In *Behavioral Medicine: Theory and Practice*, ed. O.F. Pomerleau and J.P. Brady, pp. 125–153. Baltimore: Williams & Wilkins.

Gatchel, R.J., and Price, K.P. (eds.) (1979). *Clinical Applications of Biofeedback: Appraisal and Status*. Elmsford, N.Y.: Pergamon Press.

Goldfried, M.R., and Davison, G.C. (1976). *Clinical Behavior Therapy*. New York: Holt, Rinehart and Winston.

Hatch, J.P., Gatchel, R.J., and Harrington, R. (1982). Biofeedback: clinical applications and medicine. In *Behavioral Medicine and Clinical Psychology: Overlapping Disciplines*, ed. R.J. Gatchel, A. Baum, and J.E. Singer, pp. 37–74. Hillsdale, N.J.: Erlbaum.

Jacobson, E. (1938). *Progressive Relaxation.* Chicago: University of Chicago Press.

Melamed, B.G., and Siegel, L.J. (1975). Reduction of anxiety in children facing hospitalization and surgery by use of filmed modeling. *Journal of Consulting and Clinical Psychology* 43:511–521.

Schultz, J.H., and Luthe, W. (1959). *Autogenic Training: A Psychophysiological Approach in Psychotherapy.* New York: Grune & Stratton.

Stunkard, A.J. (1979). Behavioral medicine and beyond: the example of obesity. In *Behavioral Medicine: Theory and Practice*, ed. O.F. Pomerleau and J.P. Brady, pp. 279–298. Baltimore: Williams & Wilkins.

Index